CASE MANAGEMENT FOR NURSES

Anita W. Finkelman, MSN, RN

Adjunct Associate Professor/Clinical
Nurse Consultant, Bouve College of Health Science
School of Nursing Northeastern University
University of Cincinnati
College of Nursing

Pearson

Boston • Columbus • Indianapolis • New York • San Francisco • Upper Saddle River
Amsterdam • Cape Town • Dubai • London • Madrid • Milan • Munich • Paris • Montreal • Toronto
Delhi • Mexico City • Sao Paulo • Sydney • Hong Kong • Seoul • Singapore • Taipei • Tokyo

Publisher: Julie Levin Alexander
Publisher's Assistant: Regina Bruno
Editor-in-Chief: Maura Connor
Executive Acquisitions Editor: Pamela Fuller
Editorial Assistant: Lisa Pierce
Marketing Specialist: Michael Sirinides
Marketing Assistant: Crystal Gonzalez
Managing Editor: Fran Russello
Full Service Production: Mohinder Singh/Aptara®, Inc.
Art Director: Jayne Conte
Cover design: Bruce Kenselaar
Cover photo: Fotolia: Antique ottoman gold design © Murat Cokeker
Printer/Binder: Edwards Brothers, Inc.
Cover Printer: Lehigh-Phoenix

Notice: Care has been taken to confirm the accuracy of information presented in this book. The authors, editors, and the publisher, however, cannot accept any responsibility for errors or omissions or for consequences from application of the information in this book and make no warranty, express or implied, with respect to its contents.

The author and publisher have exerted every effort to ensure that drug selections and dosages set forth in this text are in accord with current recommendations and practice at time of publication. However, in view of ongoing research, changes in government regulations, and the constant flow of information relating to drug therapy and drug reactions, the reader is urged to check the package inserts of all drugs for any change in indications of dosage and for added warnings and precautions. This is particularly important when the recommended agent is a new and/or infrequently employed drug.

Library of Congress Cataloging-in-Publication Data

Finkelman, Anita Ward
   Case management for nurses / Anita Finkelman.
     p. cm.
   ISBN-13: 978-0-13-612162-6
   ISBN-10: 0-13-612162-4
   1. Hospitals—Case management services.   2. Nursing.   I. Title.
   RA975.5.C36F56 2011
   362.11068—dc22   2010019488

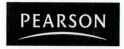

www.pearsonhighered.com

ISBN-13: 978-0-13-612162-6
ISBN-10:   0-13-612162-4

ABOUT THE AUTHOR

Anita W. Finkelman, MSN, RN, is Nurse Consultant, Bouve College of Health Science School of Nursing Northeastern University and at the University of Cincinnati College of Nursing Adjunct Associate Professor/Clinical at the University of Cincinnati College of Nursing and was on the faculty at the University of Oklahoma Health Sciences Center, College of Nursing. She served as Director of Undergraduate Curriculum and Associate Professor/Clinical Nursing at the University of Cincinnati College of Nursing. She has a master's degree in psychiatric-mental health nursing from Yale University and did post-master's graduate work in health care policy and administration at George Washington University. Additional work in the area of health policy was completed as a fellow of the Health Policy Institute, George Mason University. Ms. Finkelman's thirty-five years of nursing experience includes clinical, educational, and administrative positions. She has written many books and journal articles; lectured on administration, health policy, continuing education, and psychiatric-mental health nursing, both nationally and internationally; and served as a consultant to publishers and health care organizations and developed and managed distance education nursing programs. Other Prentice Hall publications include *Leadership and Management in Nursing*, the second edition of which is due in early 2011, *Managed Care: A Nursing Perspective* (2001), and case studies in *Critical Thinking in Nursing: Case Studies Across the Continuum* (C. Green, Ed., 1999). These are in addition to *Implementing IOM: Implications of the Institute of Medicine Reports for Nursing Education (2009) (2nd ed.)*, American Nurses Association, and *Professional Nursing Concepts* (2010), Jones and Bartlett.

PREFACE

Case Management for Nurses focuses on an important topic in health care today: how care can be improved and provided in a more effective and efficient manner. Case management is one method that is used to meet this goal. Especially in a health care system that is dysfunctional and fragmented, case management can help patients and their families meet their outcomes for care and improve care. Using the case management method, care can be coordinated and can engage the interdisciplinary health care team to focus on patient-centered care, with active involvement from the patient and family.

This book is divided into two sections. Section I provides introductory background content about case management. The topics include case management, basic information such as the status of the current health care delivery system, description of case management, discussion of case manager competencies, roles, and responsibilities, and the critical issues of ethics and legal concerns. Other topics are case management models, reimbursement, quality improvement, the consumer, and tools used by the case manager such as clinical pathways. Each chapter has objectives, an outline, critical terms, references, questions and activities for thoughts, and Internet links that relate to the chapter content. A glossary is provided at the end of the book.

The second section is a Case Management Reader. It provides published articles on case management related to case management professional issues; patient-centered care; quality improvement; costs, reimbursement, and utilization review; chronic illness; and disease management. Critical thinking questions are provided for each of the articles. This section allows the reader to explore some of the case management literature, apply what has been learned in Section I, and consider specific issues for each article.

ACKNOWLEDGMENTS

I would like to thank my husband Fred and daughters Shoshannah and Deborah Finkelman for their continued support in my career and my writing initiatives. A special thanks to Elizabeth Karle for her assistance with the manuscript and to Pamela Fuller for her consistent assistance throughout the writing and development process. The support and production staff at Pearson are responsible for turning ordinary pages and rough sketches into the final product – and the book simply would not exist without them.

Alicia L. Drew, MSN, RN, CNL, Director of Clinical Operations, Case Management, the University of Oklahoma College of Nursing, was a major contributor to Section II. Her assistance in reviewing the articles included in the Case Management Reader and development of critical thinking questions provided an important dimension to this book.

Reviewers

We extend sincere thanks to our colleagues from schools of nursing across the country who gave their time generously to help create this book. These professionals helped us plan and shape our book by contributing their collective experience as nurses and teachers, and we made many improvements based on their efforts.

Billy Michael Barbour, BSN, MSN
RN-BSN Program Faculty
Florida State University
Tallahassee, Florida

Rosalinda Haddon, MA, RN, CNE
Associate Clinical Professor
Northern Arizona University, School of Nursing
Flagstaff, Arizona

Jane Hook, RN, MN
Lecturer
California State University, Los Angeles
Los Angeles, California

Denise Isibel, RN, MSN
Lecturer
Old Dominion University
Norfolk, Virginia

Christine S. Watts, MS, RN
Clinical Assistant, Nursing Professor
Towson University
Towson, Maryland

Kristi A. Wilkerson, RN, MSN
Nursing Faculty
Southeastern Community College
West Burlington, Iowa

CONTENTS

Case Management Basics

INTRODUCTION

Section I discusses basic information that can help a case manager be successful. This content is then applied in some examples in Section II. Content that is relevant to case management includes: an overview of case management and factors that impact case management practice, including legal and ethical issues; case manager roles and responsibilities, competencies for success, the case management process, and case management delivery models; health care reimbursement; managed care, quality improvement; consumers; and case management documentation and tools for effective practice. Questions and cases found in each chapter highlight some of the critical knowledge and application of that knowledge.

CHAPTER 1

Introduction to Case Management

OBJECTIVES

After completing this chapter, the reader will be able to:

- Describe the current health care economy and health care reform.
- Discuss the relationship between collaboration and case management.
- Describe the concept of case management and its development.
- Explain the purposes and goals of case management.
- Critique the twelve characteristics of a typical case management program.
- Describe the roles and functions of the nurse case manager.
- Examine ethical and legal issues that may arise in case management.

KEY TERMS

Advance directives, p. 18
Case management process, p. 11
Case managers, p. 4
Collaborative care, p. 9
Consent, p. 17
Continuity of care, p. 11

Durable power of attorney, p. 18
Informed consent, p. 18
Liability, p. 17
Malpractice, p. 16
Negligence, p. 16
Third-party payers, p. 6

INTRODUCTION

Case management can make a difference in the quality of care that patients receive, reduce costs, and also improve consumer satisfaction (Harrison, Nolin, & Suero, 2004). The Institute of Medicine (IOM) reports on the quality of the U.S. health care system clearly support a change in focus to one of patient-centered care and the need to improve care delivery. In addition, hospitals want to control admissions and to better manage lengths-of-stay. Insurers of all types, including managed care, drive this need to control care for effective outcomes and cost containment. Case management has been used effectively to address these concerns. Typically, **case managers** are registered nurses or social workers. Given the need for case management, this book provides an introduction to nurse case management and its importance to the health care system and process of providing care.

Case management has become more important over the past few years with the growing need for greater coordination of care across the continuum of care and with the development of additional types of case management such as care management for the elderly or long-term care and nurse navigation. Case management, with its focus on care coordination, also plays a major role in the care of patients with chronic illness. The number of persons with chronic illnesses has increased, as has the number of people with more than one chronic illness. Data related to this problem include (IOM, 2003a, p. 49):

- 124 million Americans have some type of chronic condition, representing nearly half of the U.S. population.
- 1.7 million Americans die annually from a chronic illness, representing 7 out of 10 deaths.
- 60 million have more than one chronic condition.
- Chronic illnesses cause major limitations in daily living for more than 1 out of 10 Americans (25 million).
- More than 3 million American (2.5 million women and 750,000 men) live with five conditions
- Inappropriate or avoidable hospitalizations have increased from 7 per 1,000 for those with one chronic condition to 95 per 1,000 for those with five chronic conditions (appropriate ambulatory care might have prevented these hospitalizations.)
- Chronic conditions account for 70% of the $1 trillion spent on health care annually in the United States.

Based on this description of a growing need to provide services for people with chronic illness, plus all the other patients who need better care coordination, case management has the potential for growth throughout the health care sector.

The health care delivery system is complex and influenced by many factors. Critical issues to consider are identified in Box 1-1.

BOX 1-1

The Changing Health Care Environment: Critical Issues

- Changing Practice Patterns and the Physician
- Cultural Diversity
- Federal and State Governments
- Growth of Advanced Practice Nursing
- Diagnosis-Related Groups
- Health Care Consumerism
- Immigration
- Legislation
- Managed Care Backlash
- Managed Care Models
- Medical-Industrial Complex
- Mergers and Acquisitions
- Managed Competition
- Minority Health
- Move from Acute Care to Ambulatory Care
- Privatization and Corporate Health Care
- Quality Care
- Reimbursement
- Restructuring and Reengineering
- Role Changes

THE NATIONAL HEALTH CARE ECONOMY AND HEALTH CARE REFORM

National Health Care Expenditures

The health care industry is an extremely large industry, the financing of which is influenced by many factors, particularly social expectations, economic trends, technological developments, political factors, and the U.S. economy, which in the past few years has been the most critical factor. Financial issues affect all aspects of the provision of care, settings, and services, such as inpatient care, ambulatory care, home care, primary care, long-term care, public health, pharmaceutical, medical supplies, medical transportation, medical technology, medical research, and so on. Compared with other countries, the United States has the most expensive health care system with the highest living standard and economic status. Despite this, the United States has a large number of people without insurance coverage: 46 million people, which includes 9 million children, did not have health insurance as of October 2008 (Cover the Uninsured, 2009), but this number will be reduced with health care reform legislation, 2010. The largest portion of health care expenditures is found in the hospital industry despite the fact that there is a decreasing length-of-stay (LOS) rate and increasing use of nonhospital services. Health care expenditures are expected to continue to increase. An understanding of health care expenditures includes an appreciation of how the nation's health dollar is spent and also who pays for health care or the health care funding sources described in Figure 1-1. It is also important to recognize that health care expenditures change annually.

Projected health care spending for 2008–2018 is expected grow by 6.2%—2.1% points faster than average annual growth in gross domestic product (GDP) (Sisko et al., 2009). These authors also note that the health share of GDP is anticipated to rise rapidly from 16.2% in 2007 to 17.6% in 2009, largely as a result of the recession, and then climb to 20.3% by 2018. By 2016, public payers (the government) are projected to be the largest source of health care funding and by 2018 will pay for more than 50%.

Decreasing hospitalization has been greatly influenced by the need to decrease costs; however, new advances in health care and new methods for providing health care have made it easier to lower the number of hospitalization stays, LOS, and costs. Factors that have helped to decrease hospitalization costs are early ambulation of patients so that they can be discharged sooner; prep time before a patient is admitted to

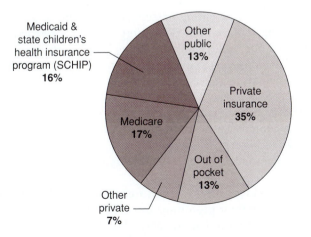

FIGURE 1-1 The Nation's Healthcare Dollar *Source:* Centers for Medicare and Medicaid Services (2006) Blue Cross Blue Shield Association, 2007 Medical Cost Reference Guide

hospital for surgery; greater use of ambulatory surgery with less use of inpatient surgery and stay; better use of medications such as antibiotics to prevent infections before they occur; greater use of home care and skilled nursing care; and more effective management of care within the hospital treatment period. Prescription costs have risen due to an increase in the cost of drugs, greater use of many new drugs that are effective but expensive, and broader health insurance coverage for prescriptions.

Health care utilization and expenditures data are used to evaluate cost control outcomes. There is, however, another perspective on health care expenditures that is more complex than these data may indicate. Is spending more on medical care worth it in terms of its impact on the length and quality of life? **Third-party payers** must view health care expenditures from many perspectives using cost-benefit analysis. Case managers are directly involved in health care expenditures when they participate in determining services and coverage.

With the worsening of the U.S. and global economies, health care has been hit hard. In a survey of Americans conducted in February 2009, the news was not positive (Henry J. Kaiser Family Foundation, 2009a). More than half of Americans (slightly more than 53%) said that they have limited their medical care due to cost in the past year. The results indicate that there is grave concern about the affordability and accessibility of health care when needed. Patients/consumers are relying more on over-the-counter drugs rather than visiting physicians (35%), and 34% are not keeping dental appointments. Twenty-one percent are not filling prescriptions, and 15% are cutting pills in half or skipping doses. Nineteen percent experienced major financial problems due to medical care that could not be put off. The survey also addressed the respondents' view of health care reform. The focus seems to be more on getting help with costs of health care and getting coverage for those who do not have coverage rather than on improving the quality of care. Given that there is considerable concern about the quality of care, as noted in recent IOM reports, it is important to keep this part of the equation in mind. A dysfunctional health care system costs more money than a functional system that provides quality care, and errors and complications are prevented.

Another area of concern is the rising cost of health insurance premiums. In 2008, employer health insurance premiums increased by 5.0%. The annual premium for an employer health plan covering a family of four averaged nearly $12,700. The annual premium for single coverage averaged over $4,700 (Henry J. Kaiser Family Foundation, 2009b). An example of how this is impacting the insured is illustrated in a 2009 survey done by the Kaiser Foundation (Henry J. Kaiser Family Foundation, 2009b). More than half of those surveyed said they decreased their use of medical care because of costs by increasing use of over-the-counter drugs and not getting prescribed medications, decreasing dental visits, putting off or not getting care recommended, and not getting needed mental health care.

Experts agree that our health care system has many inefficiencies, excessive administrative expenses, inflated prices, poor management, and inappropriate care, waste and fraud. All of these problems significantly increase the cost of medical care and health insurance for employers and workers and affect the security of families. With the growing economic crisis in 2008–2009 a greater number of families were affected. In 2008, health care spending in the United States reached $2.4 trillion and was projected to reach $3.1 trillion in 2012 and $4.3 trillion by 2016 (Keehan et al., 2008). Examples of higher employer and employee health insurance costs include (Henry J. Kaiser Family Foundation, 2009b):

- Premiums for employer-based health insurance rose by 5.0% in 2008. In 2007, small employers saw their premiums increase 5.5% on average. Firms with fewer than 24 workers experienced an increase of 6.8%.
- The annual premium that a health insurer charges an employer for a health plan covering a family of four averaged $12,700 in 2008. Workers contributed nearly $3,400 or

12% more than they did in 2007. The annual premiums for family coverage significantly eclipsed the gross earnings for a full-time, minimum-wage worker ($10,712).

- Workers are now paying $1,600 more in premiums annually for family coverage than they did in 1999.
- Since 1999, employment-based health insurance premiums have increased 120%, compared to cumulative inflation of 44% and cumulative wage growth of 29% during the same period.
- According to the Kaiser Family Foundation and the Health Research and Educational Trust, premiums for employer-sponsored health insurance in the United States have been rising four times faster on average than workers' earnings since 1999.
- The average employee contribution to company-provided health insurance has increased more than 120% since 2000. Average out-of-pocket costs for deductibles, co-payments for medications, and co-insurance for physician and hospital visits rose 115% during the same period.

The impact of rising health care costs has been dramatic as supported by the following descriptions and data.

- National surveys show that the primary reason people are uninsured is the high cost of health insurance coverage (Henry J. Kaiser Family Foundation, 2009b).
- A recent study by Harvard University researchers found that the average out-of-pocket medical debt for those who filed for bankruptcy was $12,000. The study noted that 68% of those who filed for bankruptcy had health insurance. In addition, the study found that 50% of all bankruptcy filings were partly the result of medical expenses (Himmelstein, Warren, Thorne, & Woolhander, 2005). Every 30 seconds in the United States someone files for bankruptcy in the aftermath of a serious health problem.
- About 1.5 million families lose their homes to foreclosure every year due to unaffordable medical costs (Robertson, Egelhof, & Hoke, 2008).
- Retiring elderly couples will need $250,000 in savings just to pay for the most basic medical coverage (Fidelity Investments, 2006). Many experts believe that this figure is conservative and that $300,000 may be a more realistic number.
- The United States spends six times more per capita on the administration of the health care system than its peer Western European nations (McKinsey Global Institute, 2007).

These examples illustrate how the economy is interrelated with health care, multiplying in number as the economy worsens.

The concern about the uninsured has increased over the years. "The uninsured refers to persons with any form of public or private coverage for hospital and outpatient care, for any given length of time" (IOM, 2004, p. 21). Along with this concern is the underinsured, an area that sometimes is ignored. The underinsured are "individuals or families whose health insurance policy or benefit plan offers less than adequate coverage" (IOM, 2004, p. 21). When this happens, these individuals and families are left with debt when they cannot pay uncovered care or they avoid getting care when they need it because their benefits do not cover required care. The U.S. safety net, which is the health care organizations (HCOs) that disproportionately serve the needy and uninsured, has been stretched as the number of uninsured and underinsured has increased (IOM, 2004). However, increasing the safety net services will not solve the entire problem of the uninsured and underinsured. This approach may help some, but it is not sufficient. Both of these problems are major issues in the current health care reform debate.

Health Care Reform

Early in the Obama administration, significant steps were taken to begin to address the crisis in health care, for example (The White House, 2009):

- The president signed the Children's Health Insurance Reauthorization Act on February 4, 2009, which will provide quality health care to 11 million children, 4 million of whom were previously uninsured.
- The President's American Recovery and Reinvestment Act will protect health coverage for 7 million Americans who lose their jobs through a 65% COBRA subsidy to make coverage affordable.
- The Recovery Act also invests $19 billion in computerized medical records that will help to reduce costs and improve quality while ensuring patients' privacy.
- The Recovery Act will also provide:
  - $1 billion for prevention and wellness to improve America's health and help to reduce health care costs
  - $1.1 billion for comparative effectiveness research that will give doctors objective information about which treatments work and which do not
  - $500 million for the health care workforce to help train the next generation of doctors and nurses.

The Obama administration's health care reform approach initiative goals are to (The White House, 2009):

- Reduce long-term growth of health care costs for businesses and government
- Protect families from bankruptcy or debt because of health care costs
- Guarantee choice of doctors and health plans
- Invest in prevention and wellness
- Improve patient safety and quality of care
- Assure affordable, quality health coverage for all Americans
- Maintain coverage when people change or lose their job
- End barriers to coverage for people with pre-existing medical conditions

How might health care reform impact case management? Case management might be used more to assist in controlling costs and ensuring that patients get the most appropriate care when needed. Case managers will also need to be knowledgeable about the changes that might occur in the health care system and in health care reimbursement.

WHAT IS CASE MANAGEMENT?

"Case management is not a profession but rather a collaborative and trans-disciplinary practice" (Commission for Case Management Certification, 2009, p. 1). Several health care professional organizations and experts have defined case management; however, there clearly is no universally accepted definition for case management. Case management is used in many different types of settings, and the setting also affects the definition. Case management models and settings are discussed in Chapter 2. The Case Management Society of America (CMSA) defines case management as "a collaborative process of assessment, planning, facilitation and advocacy for options and services to meet an individual's health needs through communication and available resources to promote quality cost-effective outcomes" (2002, p. 1). Case management is based on the assumption that patients with complex health problems, catastrophic health situations, and high-cost medical conditions need assistance in using the health care system effectively and that a case manager can help patients with these needs.

Case management is also an important service strategy used by third-party payers (insurers and managed care organizations to ensure cost-effective, quality care. Providers, such as acute care facilities (acute care hospitals), home care agencies, and mental health agencies, also use case management. Most case managers are nurses, but other health care professionals, such as social workers or rehabilitation counselors, also serve as case managers. This is an exciting position that provides new opportunities for nursing. As the definition of case management indicates, the case manager assesses, plans, implements, coordinates, and evaluates the patient's care. None of this is new to nursing, and this is an ideal role for nurses. The goal is quality, cost-effective outcomes. Case management is outcome driven. Coordination across the continuum of care for the individual patient is a critical component of case management and is very important in decreasing health care costs. The case manager serves as the care coordinator. A **collaborative care** process is an important element of the coordination process. Collaboration is "the process of joint decision-making among interdependent parties, involving joint ownership of decisions and collective responsibility for outcomes" (Disch, 2001, p. 275).

Stanton and Lammon (2008) discuss the impact of predicted changes on case management by identifying seven future trends. Case management experts identified these trends. The trends that are felt to be important to case management practice are (pp. 163–164):

- *Pay for performance:* There will be a greater emphasis on paying providers for performance. Case management can make a difference in performance. Recovery audit contracts are used by the Centers for Medicare and Medicaid Services to better ensure accurate payments to avoid inappropriate billing. This will impact case management.
- *Use of evidence-based practice (EBP):* As will be discussed later in this book, the IOM has identified use of EBP as a critical core competency for all health care professionals. Case managers need to understand EBP and how it impacts tools that they may use, such as clinical guidelines.
- *Transitions of care:* Transferring from different levels of care are times of great risk for errors. Case managers can help to better coordinate these periods of transitions to ensure the patient receives quality care directed at meeting the patient's expected outcomes. Collaboration is critical during these times.
- *Predictive modeling:* This method can be used to identify patients at highest risk and highest cost so that methods such as disease management can be used. Healthy People 2010, U.S. Department of Health and Human Services should be used to provide guidance about populations that require primary and secondary prevention.
- *Greater use of informatics, telehealth, and e-health:* Patients and families as consumers are much more aware of health issues and can access information quickly. Technology has also provided alternative methods to provide care such as telehealth. Case managers are involved in informatics, telehealth, and e-health.
- *The aging population:* This population requires more coordination and assistance. In addition, many nurse case managers are aging, and this will have an impact on number of case managers required.
- *Increase in the use of core measures, case-sensitive outcomes, or metrics:* These tools will be very useful in evaluation of case management services.

THE DEVELOPMENT OF CASE MANAGEMENT

Case management is not new. It has a long history beginning in the early 1900s (Powell & Tahan, 2008). Psychiatry and psychiatric social work used case management in the 1920s. In the 1930s, public health nurses and social workers began to use it. The focus during its early years was on long-term chronic illness and care in community settings, and this continues to be important today. After World War II, third-party payers became interested in case management and used nurses and social workers as case managers for veterans with complex problems. When Medicare and Medicaid were created, these programs also gravitated toward using case managers, particularly social workers, to assist in coordinating care. In the 1960s, third-party payers began to actively use case management for specific populations.

In the 1980s, nursing played a major role in the expansion of case management. Nursing focused on acute care needs with an emphasis on patient-centered care and continuous quality improvement. As Medicare grew, nursing needed to support its impact on patient care. Zander has described the stimulus for nursing's interest in case management: "We were convinced that nursing would be at risk in a diagnostic-related groups (DRGs) world and were motivated to explain first to ourselves and then others what nursing's contributions were to desired clinical outcomes (which we defined as true quality) and efficient care management" (Zander, 1996, p. 23).

A project at Carondelet Saint Mary's Hospital in Arizona is one example of a project that paved the way for a clearer concept of clinical case management rather than just an insurance- or cost-focused case management. The Carondelet project developed the concept of hospital-based nurse case managers who partnered with high-risk patients. The nurse case manager assisted in managing and accessing community services after hospital discharge. Patients in this project experienced a decreased length of stay, and patients who were readmitted exhibited less acuity. These are important outcomes in today's cost-conscious health care environment. The role of the case manager and its application in the acute care setting were further clarified at the New England Medical Hospitals' project. Primary care nurses became case managers and provided coordination and continuing care across geographic care units. In addition, clinical pathway development and implementation were important parts of these major nursing projects. More detailed content about pathways is found in Chapter 6. "As early as 1987, it became clear that nursing case management would be a classic model because it added value, consistency, quality, and accuracy to patient care, was adaptive to the environment, and both enhanced and defined the voluntary differentiation to a newly available professional level of nursing" (Zander, 1996, p. 24).

One would think by this success that all case managers are nurses, but this is not so. Third-party payers, as well as HCOs such as hospitals, long-term care, and home care, use many types of health care professionals as case managers (e.g., social workers, occupational therapists, rehabilitation counselors, and substance abuse counselors), but nurses are frequently chosen for this role. There is increasing competition for the role of case manager from many different health care professionals. In today's rapidly shifting health care environment, no health care profession is safe in assuming that it will not experience changes or that other health care professionals might not take over its functions.

CASE MANAGEMENT: PURPOSES

What does case management offer the patient and health care delivery? In order to answer this question, it is important to identify its purposes. There are many examples of purposes from case management programs that can be used when new case management programs are developed. As the health care delivery system changes, purposes and goals need to change. The CMSA identifies the following case management purposes (Powell & Tahan, 2008; NCOA, 1988; Williams & Torrens, 1993; Cohen, 1996):

- To interject objectivity and information where it is lacking in order to promote informed decision making by patients and others
- To maximize efficiency in the utilization of available resources

- To work collaboratively with patients, physicians, family members/significant others, and other health care providers to implement a plan of care that meets the individual's needs
- To promote quality, safe, and cost-effective care; ensure appropriate access to care; work collaboratively with the patient and all pertinent parties
- To make the system work more effectively in order to ensure that individuals receive assistance that is responsive to their needs
- To work directly with patients and families over time to assist them in arranging and managing the complex set of resources that the patient requires to maintain health and independent functioning
- To move the patient toward successful meeting of planned outcomes where interventions are tied to a sense of movement and constant evaluation occurs to measure progress

The key case management goal is to simultaneously promote the patient's wellness, autonomy, and appropriate use of service and financial resources (Powell & Tahan [2008]). Case management typically focuses on five major areas:

- Quality of care
- Length-of-stay (LOS)
- Resource utilization
- Continuity
- Cost control

Identification of outcomes, which is necessary for effective assessment of the quality of care, is an important component of case management. Because LOS is important to cost containment, case managers need to consider it carefully throughout the **case management process**, particularly focusing on timeliness of treatment. LOS is frequently used to determine efficiency. Resource utilization directly affects costs and is another area in which the case manager makes decisions. Inappropriate resource utilization, which includes both under- and overutilization, is always a cause for concern. **Continuity of care's** purpose is to ensure that all services required are provided at the appropriate time, over time, and across multiple health care providers and settings. This has been an integral part of case management since its inception. Cost control is critical, and it is incorporated into all of the case management focus areas.

In addition to these five focus areas, another important concern is patient satisfaction. It is important for the provider and the third-party payer to understand patient satisfaction, which has never been easy to assess. The case manager needs to assess patient satisfaction throughout the case management process. As managed care has come under increased criticism from consumers and employers, managed care organizations (MCOs) have been forced into acknowledging consumer concerns. Case managers can prevent patient dissatisfaction and can act as an important conduit between the provider and the third-party payer and often resolve problems. Patients see their case managers as their advocates and discuss their concerns and complaints with them. Advocacy is discussed in more detail in Chapter 6.

Case management is the coordination of an individual patient's health care. Other health care providers, rather than the case manager, provide the direct care. For example, telephonic case management can be used quite effectively. It can be used for screening and preventive care, such as providing health education and follow-up on compliance and outcomes. Insurers and MCOs may assess patients' needs via the nurse case management telephonic intervention. With their health care education and clinical experience, telephonic nurse case managers can identify problems and decide when patients need direct, hands-on care. It is this professional expertise that can make the difference in meeting patient needs effectively and avoiding complications. For example, high-risk pregnant women can call and discuss their concerns with a case manager, who can then assess the problems and determine if the caller/patient needs to see a physician, nurse-midwife, or requires other services. A parent with a child who has asthma can call when there is concern about a child's breathing, and the case manager can then determine with the parent the best approach to take. These calls offer excellent opportunities for health teaching and reinforcement of preventive care, but the case manager is not the direct care provider.

HEALTH CARE PROFESSIONS FIVE CORE COMPETENCIES

In 2003, the IOM discussed critical issues related to health care education and impact on patient care in its report *Health Professions Education*. The report describes five health care professions core competencies that are critical to improving care and are not currently being met by health care professions education. The IOM does not state that these competencies are the only competencies required but rather that these competencies form the core competencies for all health care professional education: Nurses, physicians, pharmacists, allied health, and health care administration. Why would these competencies be relevant to a book about nurse case management? The competencies apply to all health care professions, and nurse case managers are part of this group. The core competencies are (IOM, 2003b, p. 4):

- *Provide patient-centered care:* Identify, respect, and care about patients' differences, values, preferences, and expressed needs; relive pain and suffering; coordinate continuous care; listen to, clearly inform, communicate with, and educate patients; share decision making and management; and continuously advocate disease prevention, wellness, and promotion of healthy lifestyles, including a focus on population health. *Case managers focus on the patient/client in the services they provide; they work with patients/clients of diverse backgrounds; assist the patient/client with self-management; work with the patient's/client's family; and much more with the patient/client at the center and actively involved in the decisions.*
- *Work in interdisciplinary teams:* Cooperate, collaborate, communicate, and integrate care in teams to ensure that care is continuous and reliable. *Case managers work with multiple health care professionals and service agencies in order to ensure that the patient's/client's care is coordinated; this requires effective collaboration, communication, and interdisciplinary teamwork.*
- *Employ EBP:* Integrate best research with clinical expertise and patient values for optimum care, and participate in learning and research activities to the extent feasible. *Case managers use all four types of evidence (research results, patient/client values and preferences, patient/client assessment data, and clinical expertise) to arrive at the best case management plan for the patient/client.*
- *Apply quality improvement (QI):* Identify errors and hazards in care; understand and implement basic safety design principles, such as standardization and simplification; continually understand and measure quality of care in terms of structure, process, and outcomes in relation to patient and community needs, and design and test interventions to change processes and systems of care, with the objective of improving quality. *Case managers support the need for quality improvement and effective outcomes for their patients/clients.*
- *Use informatics:* Communicate, manage knowledge, mitigate error, and support decision-making using information technology. *Case managers use informatics daily as they assess the patient/client, determine needs, plan, implement plans, and evaluate outcomes.*

Content in this book supports each of these competencies and the need for case managers to demonstrate these competencies in their practice.

CASE MANAGER ROLES AND RESPONSIBILITES

The case manager generally focuses on specifically identified patients' (high risk, high volume, high cost) care needs across the episode or continuum of an illness. In the past, utilization review (UR) was the first and in many cases the only function that was attributed to case management. Its focus is to determine if treatment received was medically necessary, was provided in the most appropriate setting, and was of the best quality. UR is applied particularly to acute care settings, emergency departments, and psychiatric/substance abuse (behavioral health care or mental health) services. Typically, UR was done by case managers, but over time case manager functions expanded. A key issue today is that case managers need to recognize that what must be done is usually accomplished through others, requiring collaboration and negotiation. This fact affects case manager roles, responsibilities, and qualifications.

The critical case management roles and responsibilities are: Provider liaison, benefits interpreter, patient advocate, patient educator, triage coordinator, quality improvement, utilization/resource management, risk management, disease management, discharge planning, technology, case manager, and primary care provider. Some case managers are involved in all of these functions, and others are not concerned with all of them. Many of these functions are interrelated.

Provider Liaison

The provider liaison function focuses on information and interaction. All providers who work with a patient need to be cognizant of the patient's needs and treatment so that they can interact effectively to address patient-related and administrative issues. As provider functions change, it is important that the interdisciplinary team understands the functions of each team member and accepts these functions as important. Territoriality has no place in an effective team. The team's goal is to meet patient goals, not to meet individual team member needs. The four key characteristics of a provider liaison are coordination, cooperation, collaboration, and consistency. None of these are easy to accomplish. Nurses have long been involved with many different health care providers and understand the language and organization of the health care delivery system, and thus, it is easy for nurses to understand this case manager function.

Benefits Interpreter

Understanding an insurance plan and its benefits and procedures can be a major task, and if the person is sick or has a sick family member, the task can seem overwhelming. Having someone who can understand health needs and explain authorization and other plan requirements and procedures can be extremely helpful. It may even better ensure that the patient receives the most effective and efficient care when needed. Complaints and grievances cannot be avoided, and it is important to have staff who can respond with knowledge and understanding. This is a new function for nurses, but one to which nurses can bring many additional skills, such as communication, understanding of illness and stress, and knowledge of health care delivery, providers, and the continuum of care. To fulfill the responsibilities of a benefits interpreter, nurse case managers need to learn more about reimbursement, benefits, and the claims process. Chapters 3 and 6 discuss issues related to reimbursement in more detail.

Patient Advocate

Patient advocacy is not new to nurses. An advocate works with the patient or on behalf of the patient to ensure that the patient's needs are met. Nurse case managers need to help the patient and the patient's family understand the treatment options and how these options might affect the patient. Patient advocacy requires the skills of communication, negotiation, collaboration, critical thinking, problem solving, patient education, and the ability to support the patient. The case manager may act as the patient's advocate while working for an MCO, other types of insurer, or for any clinical setting, such as the hospital, primary care, home care, or long-term care. The challenge with providing effective patient advocacy is that there are times when the needs of the patient may conflict with the needs of the HCO or the third-party payer. This presents a dilemma for the nurse who is a case manager for a HCO or a third-party payer. These are situations that may lead to professional ethics and legal issues. Chapter 6 discusses patient advocacy in more detail.

Patient Educator

Nurses typically provide patients with information about their illness, treatment, and future health care needs, so the case manager's transition to this case manager function should not be difficult. Health promotion and information about prevention are usually a part of patient education, and this is included in effective case management. Providers must now become more active in providing patient education. Patient education is an important component of case management, disease management, primary and acute care, and in care provided in all types of settings. There is an increasing interest in providing education by third-party payers via the Internet, e-mail, printed material, and in many types of group settings. This is an opportunity for nurse case managers to be assertive, recognize their long history of patient education, and provide expert advice on patient education, content, teaching–learning methods, and evaluation.

Triage Coordinator

Third-party payers want patients to receive timely access to the appropriate level of health care services. Nurse case managers provide triage services to assist patients as patients work their way through the health care and reimbursement systems. Case managers may assist patients via the telephone and may provide on-site visits for patients who are having major problems. The nurse case manager who is involved in triage must listen to the patient and assess the patient's needs, review any documentation that may be available on the patient, and determine the most effective and efficient course of action to take. Often, case managers use protocols as guidelines for assessment, diagnosis, and intervention; however, clinical judgment should play a major role in decision making. Effective communication skills with the patient and/or family members and with other health care providers is critical to achieve positive outcomes for the patient. Case managers not only need to be knowledgeable about the clinical problem and the patient's psychological response to illness but also knowledgeable about the patient's/member's insurance plan, its benefits and possible treatment options, and providers.

Quality Improvement (QI)

There has been increasing concern about the quality of health care throughout the health care delivery system. The case management process needs to include QI. Accreditation and quality issues are content and activities that involve case managers. QI is discussed in more detail in Chapter 5.

Utilization/Resource Management (UR/UM)

Insurers are very concerned about the use of resources because it is a critical factor in reducing their costs. To reduce costs, it is necessary to assess appropriateness and timeliness of care and then influence decisions that are made by providers. HCOs are also very interested in UR and use UR activities, which are often coordinated by case managers. Typically, utilization/resource management or UR focuses on LOS or length-of-treatment, use of services, complications, readmission rates, number of transfers, number and type of prescriptions, number of referrals to specialists, number of procedures, and so forth. Nurse case managers have the necessary skills for utilization/resource management: clinical knowledge, understanding of HCOs, nursing process, communication and collaboration within interdisciplinary teams, and understanding of documentation. The UR function also requires the nurse to be knowledgeable about reimbursement, provider options, benefits, and costs. Case managers are very involved in resource management. Authorization of services is the key task in resource management. UR is discussed in more detail in Chapter 4.

Outcomes Management

There is greater interest in and need for health care decisions driven by outcomes. A major concern with outcomes management is the need for nurses and other health care professionals to learn more about outcomes; what influences them; how to identify them; and how and when to measure them. With the primary care provider as the direct link, this may make it easier to track a patient's care. Managed care requires better information systems, and this should make it easier to collect outcomes data. MCOs are providing reports to providers about their patients and outcomes, and this can influence decision-making. In some cases, there has been concern that this might lead to negative results (e.g., decreasing treatment when needed); however, the data can be used positively to improve care. Managed care has influenced all types of insurers so that all insurers are more concerned with outcomes management and performance. Outcomes management is discussed in more detail in Chapter 4.

Discharge Planning

With the need to discharge patients from hospitals earlier than they were in the past and the pressure this puts on staff, it is important that hospitals have staff who can focus on the discharge needs of patients and their families. Many staff nurses have less and less time to do this. Some hospitals have identified specific nurses who provide patient discharge planning. These nurses need to work closely with unit staff, the patient's physician or primary care provider, utilization/resource management staff, case managers, and the patient's insurer. In some HCOs case managers serve as the discharge planner. Patients are discharged earlier in their recovery than they were in the past and thus have complex needs when they return home. The discharge planner must identify these needs and the community resources available to the patient that will be covered by the patient's third-party payer. Discharge planning is also very important in home care. Reimbursement for home care services is usually not indefinite. Patients and their families need to be prepared for self-care. Knowledge of discharge planning and involvement in the process may be a function important to some case managers, depending on their specific job. There is also an increasing number of patients with chronic illness who often have complex care issues.

LEGAL AND ETHICAL ISSUES

Legal and ethical issues are important aspects of the case management roles and responsibilities. Case managers need to understand these issues and their implications to their practice.

Legal Issues

Nurse case managers confront legal issues daily in their practice, although often it may not be obvious. Documentation is critical to any legal issue that may arise. The statement "if it isn't documented it didn't happen" is highly relevant to any **malpractice** suit. Case managers need to keep records of their plans and work. What do nurse case managers need to know about the legal issues? They certainly do not have to be attorneys, but they should seek the advice of an attorney when they are involved in a serious legal issue. Some issues, however, bear some review so that nurses have a basic understanding of the critical issues. Prior to reviewing these issues, it is important to clarify the definition of a law. The law is the formal organization of societal values that are demonstrated through individual laws that are passed and then implemented on the local, state, and federal level, and in some cases, even internationally.

BASIC LEGAL TERMINOLOGY.   Laws are developed and implemented through organizations within society. State legislatures, state and local governments, and Congress develop these laws. Laws are then implemented by state and federal law enforcement agencies or other agencies such as the state board of nursing. There are several types of laws. Common laws are rules and principles that were derived from past legal decisions that were developed in England and then brought to the United States. Criminal laws deal with offenses against the general public, and the public's response to criminal offenses is directed at deterrence, punishment, and/or rehabilitation of the person who committed the crime. Examples of criminal offenses are murder, robbery, and rape. Criminal law can also apply to health care situations because it covers assault and battery, which can occur in the health care setting. Civil law relates to the rights of individuals. Remedies typically involve payment of money or some type of compensation for **negligence**, personal injury, and medical malpractice.

NEGLIGENCE AND MALPRACTICE.   *Negligence* and *malpractice* are terms that are often heard together. What is the difference between malpractice and negligence? "**Negligence** is a general term that denotes conduct lacking in due care. Thus, negligence equates with carelessness. . . . Malpractice is a more specific term and looks at a professional standard of care as well as the professional status of the caregiver . . . the failure of a professional person to act in accordance with the prevailing professional standards or failure to foresee consequences that a professional person, having the necessary skills and education, should foresee" (Guido, 2001, p. 79). It is the failure to act as an ordinary prudent person would under similar circumstances, which is based on that person's education and training. The standard in negligence is average level of care. Sources for standards include expert witness testimony, accreditation requirements, publications by experts, clinical practice guidelines or pathways, statutes and regulations, advertising for services, contracts, and professional standards). There are four elements required to prove negligence.

1. There was a duty owed to the patient.
2. There was a breach of duty or standard by the health care professional.
3. There was harm caused by the breach of duty or standard.
4. The person (plaintiff) experienced damages or injuries.

Figure 1-2 describes the four elements.

An exception to meeting all four elements is the doctrine of *res ipsa loquitor*, which means that the "thing speaks for itself." This rule of evidence indicates that although a person may not be able to prove that an individual did something to cause harm or injury, because there is harm or injury the negligence can be inferred.

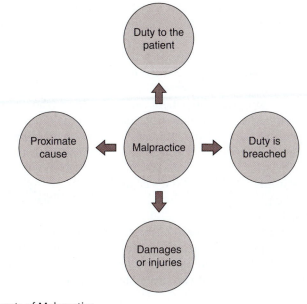

FIGURE 1-2   Elements of Malpractice

When negligence occurs damages or injuries may be physical, emotional, loss of job, loss of present and/or future earnings, disfigurement, disability, pain and suffering, and/or loss of enjoyment of life. There are two types of negligence. Unintentional negligence occurs when no harm was intended. Intentional negligence occurs when there is invasion of privacy or false imprisonment, although these are rare in health care. These situations can occur in health care when a patient's privacy is not maintained or when a patient is held against his or her wishes without legitimate medical reasons.

The elements that must be met for malpractice are the same as those for negligence, but there is greater emphasis on what would be expected from a professional. Some examples of common potential areas that might lead to negligence are failure to adequately assess, monitor, and communicate; failure to act as the patient's advocate; failure to provide patient education that leads to adjustment; and failure to protect a patient such as when the patient is at risk for falls or is suicidal.

A question that often comes up is, who is responsible for negligence? Is it the staff member (such as case manager) or the case manager's employer? If at the time the negligence occurs, the case manager is functioning in the employee role in a situation where the employer controls the case manager, then the doctrine of *respondent superior* applies. This means that both the case manager's employer and the case manager could be sued. This is also referred to as vicarious **liability.**

The following terms about consent are relevant in daily case management practice.

CONSENT.

- **Consent** may be one of three types: oral, implied by law, or apparent. This can be as simple as the patient orally consenting to talk to the case manager or it may be the patient signs a consent form for services or treatment. Consent implied by law is consent that may occur in emergency situations when, even though the patient may not be able to provide consent for emergency treatment, emergency treatment can be given. The patient is unable to give consent due to his/her condition, and there is a belief that the patient would give consent if the patient could. In other words, the patient would do what a reasonable person would do in a similar medical situation.

- *Informed consent* takes place when the provider has explained the facts to the patient in a manner in which the patient can understand so that the patient can make a decision. This is an interactive process in that the health care provider is required to tell the patient in language the patient can understand who will perform the procedure or treatment; discuss available alternatives to the recommended treatment; and identify possible harm. Patients must be informed that they have the right to refuse treatment. If there is no informed consent, the health care provider is at risk for negligence. Informed consent can be given orally or in writing. Informed consent can also be implied by the patient's behavior, or in emergency situations it can be presumed. The physician or the independent practitioner is accountable for obtaining informed consent.

- Informed consent for human research is very important. Case managers may have patients that participate in research in a variety of settings such as hospitals, clinics, and research institutes. The patient as the research participant needs to be informed in language the patient can understand. The key elements of consent for research include:
  1. Nature, purpose, procedures, drugs, or devices involved
  2. Identification of any experimental procedures
  3. Potential benefits, risks, and discomforts to participant
  4. Identification of privacy, confidentiality, and anonymity issues and how addressed
  5. Compensation if injury occurs and any compensation to participate
  6. Participation in research should be voluntary, and if the patient chooses to withdraw, which the patient can do, there is no negative impact on care needed.

PATIENT RIGHTS.

- **Advance directives** are now part of the health care system. The Self-Determination Act of 1990 resolved issues about the use of living wills and other similar documents. Health care providers must now ask patients if they have living wills and durable powers of attorney or advance directives. The goal of this law is to make individuals more aware of their rights and the importance of making informed decisions that give some consideration to costs of care. Case managers must follow their organization's policies and procedures related to any of the advance directives. Typically, the advance directive, which is a legal document, describes what the person wants done related to his or her end-of-life needs. These documents are often referred to as living wills. When a patient presents this document to the health care provider, it must be followed. There are no set requirements for content, but typical interventions that reincluded are: (1) use of life-sustaining equipment such as ventilators, respirators, or dialysis, (2) artificial hydration and nutrition (tube feeding), (3) "do not resuscitate" or "allow a natural death" orders, (4) withholding of food and fluids, (5) palliative care, and (6) organ or tissue donation. If a person is competent and able to speak for himself or herself, an advance directive serves no purpose, but it is recommended that individuals have this document for possible use in the future. If an advance directive is in place or applied, the patient always has the right to rescind it.

- **Durable power of attorney** (medical power of attorney) is another method that allows an individual to determine the individual's preferred care. A competent person may appoint a surrogate (often several are identified in priority order) to make health care decisions for that person when the person is not able to do so. This solves some of the issues with the advance directives or living will because there is a person who is actually making the decisions for the patient in case the patient cannot do so. Typically, individuals select someone whom they trust will carry out their wishes, and these wishes are discussed while the individual is competent to do so. The surrogate does not have to be a family member, although it is highly advisable that family members be informed about these documents and decisions prior to needing them.

• The do-not-resuscitate (DNR) directive is another form of advance directive that patients may request when they are receiving care. The physician may be implementing advance directives when writing a DNR order; for example, the patient has stated in the advanced directive that he or she does not want resuscitation. DNR orders also can be written without an advance directive; however, family members should also be consulted to prevent increasing family stress and possible legal actions. HCOs have policies and procedures to follow when patients request DNR and physicians write DNR orders, which should be followed. If the patient is able to participate, there must be some discussion between the physician and patient about the decision. There should also be specific intervals for reevaluation. End-of-life decisions are not easy to discuss. Palliative care is "care given to improve the quality of life of patients who have a serious or life-threatening disease. The goal of palliative care is to prevent or treat as early as possible the symptoms of a disease, side effects caused by treatment of a disease, and psychological, social, and spiritual problems related to a disease or its treatment. Also called comfort care, supportive care, and symptom management" (National Cancer Institute, 2009). The decision not to receive "aggressive medical treatment" is not the same as withholding all medical care. A patient can still receive antibiotics, nutrition, pain medication, radiation therapy, and other interventions when the goal of treatment becomes comfort rather than cure. At any time patients can change their minds and ask to resume more aggressive treatment. If the type of treatment a patient would like to receive changes, then it is important to be aware that such a decision may raise insurance issues that will need to be explored with the patient's health care plan. Ideally, all patients should have advance directives. The case manager should discuss advance directives, living wills, medical power of attorney, and DNR orders with patients/clients and find out if the patient has these documents and how they may impact current care needs.

REIMBURSEMENT LIABILITY. There is a difference in liability between traditional insurance and managed care. The critical difference is that some managed care organizations may be directly involved in the provision of care and very involved in the selection of providers, whereas traditional third-party payers usually are not involved in these two activities. Discussions about liability have focused on two major areas: Provider contracting and medical management program and activities. Provider contracting liability is primarily concerned with provider selection and provider termination. Provider–insurer contracts and their implementation are important to the provider–insurer relationship. They also have an impact on care delivery (e.g., authorization requirements, performance-based evaluation, and incentives). Medical management liability focuses on benefit decisions. Liability suits consider the cause and effect between denial of services and harm to the patient. In some cases, MCOs have declared that they do not provide care, and consequently, malpractice does not apply. MCOs, however, are more directly involved in the provision of care, which makes the issue of liability more complex. Early discharge and negligent referrals also expose MCOs to legal problems.

Malpractice suits against MCOs have been problematic. To win a negligence case against an MCO, the enrollee must demonstrate the major elements that must be found in any negligence suit:

- The MCO was under a *duty of care* to the enrollee to carry out the activity in conformance with a particular standard or to see that another entity did so on its behalf; level of care that would be provided by a reasonably prudent MCO.
- The MCO failed to meet the required *standard of care.*
- There was a *reasonably close causal connection between the failure and an injury.*
- The enrollee *suffered an actual loss or damage.*

The duty of care depends on the agreement between the insurer and the purchaser of the care. Was the harm to the patient a foreseeable consequence of the breach of the agreement? For example, an MCO agrees to screen providers prior to contracting with them to provide care to its enrollees. If a provider is not competent and the MCO selected that provider, is there a potential legal risk to the MCO if that provider provides or denies care that causes harm to the enrollee/patient? A key to this question is the MCO's knowledge of the provider's qualifications. It would be unrealistic to expect that the MCO could guarantee that every MCO provider will always provide quality care without errors.

Case managers can get involved in these lawsuits. An example is a case manager offers telephonic advice and does not follow the standard protocol. When the case manager is involved in making decisions about coverage and intervention choices there is greater risk. Both of these examples involve typical case management functions. It is important for the case manager to follow standard guidelines, protocols, policies, and so on. The case manager should be knowledgeable about the patient's medical history and needs, the patient's care, and as necessary, insurance factors.

Informed consent is always an area of risk. If there has been noncompliance with the case management plan by any member of the interdisciplinary team and this can be proven, there may be a claim for mismanagement of care. As the patient is part of the decision-making process (patient-centered care), it is important that the patient and family are told at the beginning that complications and undesired outcomes may occur. Case managers are involved in the informed consent process and need to be aware of the organization's requirements.

NEGLIGENCE AND MALPRACTICE AND THE CASE MANAGER.   There are also legal risks for the practicing case managers that are important to consider. Negligence and malpractice can occur in case management. Negligence occurs when standards are not met. For example, if a case manager does not review pertinent patient records with the MCO or insurer, and then the patient's surgery is denied due to inadequate review and the patient suffers serious consequences. In this case, both the case manager and the case manager's employer may be sued. Malpractice or professional misconduct and negligent care or failure to meet the standard of care that results in patient harm must be considered when care is provided and during the case management process.

Ethical Issues

Ethics focuses on what ought to be done in relation to what is done. Today, ethical conflict is present in all areas of health care. Even patient advocacy causes ethical dilemmas for the case manager. Some experts suggest that the case manager cannot truly resolve this dilemma. Case managers allocate resources daily and must at the same time consider patient needs. What happens when the case manager knows that a patient requires a particular service, but it is not covered by the patient's benefits or the service is denied? This can certainly lead to case manager stress and to an ethical dilemma. The case manager must consider ways to meet the need ethically and legally. In some cases, it may be impossible to meet the patient's needs. Knowledge of benefits, finances, and resources are critical at this time and are part of the following conflicts. The issue of insurance or healthcare organization profit is often present when case managers provide their services. Confidentiality is also important, and sometimes there is a dilemma in deciding what information might be revealed, such as information that might mean the patient would not receive coverage for care. Resource allocation often means choices have to be made, and sometimes the choices are far from ideal.

At the beginning of the case manager–patient relationship, the patient needs to be told about the case manager's limitations, availability, and responsibilities, such as assisting in managing benefits and costs. Patients and their families need to understand that the case manager does not provide direct care and must seek others to do this unless there is a medical emergency requiring immediate attention. In this case, the case manager can provide emergency care under the Good Samaritan Act; providing care to the best of ability until other care providers can assume responsibility. Patients can be confused about the role of the case manager, particularly if the case manager is a nurse.

Confidentiality is also important. Case managers inform their patients about the type of information they can keep confidential and what must be shared with the case manager's supervisors/employers or health care providers. For example, if the patient is not supposed to be working in order to receive reimbursement and the case manager learns that the patient is working, the case manager must report this to his or her employer or the insurer. The case manager must report all relevant information, and the patient has to understand that this is what the case manager must do. There is no doubt that the roles of gatekeeper and advocate often result in conflict. This requires that the case manager step back, consider the facts, use critical thinking, and then arrive at the best decision possible for the patient and the case management program or insurer.

The Commission for Case Management Certification (CCMC) describes the underlying case management values (2009, p. 1).

- Belief that case management is a means for improving client health, wellness and autonomy through advocacy, communication, education, identification of services resources, and service facilitation
- Recognition of the dignity, worth, and rights of all people
- Understanding and commitment to quality outcomes for clients, appropriate use of resources, and the empowerment of clients in a manner that is supportive and objective
- Belief in the underlying premise that when the individual(s) served, their support systems, the health care delivery systems, and the various reimbursement systems
- Recognition that case management is guided by the principles of autonomy, beneficence, non-malfeasance, and justice

Ethics, case management, and reimbursement issues are complex. For example, were inappropriate financial incentives given to providers, which is also a legal issue, or how was care resource allocation determined? The case manager needs to recognize that health care reimbursement and case management programs are businesses. It is recognized that some third-party payers are "good" ones, and this must imply that some type of standard has been used to compare one with the other to arrive at this conclusion. Are there standards? Can conflicts between business ethics and medical ethics within the same organization be resolved? Health care professionals want to apply medical ethics to insurers, particularly MCOs, because MCOs are involved in health care delivery services, which are viewed by many as being somewhat different from other business "products." Do the same ethical obligations that apply to health care professionals also apply to MCOs? There is no clear answer to this question.

Business ethics that promote fair competition when people are free to make voluntary choices to buy or sell goods or services do not fully apply to the managed care business. Depending upon an individual's insurer, the person may have limited health care provider choice in a system where the employers select insurance plans and employees must then choose from the employer list of plans. Investor-owned insurers and MCOs have a very important relationship with their stockholders, who expect a financial return on their investment. This can set up conflicts between their business needs to control costs and meet their budgetary requirements and their contractual obligations to provide health care services to the purchasers of their services, typically the employer.

The relationship between the insurer and the patient/enrollee is a contractual one, and this is very different from a fiduciary relationship. The third-party payer is responsible only for meeting the requirements of the health plan contract, and there is no requirement that all contracts must be the same. There is inequality in insurer contracts and benefits, and this is not considered to be an ethical problem. Lack of choice is a common complaint about managed care; however, the very nature of managed care denies some choice. Choice comes into play in the patient/enrollee's decision to join a health plan, and even this is limited by the employer's selection of plans. Patients rarely have complete information about the plan when they join, and many do not really become interested in these details until they need services. The ideal situation is the patient/enrollee who reviews each health plan option, including all of the details related to benefits, providers, outcome data, and the like, and then decides on the best plan based on the individual's and dependents' health status and needs. Choice is more operable in this scenario, but this rarely occurs.

If one could identify third-party payer ethical standards, what might be included? These standards would include accountability for the scope and quality of the patient care delivered. Fairness, honesty, truthfulness, respect for persons, and justice. These standards, however, are sometimes difficult to meet. For example, allocation of resources may conflict with many of these standards. Since a third-party payer wants to ensure that all of its enrollees receive care, there will be decisions made that will be unfair or unjust for some enrollees but fair and just to others. Patient satisfaction is directly affected by decisions that the insurer makes, and sometimes insurers make decisions that dissatisfy enrollees but meet the insurer's financial goals. The insurer makes a choice and decides what approach will result in the most benefit; however, this is a delicate decision because patient satisfaction is very important to insurer survival. Too much patient dissatisfaction can lead to the loss of employer health contracts.

ETHICAL DECISION MAKING.   Ethical decision making involves ethical dilemmas, which occurs when a person is forced to choose between two or more alternatives, none of which is perfect, but a decision must be made. Four of the primary principles used to make ethical decisions are those of autonomy, beneficence, justice, and veracity. Autonomy is a principle that has always been important to nurses. Patients have the right to determine their own rights. The second ethical principle is beneficence or doing something good. Health care providers should not inflict harm and need to safeguard the patient. Patients should also be treated fairly or with justice. This, of course, is a problem when decisions are made as to which patients will receive treatment. The fourth of the primary principles is veracity. Truth telling is critical to effective communication with patients. Figure 1-3 describes the ethical decision-making principles.

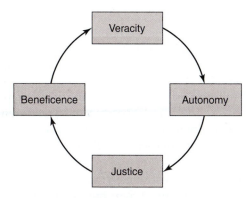

FIGURE 1-3   Ethical Decision-Making Principles   *Source:* Authors

Within any organization, individual staff have their own personal ethics, such as the ethics of the individual nurse case manager. Frequently, when ethical dilemmas are experienced, there is conflict between individual or personal ethics and organizational ethics. Knowing what is right and then doing what is right can be very difficult, and sometimes it is even difficult to determine what is right. Case managers confront this frequently when they advocate for the patient and yet still must meet requirements of their case management position and their employer. When a nurse case manager is faced with an ethical dilemma, the critical questions that need to be considered during decision making are:

- What is the problem? Are there different perspectives of the problem?
- Who are the people involved? (Directly or indirectly; what are their histories and involvement in the situation?)
- What are the choices for the patient/family, case manager, and health care provider?
- Who should decide and why?
- What are the causes and consequences?
- What degree and type of patient consent is required?
- How does the problem relate to personal and professional ethical codes?
- What are the costs and benefits of each possible solution? Who will receive the benefits? Who will pay the costs? (Costs can be more than financial.)

Each of these questions requires thought and data. Discussing them with peers can be very helpful, since peers can provide additional information and support. Nurse case managers need to be aware that there may be times of "disconnect" between what they think may be professionally relevant and what the organization that employs them thinks is relevant (O'Donnell, 2007). This can lead to ethical dilemmas.

Advocacy is an important part of case management. This topic is discussed more in Chapter 5. It is tied to ethical issues and the daily practice of case managers. The CCMC defines advocacy as: "A process that promotes beneficence, justice, and autonomy of clients. Advocacy especially aims to foster the client's independence. It also involves educating clients about their rights, health care and human services, resources, and benefits, and facilitating appropriate and informed decision making, and includes considerations for the client's values, beliefs, and interests" (2009, p. 3). Advocacy is also noted by the IOM to be an important component of patient-centered care.

HEALTH CARE FRAUD AND ABUSE.   Health care fraud and abuse are not so uncommon. Legal and ethical issues are found in both fraud and abuse experiences. Since the 1980s, there have been some serious, major fraud problems in health care, particularly in psychiatric care, home care, long-term care, and large corporate HCOs. In the United States in 2007, $2.26 trillion was spent on health care, and more than 4 billion health insurance claims were processed. "It is an undisputed reality that some of these health insurance claims are fraudulent. Although they constitute only a small fraction, those fraudulent claims carry a very high price tag. The National Health Care Anti-Fraud Association (NHCAA) estimates conservatively that 3% of all health care spending—or $68 billion—is lost to health care fraud" (National Health Care Anti-Fraud Association, 2009). This is more than the gross domestic product of 120 different countries, including Iceland, Ecuador, and Kenya (International Monetary Fund, 2008). Other estimates by government and law enforcement agencies place the loss due to health care fraud as high as 10% of our nation's annual health care expenditure—or a staggering $226 billion—each year (Federal Bureau of Investigation, 2007). And the cost of health care will only continue to rise, which means the price tag associated with health care fraud will rise too unless there is increased prevention of fraud (Centers for Medicare and Medicaid Services, 2007).

Fraud is a legal term that means a person deliberately deceived another for personal gain. In doing this, a health care professional is also breaking professional ethical principles. How does this happen in health care? Usually it involves money and reimbursement. For example, a patient is charged for care he or she did not receive or is charged more than the usual fee. Fraud cases have involved third-party payers, physicians, pharmacists, medical equipment companies, and HCOs. The False Claims Act (FCA) is a very old law that was amended in 1982. The law was passed during the Civil War to award citizens who exposed fraud against the government; however, it became a more useful law after it was amended in 1982. This is the federal law that protects whistle-blowers—those who expose fraud. Health care fraud, as is true of most fraud, is very difficult to prove. Having people on the inside of the organization who are willing to share information is often critical to successfully prove fraud. If a case manager or staff member decides to file a suit and report fraud and the government decides to intervene in the staff member's case, the staff member is entitled to a percentage of the government's ultimate recovery. It is not easy to report an employer and presents the person with a major ethical dilemma. Employees have concerns about retaliation, and there is no doubt that this is a highly stressful, long-drawn-out process. Examples of FCA cases that would have relevance to case managers concern falsely reporting services related to Medicare; up coding (deliberately changing a procedure classification to obtain greater reimbursement) and unbundling (separating procedures in order to get paid for each of them to increase the total cost); and falsifying cost reports. Other examples of health care fraud as reported by NHCCA are: Billing for services never rendered; billing for expensive services or procedures than performed (up coding); performing medically unnecessary services; misrepresenting non-covered services as medically necessary, falsifying diagnosis to justify tests, procedures, surgery, and so on; unbundling; accepting kickbacks for referrals, waiving patient co-pays or deductibles and over-billing for services that were prepaid or paid in full by the benefit plan.

PROFESSIONAL ETHICS.   The appropriate allocation of scarce resources to reduce costs is a complex problem that is experienced every day by HCOs and all types of third-party payers. Nurse case managers are very involved in allocation of resources. Examples of typical ethical decisions that a nurse case manager may encounter are:

1. Cost containment issues that may jeopardize patient welfare
2. End-of-life decisions
3. Informed consent
4. Incompetent, unethical, or illegal practices of health care professionals

5. Access to health care
6. Denial of care or providing care that is not the patient's preference

Case managers confront ethical dilemmas in all practice settings and a wide variety of locations. They may feel unprepared to cope with ethical dilemmas. Conflicts come from differences in professional roles and responsibilities and what the employer may expect of the nurse case manager, leaving the nurse case manager feeling powerless.

THE ETHICAL ROLE OF PROFESSIONAL ORGANIZATIONS.   Since nurse case managers are nurses they do have a responsibility to follow the nursing profession code of ethics organizations. The American Nurses Association (ANA) *Code for Nurses with Interpretive Statements* (2001) is the primary source or guide for nurses when ethical issues are encountered. "Individuals who become nurses are expected not only to adhere to the ideals and moral norms of the profession but also to embrace them as part of what it means to be a nurse. The ethical tradition of nursing is self-reflective, enduring, and distinctive. A code of ethics makes explicit the primary goals, values, and obligations of the profession" (American Nurses Association, 2001, p. 5). The code includes the following principles (American Nurses Association, 2001).

1. The nurse, in all professional relationships, practices with compassion and respect for the inherent dignity, worth, and uniqueness of every individual, unrestricted by considerations of social or economic status, personal attributes, or the nature of health problems.
2. The nurse's primary commitment is to the patient, whether an individual, family, group, or community.
3. The nurse promotes, advocates for, and strives to protect the health, safety, and rights of the patient.
4. The nurse is responsible and accountable for individual nursing practice and determines the appropriate delegation of tasks consistent with the nurse's obligation to provide optimum patient care.
5. The nurse owes the same duties to self as to others, including the responsibility to preserve integrity and safety, to maintain competence, and to continue personal and professional growth.
6. The nurse participates in establishing, maintaining, and improving health care environments and conditions of employment conducive to the provision of quality health care and consistent with the values of the profession through individual and collective action.
7. The nurse participates in the advancement of the profession through contributions to practice, education, administration, and knowledge development.
8. The nurse collaborates with other health professionals and the public in promoting community, national, and international efforts to meet health needs.
9. The profession of nursing, as represented by associations and their members, is responsible for articulating nursing values, for maintaining the integrity of the profession and its practice, and for shaping social policy.

These principles also relate to the work of the nurse case manager for example in areas of patient choice, contracts, conflicts of interest, denial of coverage, application of standards, access to care, uninsured, and information, information systems and privacy.

The Commission for Case Manager Certification identifies the specific case management ethical principles in its *Code of Professional Conduct for Case Managers* (2009, p. 1) by identifying case manager certificants' expectations as:

1. Place the public interest above their own interest at all times.
2. Respect the rights and inherent dignity of all their clients.

3. Maintain objectivity in their relationships with clients.
4. Act with integrity in dealing with other professionals to facilitate their clients' achieving maximum benefits.
5. Keep their competency at a level that ensures each of their clients will receive the benefit of services that are appropriate and consistent for the client's conditions and circumstances.
6. Honor the integrity and respect of the limitations placed on the use of CCM designation.
7. Obey all laws and regulations.
8. Help maintain the integrity of the Code.

The basic objective of the Code is to protect the public, which is the same as the basic objective of Nurse Practice Acts and the ANA *Code for Nurses* (2001).

ORGANIZATIONAL ETHICS.   Utilization Review Accreditation Commission (URAC), one of the accrediting organizations for insurers, emphasizes the need for organizational ethics and confidentiality. Corporate compliance programs are more common today due to greater emphasis on ethics resulting in more methods of insurance fraud. The organization may be an insurer, MCO, or an HCO such as a hospital. Each must establish policies and procedures to protect the "confidentiality of individually identifiable health information and to protect the welfare and safety of consumers and case managers" (Utilization Review Accreditation Commission, 2009). These policies and procedures need to also include consumer and family autonomy in decision making, respecting patient rights. Policies and procedures important to the case management planning process in such areas as patient participation in the planning, refusal of treatment or services, and obtaining information to determine criteria for case closure.

The quality and commitment of compliance ethics programs must be monitored. Monitoring can become only another process that might look good on paper but does not truly reflect the organization's culture and the behavior of its employees and has no impact on quality improvement. Some of these organizations also have ethics officers or compliance officers. What is their authority, and how can they really effect change? These are critical questions that should be asked by organizations. It is not easy to change organizational culture, and it takes time. Is there true commitment to improve, or is this being done to put the organization in a better legal position in case there are problems? What are some of the activities of these compliance programs? Employee education is one important activity. Topics that might be covered include the organization's mission and values, code of conduct, compliance plan, roles and responsibilities of the compliance officer, compliance with laws and regulations, conflict of interests, financial and accounting records, fraud and abuse, professional standards and codes of ethics, confidentiality of patient information and organization information, physician relations, patient rights, respect and concern for others, and anti-trust issues. Some of these topics are not applicable to all staff. For example, not all staff need an understanding of financial and accounting records. But all staff need to know the procedure for reporting their concerns. Staff may see the compliance program as another "change" that will have little impact on the organization. If an organization really wants to change the organizational culture and commit itself to a more ethical work environment, this type of staff attitude needs to be addressed by the organization. Organizational leaders must be role models for all of the staff.

SPECIAL ETHICAL ISSUES.   There are two special ethical issues that are important in case management practice: Patient privacy and HIPAA and organ transplantation.

The Health Insurance Portability and Accountability Act (HIPAA), 1996, has had a major impact on information technology and patient information. It identifies the first comprehensive privacy federal standards (U.S. Department of Health and Human Services, 2009). Case managers are required to follow this law to protect patient privacy. Patients are informed about HIPAA when they enter a hospital or when they receive other types of health care. Regulations about patient privacy were added to HIPAA and went into effect in April 2003. HIPAA impacts policies and procedures related to oral, written, and electronic patient identifiable data set up by the HCO; however, there are some key areas that are affected by these new privacy regulations.

- Patients must be informed of their privacy rights.
- Patients must be informed as to who will see their records and for what purpose.
- Patients have the right to inspect and obtain a copy of their medical records. (There are some exceptions to this that each organization should make clear to staff.)
- Valid authorization to release health information must contain certain information, such as a copy of the signed authorization given to the patient, use of understandable language, and how the patient may revoke authorization.
- Although information may be used for research purposes to assess outbreak of a disease, all individual identifiable data must be removed.
- Personal data may not be used for marketing (for example, pharmacies may not share this information with others for this purpose).

These privacy standards are complex and require HCOs to make changes in how they manage information. It also requires that staff are trained and updated about the changes. The standards give patients more control while at the same time makes providers more accountable for keeping information private. This is federal law, but if a state has more rigorous privacy requirements then the state requirements would have to be followed.

Organ Transplantation.   Organ transplantation is a form of resource allocation, and case managers may be involved with patients and families around these issues either in a donor or recipient situation. Both of these situations are stressful and complex. There are specific criteria to be followed for each type of organ donation that HCOs must implement. Specific criteria should determine who gets a transplant and when, though it is not always clear as to who gets a transplant through organ transplantation registries. Criteria include factors such as age; other illnesses; what the person might be able to contribute over his or her lifetime; single or married with children; comorbidities such as substance abuse; and the patient's ability to comply with follow-up treatment. Transplantations are expensive and may not be covered by health insurance or may only be partially covered. This, of course, makes it complicated for case managers. Why might transplantation be denied? The patient requires lifetime specialized care, which is also costly. The other aspect of transplantation is organ donation. For some donors the decision to donate is made when the person is healthy, such as by identifying future intent through driver's license organ donor program. The case manager may learn of this decision when working with the family after a traumatic injury to the patient. It is not unusual for families to be hesitant and very upset over the decision that needs to be made, even if the injured and terminal family member requested this action. Health care providers also ask for organ donations, which are complex ethical and legal experiences. With organ donation and transplantation, time is a critical element to maintain organ viability. Case managers may be involved in this decision-making process.

Summary

This chapter serves as an introduction to case management. The health care delivery system and insurers are using case management more as they strive to improve care and control costs. Case management has been changing and has expanded its functions. The IOM five health care professions core competencies also apply to case managers. Case managers encounter legal and ethical issues in their daily practice.

Chapter Highlights

1. The U.S. health care economy has struggled for many years. The cost of health care is high and continues to increase. This has had a major impact on the health status of individuals and an economic impact.
2. Health care reform is a critical need; however, at this time it is not clear where it will lead and what changes will be made.
3. Case management is not a profession as several different health care professions may serve as case managers, for example nurses and social workers. Case management is a collaborative process with the case manager serving as the care coordinator.
4. Case management has a long history, and the role has changed over time.
5. There are multiple purposes for case management. The key goal is to simultaneously promote the patient's wellness and autonomy and ensure appropriate use of service and financial resources.
6. The IOM five core competencies are important to case management. The competencies are: deliver patient-centered care, work in interdisciplinary teams, apply EBP, employ QI, and utilize informatics.
7. The key case manager functions and responsibilities are provider liaison, benefits interpreter, patient advocate, patient educator, triage coordinator, quality improvement, utilization/resource management, outcomes management, and discharge planning.
8. Case managers need to be aware of legal issues as they pertain to case management. Many of these issues are the same as they are for nursing practice. Case managers need to be particularly concerned about patient rights and consents.
9. Ethics has become a critical issue in the health care environment, with providers struggling with the dilemma of quality versus cost. There have been major fraud and abuse scandals in psychiatry, home care, and long-term care that have resulted in congressional hearings and programs to combat health care fraud. Case managers must continue to openly discuss ethics, maintain an ethical code, and provide content on ethics at all levels of nursing education.

References

American Nurses Association. (ANA). (2001). *Code for Nurses with Interpretive Statements.* Silver Springs, MD: Author.

Case Management Society of America. (CSMA). (2002). *Standards of practice for case management.* Little Rock, AR: Author.

Centers for Medicare and Medicaid Services (CMS), Office of the Actuary. *National health expenditure projections 2007–2017.* Retrieved from http://www.cms.hhs.gov/NationalHealthExpendData/Downloads/proj2007.pdf

Cohen, E. (1996). *Nurse case management in the 21ˢᵗ century.* St. Louis, MO: Mosby Year Book.

Commission for Case Management Certification. (CCMC). (2009). *Code of Professional Conduct for Case Managers.* Mt. Laurel, NJ: Author.

Cover the Uninsured. (2009). Current Data. Retrieved from http://covertheuninsured.org/ on July 8, 2009.

Disch, J. (2001). Strengthening nursing and interdisciplinary collaboration. *Journal of Professional Nursing, 17*(6), 275.

Federal Bureau of Investigation. (FBI). (2007). *Financial crimes report to the public, fiscal year 2007.* Retrieved from http://www.fbi.gov/publications/financial/fcs_report2007/financial_crime_2007.htm

Fidelity Investments, (2006, March 6). Press release. Retrieved from http://www.fidelity.com on June 10. 2009.

Harrison, J., Nolin, J., & Suero, E. (2004). The effect of case management on U.S. hospitals. *Nursing Economics, 22*(2), 64–70.

Henry J. Kaiser Family Foundation. (2009a). News release. Retrieved from http://www.kff.org/kaiserpolls/kaiserpolls022509nr.dfm on February 27, 2009.

Henry J. Kaiser Family Foundation. (2009b). Health insurance. Retrieved from http://www.kff.org/ on June 27, 2009.

Himmelstein, D., Warren, D. Thorne, D., & Woolhander, S. (2005, February). Illness and injury as contributors to bankruptcy. *Health Affairs*, Web Exclusive W5–63, 02.

Institute of Medicine. (IOM). (2003a). *Priority areas for national action: Transforming health care quality.* Washington, DC: Author.

Institute of Medicine. (IOM). (2003b). *Health professions education. A bridge to quality.* Washington, DC: Author.

Institute of Medicine. (IOM). (2004). *Insuring America's health.* Washington, DC: Author.

International Monetary Fund. (IMF). World Economic Outlook Database. (2008, April). Nominal GDP list of countries. Data for the year 2007. Retrieved from http://www.imf.org/external/pubs/ft/weo/2008/01/weodata/index.aspx

Keehan, S., et al. (2008, February). Health spending projections through 2017. *Health Affairs* Web exclusive W146: 21.

McKinsey Global Institute. (2007, January). Accounting for the cost of health care in the United States. Retrieved from http://www.mckinsey.com/mgi/rp/healthcare/accounting_cost_healthcare.asp on July 6, 2009.

National Cancer Institute. (NCI). (2009). Retrieved from National Cancer Institute at http://www.cancer.gov/Templates/db_alpha.aspx?CdrID=269448 on February 12, 2009.

National Council on Aging. (NCOA). (1988). *Care management standards.* Washington, DC: Author.

National Health Care Anti-Fraud Association. (NHCAA). (2007). The problem of health care fraud. Retrieved from http://www.nhcaa.org/eweb/DynamicPage.aspx?webcode=anti_fraud_resource_centr&wpscode=TheProblemOfHCFraud on June 11, 2009.

O'Donnell, L. (2007). Ethical dilemmas among nurses as they transition to hospital case management: Implications for organizational ethics, part II. *Professional Case Management, 12*(4), 219–231.

Powell, S. & Tahan, H. (2008). *CMSA© core curriculum for case management.* Philadelphia: Lippincott Williams & Wilkins.

Robertson, C., Egelhof, R., & Hoke, M. (2008). Get sick, get out: The medical causes of home mortgage foreclosures," *Health Matrix: Journal of Law-Medicine, 18*(65).

Sisko, A., et al. (2009). Health spending projections through 2018: Recession effects add uncertainty to the outlook. *Health Affairs, 28*(2), 346–357.

Stanton, M. & Lammon, C. (2008). The "wins" of change. Evaluating the impact of predicted changes on case management practice. *Professional Case Management, 13*(3), 161–168.

The White House. (2009, February). Health Reform. Retrieved from http:www.whitehouse.gov on May 10, 2009.

U.S. Department of Health and Human Services. (DHHS). (2000). *Healthy People 2010.* Retrieved from http://www.healthypeople.gov/ on May 10, 2009.

U.S. Department of Health and Human Services. (DHHS). (2009). Health Insurance Portability and Accountability Act (HIPAA), 1996. Retrieved from http://www.hhs.gov/ocr/hipaa on May 29, 2009.

Utilization Review Accreditation Commission. (URAC). (2009). FAQ and interpretations. Retrieved from http://www.urac.org/accreditation/faq.aspx#core23 on June 3, 2009.

Williams, M. & Torrens, P. (1993). *Introduction to health services.* (4th ed.). Albany, NY: Delmar Publishers.

Zander, K. (1996). The early years: The evolution of nursing care management. In D. Flarey & S. Blancett (Eds.), *Handbook of nursing case management* (pp. 23–41). Gaithersburg, MD: Aspen Publishers, Inc.

Questions and Activities for Thought

1. What is the current status of the U.S. health care economy and health care reform?
2. How do the IOM's five healthcare professions core competencies relate to case management?
3. Review each of the case manager functions and describe how you would apply that function in case management practice. Provide examples and discuss in class.
4. What is the difference in liability for traditional third-party payer insurance and MCOs?
5. How does the American Nurses Association's *Code for Nurses* relate to case management ethics? What are the ethical code issues for case managers?
6. Examine the examples of problems in health care organizational ethics that have occurred in the past 10 years. What could be their long-term effects?

Case

You have been hired as a consultant by a hospital that is going to begin using case managers. When you go in for your initial meeting with the vice president of patient services. The VP identifies one of the key problems. She tells you that the hospital tried to use case managers 3 years ago, and the project failed. She believes one the major reasons it failed is there was no effective position description that was understood by the staff. The first activity she wants you to help the hospital accomplish is to develop an effective case manager position description. Two weeks later you return with your draft of the position description to discuss it with the VP and with other key stakeholders. Develop the position description you would submit and then identify the key points you would discuss with the group to clarify the role and open a discussion on the role.

Internet Links

1. URL: http://www.aoa.dhhs.gov
   Is there information about health care antifraud initiatives on this site? Why would this information be on this site?
2. URL: http://www.medicare.gov
   Visit this site and click on "Fraud and Abuse." How should fraud and abuse be reported? What fraud tips are provided? Why is it important to involve the consumer in fraud and abuse detection?
3. URL: http://www.hcfa.gov
   What are some of the legislative and regulatory issues that are of interest to the Health Care Financing Administration at this time?
4. URL: http://www.aahp.org
   What is included in the code of conduct for the American Association of Health Plans? Is this an adequate code of ethics? To whom does it apply? Do you think it is followed?

CHAPTER 2

Case Management Models

OBJECTIVES

After completing this chapter, the reader will be able to:

- Describe the four key case manager functions.
- Discuss critical competencies required to provide effective case management services.
- Identify red flags for case management.
- Apply the phases of the case management process.
- Apply key case management program characteristics.
- Compare and contrast case management models and settings.

KEY TERMS

INTRODUCTION

Collaborative care or cooperative effort among health care professionals is central to the success of efficient, outcome-driven care. With the complex health care system, specialization of many health care professionals, variety of health care settings, complex reimbursement systems, technology, and new drugs, collaboration is critical to ensuring that patients receive quality care that is cost effective. Today, the health care system is an interdependent system, and case management supports collaborative care in this type of system. This care requires flexibility to adjust to the changing needs of the complex health care environment. All of these activities are integral to successful case management. The nurse case manager works with many different health care providers, within many different health care settings, and with the patient and family to ensure quality care that is cost effective for the patient. Case management is an important component of the health care system today. Its increased use is primarily due to increased health care costs, prospective payment systems, and the growth of managed care as well as an increasing concern about fragmented care. Case management is a strategy that is used by most insurers/third-party insurers and health care organizations (HCOs) such as hospitals. This chapter discusses case management, models, and settings, and further explores the case manager roles and functions. Many experts advocate that the nurse is the best candidate for the case manager position.

CASE MANAGER KEY FUNCTIONS

The Case Management Society of America (CMSA) (2002) identifies four major case manager functions.

1. *Assessor.*   The case manager gathers all relevant data and obtains information by interviewing the patient/family and performing a careful **evaluation** of the entire situation. All information related to the current treatment plan should be evaluated objectively and critically to identify barriers, clarify or determine realistic goals and objectives, and seek potential alternatives.
2. *Planner.*   The case manager works with the patient and family to develop a treatment plan that enhances patient outcome and reduces the payer's liability. The planning process includes the patient and family as the primary decision makers and goal setters. Contingency plans are incorporated for each step in the process to anticipate treatment and service complications. The case manager initiates and implements plan modifications as necessary through monitoring and reevaluation to accommodate changes in treatment or progress.
3. *Facilitator.*   The case manager actively promotes **communication** among all team members, patient/family, providers, and all parties involved. Collaboration between the patient and the health team is enhanced, which maximizes outcomes. The health delivery process is streamlined to focus on the best treatment or approach for the patient and to minimize or eliminate unnecessary steps, thus promoting the timely provision of care and use of resources. This is accomplished via **coordination** of the delivery of services and frequently requires negotiation skills. Financial analysis is also important as cost–benefit is assessed.
4. *Advocate.*   The patient's individualized needs and goals are incorporated throughout the case management process. The case manager, however, does not assume patient responsibilities or take over control. The patient is supported and educated to become empowered and self-reliant in self-advocacy. The consensus of all parties is obtained to achieve optimal outcomes. Early referral is promoted to provide the greatest degree of quality care and cost containment. The patient's best interests are represented by the case manager's advocacy for necessary funding,

treatment alternatives, timelines and coordination of health services, and frequent reevaluation of progress and goals. Other functions that are very important are **discharge planning,** resource management, and outcome management.

BOX 2-1

Case Manager Key Functions

- Assess
- Plan

- Facilitate
- Advocate

Case manager functions are highlighted in Box 2-1. (CMSA standards are under revision. When new standards are available, they can be found at http://www.cmsa.org.)

Case managers must be people who "possess a sense of humor, perseverance, optimism, and confidence, are not risk adverse, and above all, are good communicators" (Mullahy & Boling, 2008, p. 287). Throughout the case management process, the case manager uses communication skills, works collaboratively with the patient/family to make informed decisions, and views the patient and family/significant others as a functional unit. The case manager needs to be knowledgeable about many topics as well as demonstrate many skills. Critical skills are communication, decision making, brokering, negotiation, conflict resolution, creative persuasion, and **delegation. Critical thinking** is a very important part of all of these skills.

Most nurses who have had some clinical experience have most of the qualifications and some of the competencies required to be a case manager. The problem is that most nurses lack knowledge about reimbursement, claims management, managed care, and health care financial issues. Understanding this information is critical to the role because the case manager needs to demonstrate direct accountability for managing outcomes and reducing patient care costs.

CRITICAL CASE MANAGEMENT COMPETENCIES

Nurse case management requires improved and new competencies to be successful. The five core health care professions competencies were described in Chapter 1 and apply to case managers. The following discussion highlights additional critical competencies and their relationship to case management. Case management competencies are listed in Box 2-2.

Critical Thinking

Critical thinking is very important in all aspects of case management. Why is it so important? Dichotomous thinking, which is the tendency to view things as polarized, gets case managers into trouble. Change is evident throughout the health care delivery system. Dichotomous thinking limits thinking to two alternatives to which values are assigned, good or bad. This type of thinking is very limiting and is not the type of thinking that will be successful today. However, critical thinking is helpful.

Critical thinking is the "purposeful, informed, outcome-focused (results-oriented) thinking that requires careful identification of key problems, issues, and risks involved" (Alfaro-LeFevre, 2006, p. 30). This type of thinking allows the case manager to develop a clearer view of an issue. Critical thinking skills that are important to develop are: affective learning; applied moral reasoning and values (relates to ethics); comprehension; application, analysis, and synthesis; interpretation; knowledge,

---

BOX 2-2

Case Manager Competencies

- Patient/client-centered care
- Assessment
- Case management planning
- Outcome development
- Discharge planning
- Communication skills
- Collaboration
- Coordination
- Critical thinking and clinical reasoning and judgement
- Documentation
- Interdisciplinary team roles and responsibilities
- Team building and collaboration
- Reimbursement
- Managed care
- Claims management

- Retrieval and interpretation of data (e.g., clinical, financial)
- Resource management
- Utilization review
- Legal issues
- Ethical issues
- Negotiating skills
- Disease management
- Implementation of clinical pathways
- Patient/family education
- Medication management/compliance
- Knowledge of community resources
- Quality improvement
- Knowledge of standards and regulations
- Healthcare informatics
- Evidence-based practice

---

experience, judgment, and evaluation; learning from mistakes when they happen; and self-awareness (Finkelman, 2001). Problem solving is not critical thinking, but effective problem solving requires critical thinking; as an example, use these methods (Finkelman, 2001, p. 196):

1. Seek the best information and data possible to allow you to fully understand the issue, situation, or problem. Questioning is critical. Examples of some questions that might be asked are: What is the significance of _____? What is your first impression? What is the relationship between _____ and _____? What impact might_____have on_____? What can you infer from the information/data?
2. Identify and describe any problems that require analysis and synthesis of information—thoroughly understand the information and data.
3. Develop alternative solutions—more than two is better because this forces you to analyze multiple solutions even when you discard one of them. Be innovative and move away from proposing only typical or routine solutions.
4. Evaluate the alternative solutions and consider the consequences for each one. Can the solutions really be used? Do you have the resources you need? How much time will it take? How well will the solution be accepted? Identify pros and cons.
5. Make a decision—choosing the best solution though there is risk in any decision making.
6. Implement the solution but continue to question.
7. Follow up and evaluate; plan for evaluation from the very beginning.

Decision making, which occurs daily in case management, is not equivalent to critical thinking. It is the end point of using critical thinking, but critical thinking is also part of each step of the decision-making process. For a long time nursing has emphasized critical thinking, while clinical reasoning and judgment have been ignored, but they are actually more important than critical thinking. Clinical reasoning is the ability to assess a patient's problems and needs, and then to analyze the data to accurately identify the problem(s) within the context of the patient's enviroment, which relates to patient-centered care. Clinical judgment is the process the case manager uses to understand the patient's (and family's or significant other's) problems, issues, and concerns, to focus on critical information, and to respond in order to work to resolve the problem using conscious decision making and intuitive response. Technology is discussed in Chapter 6, and of particular importance to decision making are electronic decision support systems (DSS) that a case manager might use through an electronic medical record system. Throughout the process the case manager needs to be focused on outcomes, not tasks. The case manager may need to use creativity to arrive at innovative solutions but still needs to consider the required parameters of effective benefits and costs.

Collaboration and Interdisciplinary Relationships

The American Nurses Association (ANA) defines collaboration as "recognition of the expertise of others within and outside the profession, and referral to those other providers when appropriate. Collaboration involves some shared functions and a common focus on the same overall mission" (2003, p. 8). This is a critical competency required to practice in any health care setting today or to participate in any aspect of health care delivery. The increased emphasis on interdisciplinary teams that can meet the patient's needs across the continuum of care requires collaboration. Team members and different health care providers must be able to work together, recognize strengths and limitations, respect individual responsibilities, and maintain open communication.

Nurses have long worked on teams, and nurse case managers should be familiar with teamwork. Despite this, there continues to be a separation between physicians and nurses, and this is very destructive in the managed care environment. Nurse case managers and physicians can work together to ensure that the patient receives the care that is required when it is required. Collaboration requires cooperative effort among all health care providers providing care for a patient. All need to work together to accomplish the identified goals and reach identified outcomes. This is not easy to do. There are professional issues, territory issues, conflicting goals, inadequate communication, and multiple differences; however, despite all of this, effective and efficient care requires collaboration. The system is just too complex to function well without collaboration. The case manager is often the person who must lead the effort to ensure collaboration occurs.

Coordination

The Institute of Medicine (IOM) identifies care coordination as one of the critical priority areas of care that need to be monitored and improved. The purpose of care coordination is "to establish and support a continuous healing relationship, enabled by an integrated clinical environment and characterized by a proactive delivery of evidence-based care and follow-up" (IOM, 2003a, p. 49). The Commission for Case Manager Certification (CCMC) defines coordination as "organizing, securing, integrating, modifying, and documenting the resources necessary to accomplish the goals set forth in the **case management plan**" (2005, p. 6). There needs to be greater attention on how care is coordinated across people, functions, activities, and sites so that the outcome is effective and efficient care that meets the patient's specific outcomes. How the pieces are put together to reach desired outcomes is an important part of case management. Coordination requires that the nurse case manager understands patient needs and the resources that are available to meet these needs. An awareness of the association of costs and services is part of coordinating patient care.

In addition, coordination is not only very important in case management but also within the health care delivery system. This system has become more complex, which has made communication and coordination more complex, all of which leads to increased errors. There is greater need for interdisciplinary teams. Team members may not always view the patient, problems, or priorities in the same way, yet it is critical that the team find a way to work collaboratively to provide coordinated patient care. Team members need to have a better understanding of individual responsibilities and stress in order to appreciate each other and develop more realistic working relationships. As noted by the IOM health care core competency, all health care professionals need to know how to work in interdisciplinary teams (IOM, 2003b). Recognizing this will make coordination less frustrating, and the case manager has a major role in health care teams.

"With pressure being mounted by the Centers for Medicare and Medicaid Services, the Office of the Inspector General and the general public, the role of the case manager (in all practice settings) will become increasingly more crucial. Through development of a network of local venues of care, the case manager can facilitate care transitions throughout the health care system with the goal of improved outcomes for the patient regardless of setting. Providing the right care, in the right setting to improve patient care, can only benefit our aging and declining populations" (Thomas, 2008, p. 220).

Communication

Communication is a complex process that should not be ignored. Case managers need this skill daily in their work as they communicate with patients, families, coworkers, physicians and other providers, insurers, administrators and managers, support staff, other case managers, utilization management staff, and so on. Case managers may provide inadequate communication and certainly encounter poor communication from others daily. The transmission of information and understanding takes place on many different levels: individual to individual, in small teams, in large organizations, and between large organizations. Each level of the communication process requires:

- Encoding, or translation of the communicator's ideas into language
- Message, or the result of the encoding process
- Medium, or the carrier of the message (e.g., face-to-face, memo, medical record, group meeting, computer, policy statement, or can be unintended message that is sent by silence or inaction)
- Decoding, or the process the receiver goes through to receive and interpret the message
- Feedback, an important component of two-way communication

Reimbursement with its complexities has made communication in health care even more problematic. Sometimes just trying to get approval for a patient procedure can strain a physician or staff member's patience so that when the physician or staff member interacts with the case manager tempers flare, and effective communication is blocked. There may need to be telephone calls, written documentation of needs, and in some cases, actual face-to-face contact. The result may still be unsatisfying.

Improving communication is important for all concerned. Several strategies may be used to improve it. Follow-up helps to determine if the message that a person intended to send was actually received. It is easy to make assumptions, which can lead to problems when the assumption is incorrect. Regulating information flow during a time of excessive information from computers, different providers, e-mail, memos, policies, insurers, and so forth can make a big difference. What information is really necessary to assist staff in providing care and making decisions? This question is frequently ignored as staffs are flooded with more information. Feedback is a critical component. It is important for all staff to feel that their feedback is respected. Patients and families and all types of consumers expect that their feedback will be considered. Empathy is often something that gets left out as staff become consumed with excessive information and have less and less time to cope with it. The communicator needs to be receiver oriented to anticipate how the message may be decoded or interpreted.

Mutual trust is something that is not always so easy to accomplish today. Poor or inconsistent communication, inadequate staff input during the change process, and fears (e.g., job loss) can damage mutual trust. This trust is a critical component of communication. Case managers who communicate effectively—responding to others clearly and also anticipating issues to prevent communication blocks—will be more successful and their patients will receive better care.

Developing strategies to build mutual trust is also important. Effective timing is something that should be considered for any important communication. With so much information coming at a person, it is easy to miss the important information. E-mail has made it easier to communicate and made memos less necessary; however, e-mail also increases information because it is too easy to send. Case managers who do not use effective listening will soon find that they are not communicating. There seems to be increasingly less staff to listen to patients and their families. Listening with all senses is very important, and there is less time for this, too. In general, improving communication requires constant effort and effective strategies to send and receive communication effectively.

Assertiveness is a communication style that case managers need to develop. Assertiveness is not aggression, though sometimes people confuse the two. Assertiveness is a constructive communication style. In using this style the case manager is standing up for what the case manager believes. How does this work? An assertive case manager uses "I" statements when communicating thoughts and feelings and uses "you" statements to persuade others (Fabre, 2005). Fabre identifies the following guidelines for effective assertiveness (2005, p. 78).

- Intervene in situations calmly and confidently.
- Respond to problems in a timely way to avoid accumulation of negative feelings. Those who are passive for a long time run the risk of overreaction to small incidents.
- Clearly articulate your perspectives.
- Use language that others understand (the audience, for example, the team, management, and so forth).

Case managers often work with physicians, and in many cases in situations where the case manager has different goals and needs from the physician. Nurse case managers have had experience working with physicians in their nursing role. In a study done by Burke, Boal, and Mitchell (2004), nurse–physician communication was explored. The methods identified to improve this communication also apply to nurse case manager–physician communication. These methods include:

1. Develop a personal connection helps to increase colleagueship.
2. Use humor.
3. Make the assumption that you are on the same team.
4. Recognize that team members are equal in expertise that can be important to patient care.
5. Arrange to meet in person with physicians you speak to frequently over the telephone.
6. Report good news about patients—improvements, not just problems.
7. Recognize that conflict will occur, but this does not mean that communication and collaboration cannot be maintained.
8. Discuss preferred methods of communication (telephone, e-mail, pager, in person, voice message) and under what circumstances these should be used.
9. Ask for parameters as to when the physician wants to be called.
10. Plan ahead for meetings or times of contact so you are prepared with information and what you want to communicate.
11. Provide clinically pertinent information.

Working with the physician to determine best communication methods to use can help the case manager to meet the needs of the patient. Allowing time to discuss issues rather than sounding pressured to end conversation increases the chance of positive results and mutual agreement.

Conflict and Negotiation

Negotiation becomes important when two or more people or organizations disagree or have opposing views about a problem or solution. **Conflict** is inevitable. It cannot be avoided, but in many cases it can be prevented. It is important to recognize causes of conflict. Typical issues that lead to conflict are conflicts of interest, for example between the insurer, health care provider, case manager, and HCO; unresolved past conflicts; lack of trust; lack of resources; conflicts in sharing resources (territoriality); insufficient information that leads to confusion about roles and responsibilities; questioning performance; unexplained changes; stress; unclear or conflicting goals; and inability to view different perspectives or to step back and see the whole or to see another's perspective. Conflict prevention strategies include:

- Open, clear, timely communication
- Presentation of willingness to listen and consider other options
- Recognition that compromise is required in many situations
- Clear perspective of goals and desired outcomes

In order to resolve conflict, those involved in the conflict must discuss how to resolve it in a way that is acceptable to all parties. This process is negotiation or bargaining. It does not have to take long, but in some cases the process may be very long, such as during a union–employer negotiation for a contract. What are the points of resistance and areas that might lead to compromise? Each side should have the opportunity to express its concerns and viewpoint; then compromise will have to occur. Both sides will not be able to get everything they want. Negotiation requires leadership. There are several conditions that are important to consider in negotiation. Conflict should be dealt with as soon as possible but not when emotions are high. Negotiation involves offers and counteroffers, and this inevitably leads to emotions, which are often present before negotiation even begins. The relationship between the parties in the negotiation must be voluntary, which means all must recognize that anyone may remove himself or herself from the negotiation process at any time. The goal should be to arrive at a win–win situation. This is not always easy to accomplish because often people go into negotiation with the attitude of obtaining a win–lose result. Strategies that improve the negotiating process include willingness to listen to the other viewpoint, establishing a cooperative climate, describing your viewpoint clearly without emotion, supplying information that supports a viewpoint or proposal, appealing to fair play, treating all involved with respect, and rewarding work rather than making threats. Nonverbal communication can provide important information as the negotiation progresses. Emotions can interfere, and if they get high, all parties should step back and take a break. When a compromise is reached, the approach should be one of respect for all viewpoints and not an attitude of "I beat you."

Why is negotiation identified as a critical competency for case managers? Conflicts are present daily in all types of health care settings. Patients should not become part of staff or organizational conflicts. These conflicts need to be resolved, or patient care may suffer negative consequences. Negotiation takes practice. Consider these examples: The interdisciplinary team cannot agree on a treatment approach, and a decision must be made by the end of the team meeting. A patient's insurer refuses to extend the patient's hospital stay two more days based on the patient's insurance plan benefits.

As the hospital's nurse case manager, you must work with the insurer's representative to reach a compromise. Or it could be a situation in which the insurer's case manager informs the physician that a patient's hospitalization cannot be extended or that certain treatment will not be covered. This often leads to conflict. Developing negotiation skills makes conflicts easier to handle and less stressful, and this helps the case manager to provide more effective case management.

Leadership

As health care changes, leadership must also change. Organizational management and involvement in preparing the organization for the future, which includes working with the community, consumers, insurers, and any other organizations, continually experience changes. A critical characteristic is the ability of the leader to step back and see the whole picture with a willingness to change and take calculated risks. Case managers need to lead and be effective leaders in order to ensure that their role and responsibilities are met. Leaders may be formal leaders (leaders because of their position) or informal (leaders because others seek their advice and experience). **Transformation leadership** is recommended as the important leadership style for today's health care system by the IOM (2003b). This style emphasizes:

- Developing a vision of what could be and working toward it
- Viewing the total picture
- Accepting change and seeing it as an opportunity
- Guiding and rewarding staff you work with
- Encouraging the team to be self-aware and to take risks; learning from mistakes

"The essence of leadership is the ability to influence other people" (Tappen, Weiss, & Whitehead 2004, p. 4). This is something case managers have to do daily. Leaders need to understand themselves and increase their self-awareness. This will assist them in understanding the people with whom they work and improve their communication. Assertiveness is also vital for success, and it is required for the leader who initiates action, provides feedback, and includes staff in the development of goals and plans. This all requires critical thinking. Leaders must also be knowledgeable, or the people they work with will not respect them. It is easy for nurse case managers to forget about their own needs for continued learning while at the same time requiring that their staff continue their learning. Effective transformational leadership requires a new vision and new frameworks for thinking about strategy, structure, and people. A transformational leader does not function in isolation. Descriptors of leadership roles are: decision maker, communicator, evaluator, facilitator, risk taker, teacher, coach, critical thinker, advocate, creative problem solver, diplomat, and change agent.

Delegation

Delegation is important in the case management process and to care coordination. Why is it important? A case manager cannot do everything. Nurse case managers are familiar with delegation from their nursing role. The process of delegation is no different regardless of the perspective. Delegation is "transferring to a competent individual authority to perform a selected task in a selected situation" (Hansten & Washburn, 2004, p. 2). *Transferring* implies a process and indicates that the task, activity, or intervention is something the nurse would do but is giving the responsibility to someone else. *Competent* means the person who will do the task has the required skills and experience. The nurse case manager must be able to determine that the delegatee can do the task. *Authority* or the power to act is given to the delegatee. *Perform* means that some action must take place, and this action is described as *a selected task in a selected situation*. The case manager (delegator) must inform the delegatee what is to be done. Hansten and Washburn describe delegation as a cyclical process (Hansten & Washburn, 2004, pp. 4–8).

1. The **assessment** phase focuses on knowing your world, which includes your practice area and your organization; knowing yourself, your strengths and limitations; and knowing your delegate. You need to have an understanding of the delegatee's competency level and motivation. Neither of these is easy to assess, but both are critical to ensure patient safety and quality of care.
2. The plan requires that you know what needs to be done. If you do not, you will not be able to clearly define the task for the delegatee. This requires that you have professional and technical skills and that you acknowledge the importance of customer service.
3. Intervention means that you are able to prioritize and match the job to the delegatee. Communication, which includes the initial directions and follow-up, plays a critical role. If the delegatee does not understand what needs to be done, when, where, to whom, and how, then the task will not be completed as you expected. Conflicts may arise as you delegate, which require collaboration and negotiation.
4. Evaluation is ongoing throughout the care process. You need to know how to give constructive feedback. It can be a powerful motivator. Evaluation does require problem solving, particularly if the results or outcomes were not what you expected.

Case managers need to be able to use the delegation process when they delegate work to others.

The National Council of State Boards of Nursing identified five delegation rights that can also apply to delegation used in case management. These rights are familiar to nurses (National Council of State Boards of Nursing, 1995, American Nurses Association, 2006; Finkelman & Kenner, 2010).

1. *Right Task:*   The task must be delegatable for a specific patient or situation. What is the task? If the case manager or delegator is not clear about the task, then the case manager will not be able to clearly identify what needs to be done and by whom.
2. *Right Circumstances:*   Appropriate setting, available resources, and other relevant factors need to be considered. Where should the task be done? What is needed to complete the task? It may be that the case manager will need to tell the delegatee where to complete the task and identify what is needed to complete the task effectively.
3. *Right Person:*   The right person is delegating the right task to the right person to be performed by the right person. The case manager must consider who is the best person (type of staff, experience and skills, has time to complete task without negatively impacting other required work, and so on) to complete the task.
4. *Right Direction/Communication:*   Clear, concise description of the task, including the objective, limits, and expectations is part of effective delegation. The delegator (case manager) must explain to the delegatee what is to be done, how to do it if it is not clear, timeframe, outcomes, and so on. The delegatee needs to feel comfortable in asking questions for clarification or expressing concern about inability to complete the task. The delegator must be an effective communicator and also sensitive to concerns and issues—to establish a communication environment that allows for open discussion. This is critical to ensure patient-centered care that is focused on safety and quality. If the delegatee is afraid of speaking up and saying, "I do not know how to do something," or "Would you explain more about what you want done?" then this is an ineffective delegation process that can harm the patient. The delegatee may need help in organizing work and setting priorities

or may need to be told what to report to the case manager and when to report. The delegator needs to ask directly if there are questions or concerns and be open to the response. All of this is part of providing clear directions.

5. *Right Supervision:*   Appropriate monitoring, evaluation, intervention (as needed), and feedback are important in effective delegation. The case manager as a delegator does not just delegate a task and then forget about it. The case manager needs to supervise as needed. Monitoring methods include observation, verbal feedback, written feedback, and review of records where the delegatee documents what has been done. In some situations supervision may be minimal. In other situations, there may be a greater need to monitor. Factors such as the expertise of the delegatee, the patient's status, the complexity of the task, and timing may all impact the monitoring process. Another factor that cannot be ignored is how comfortable the delegator feels in delegating and how well the delegator knows the delegatee.

Evaluation

Evaluation serves many purposes. It clarifies performance expectations, reinforces constructive behavior, corrects unsatisfactory behavior, provides recognition, increases self-awareness, and promotes growth and change. One can view evaluation from perspective of performance evaluation; evaluation of meeting a patient's outcomes; and evaluation of a program such as a case management program. Informal evaluation occurs daily during the work process. Ongoing feedback is important because it is usually more relevant to the person than it would be months later. Formal evaluation usually occurs at specific times for specific purposes, such as annual performance review. Evaluation occurs constantly as patient care is delivered, and in many cases is not even done consciously. Quality improvement (QI) is an organized or structured form of evaluation required by HCOs, including insurers. Evaluation from quality improvement perspective is discussed in detail in Chapter 4. It is mentioned in this chapter because it is an important case manager competency.

Entrepreneurship

An **entrepreneur** is a person who sees things differently and takes the opportunity to make a difference. Entrepreneurs are not overwhelmed by barriers. Why is this a topic in a textbook on case management? Case management offers many opportunities for entrepreneurs. For example, a proactive nurse case manager can take advantage of the changing environment and step into a new role. To be entrepreneurs, case managers must be knowledgeable about changes in the health care environment, health care reimbursement and financial skills, managed care, quality issues, and changes in health care policy and legislation. Conformity is not a characteristic of an entrepreneur; rather, the entrepreneur moves away from "either–or" thinking to looking at many options creatively. Entrepreneurs must also be willing to work collaboratively and communicate with others. The future is where the entrepreneur will find opportunities for new roles and new professional experiences, but risk is inherent in this process. The entrepreneur often has to convince others in risky situations that the entrepreneur's recommendations will be successful. Nurse case managers are opening their own businesses, either in solo situations or groups. This increases opportunities and expands access to case management services.

Case managers need to continue with their own professional learning and maintain their professional licensure, such as registered nurse licensure. Joining the CMSA provides opportunity for professional dialogue with colleagues. Reading current health care and case management literature is critical in maintaining current practice standards.

THE CASE MANAGEMENT PROCESS

The nursing process and the case management process include the same major phases:

- Assessment
- Planning
- Implementation
- Intervention
- Evaluation

These five phases are found in all types of case management; however, how they are implemented may vary depending on the setting and patient/family needs. The case management process has four phases, which are discussed later in this section. The first critical issue in the case management process is identifying patients who require case management services.

Red Flags: Who Needs Case Management?

For years it has been known that the greatest portion of health care costs is generated by the three percent to five percent of the patient population that is high risk, critically injured, or suffering from chronic illness (Mullahy, 2001). As was discussed in Chapter 1, more people are living longer and often with chronic illnesses, mostly because of advances in medical science and technology. It is not uncommon for these patients to have comorbid conditions, increasing the complexity of their problems and requiring more collaboration and coordination. Many people are in relatively good health, though chronic illness is a problem. Patients over 75 average three chronic conditions and may take four or more medications (Institute of Medicine, 2008). Given the growing number of people with chronic illnesses, which in 2004 accounted for more than two thirds of the United States' $1.6 trillion medical bill, and the increasing need to respond to the growing number of persons with chronic illness, the need for effective services for this population is critical. From 2003 to 2004, employer-sponsored health plans that included a disease management service increased from 41% to 58% (Landro, 2004). Typical disease management goals are to improve quality of life, decrease disease progression, and reduce hospitalizations. Chronic illnesses that are typically monitored are: diabetes, heart disease/hypertension, asthma, cancer, depression, renal disease, low back pain, and obesity. Disease management is discussed in more detail in Chapter 6. In general, key **red flags** identify care that is the most expensive, high frequency of admissions in a short time period, and long length-of-stay (LOS). Specific examples of red flags include (Mullahy, 2001):

- *Diagnoses:*   For example, cancer, AIDS, stroke, transplant, neuromuscular diseases, spinal cord injuries, alcohol and substance abuse, cardiovascular, head injury, severe burns, high-risk pregnancy, chronic respiratory illness, psychiatric, multiple traumas, and high-risk infant
- *Potential Treatment:*   For example, ventilator dependent, IV antibiotics, TPN/enteral, extended ICU
- *Frequent Hospitalizations:*   For example, same year/same or related problem
- *Location of Claim:*   For example, complex care delivered in rural setting, small hospital or facility with poor outcome history/diagnosis history
- *Patterns of Care:*   For example, failed or repeated surgeries, hospital-acquired infections, malpractice concerns

The leading causes of death might also be used to guide identification of patients for case management services. Table 2-1 provides an example of leading causes of death. Data are available at the government website for National Vital Statistics. LOS also is

TABLE 2-1   Leading Causes of Death

| | | | | | | Age-adjusted death rate | | | |
| | | | | | | Percent change | | Ratio | |
Rank	Cause of death (based on ICD-10, 1992)	Number	% of total deaths	2005 crude death rate	2005	2004 to 2005	Male to Female	Black to White	Hispanic to non-Hispanic white
. . .	All causes	2,448,017	100.00	825.9	798.8	−0.2	1.4	1.3	0.7
1	Diseases of heart	652,091	26.6	220.0	211.1	−2.7	1.5	1.3	0.7
2	Malignant neoplasms	559,312	22.8	188.7	183.8	−1.1	1.4	1.2	0.7
3	Cerebrovascular disease	143,579	5.9	48.4	46.6	−6.8	1.0	1.5	0.8
4	Chronic lower respiratory diseases	130,933	5.3	44.2	43.2	5.1	1.3	0.7	0.4
5	Accidents (unintentional injuries)	117,809	4.8	39.7	39.1	3.7	2.2	1.0	0.8
6	Diabetes mellitus	75,119	3.1	25.3	24.6	0.4	1.3	2.1	1.6
7	Alzheimer's disease	71,599	2.9	24.2	22.9	5.0	0.7	0.8	0.6
8	Influenza and pneumonia	63,001	2.6	21.3	20.3	2.5	1.3	1.1	0.8
9	Nephritis, nephritic syndrome and nephrosis	43,901	1.8	14.8	14.3	0.7	1.4	2.3	0.9
10	Septicemia	34,136	1.4	11.5	11.2	0.0	1.2	2.2	0.8
11	Intentional self-harm (suicide)	32,637	1.3	11.0	10.9	0.0	4.1	0.4	0.4
12	Chronis liver disease and cirrhosis	27,530	1.1	9.3	9.0	0.0	2.1	0.8	1.6
13	Essential (primary) hypertension and hypertensive renal disease	24,902	1.0	8.4	8.0	3.9	1.0	2.6	1.0
14	Parkinson's disease	19,544	0.8	6.6	6.4	4.9	2.2	0.4	0.6
15	Assault (homicide)	18,124	0.7	6.1	6.1	3.4	3.8	5.7	2.8
. . .	All other causes (residual)	433,800	17.7	146.4	. . .	. . .	. . .	. . .	. . .

Source: National Vital Statistics Report. Volume 56, Number 10, April 24, 2008. Retrieved from http://www.cdc.gov/nchs/products/pubs/pubd/nvsr/nvsr.htm#vol56 on May 28, 2008

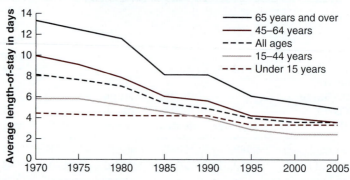

Average length-of-stay in days by age:
United States, selected years 1970–2005

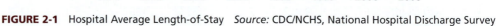

FIGURE 2-1 Hospital Average Length-of-Stay   *Source:* CDC/NCHS, National Hospital Discharge Survey
http://www.cdc.gov/nchs/data/ad/ad385.pdf

considered in the analysis of the best red flags for case management. LOS data are found in Figure 2-1.

Despite the fact that these patients could benefit from better care coordination of their complex needs, little was done to focus on these patient populations until case management became more acceptable. Case finding or identification of patients who require case management based on the red flags criteria is used to begin the case management process. Each case management program should develop its own list of red flags considering its case management model and its services. The red flags list targets patients with specific characteristics and needs. The case manager focuses on patients who or problems that are high volume, high risk, high cost, or all three. For example, if an MCO has a large number of enrollees with diabetes, MCO case managers might be assigned to these enrollees. Diabetes also has a high risk of complications and thus high costs; therefore, this is a particularly important group to assess for case management. Hospital case managers might focus on patients who tend to have a longer stay in order to decrease their LOS, which decreases hospital expenses. Each organization that uses case management must clearly identify in its policies the criteria and methods it uses to identify or refer patients for case management or its red flag patients. The identification system needs to be efficient. The longer it takes to identify patients who can benefit from case management, the greater the financial risk. Case management can decrease patient costs; however, it is not cost-free. There are expenses in operating a case management program. Providing case management to all patients or to patients that really do not need case management is not an effective, efficient approach. Box 2-3 identifies some red flags.

Case Management Process Phases

PHASE I: ASSESSMENT AND PROBLEM IDENTIFICATION.   After the patient is identified as appropriate for case management, the case manager further assesses the patient to identify the patient's problems and needs. The case manager develops a relationship with the patient/family or at least begins to establish one. This relationship can be quite different from the typical nursing relationship, particularly if the case manager never sees the patient and all contact is via the telephone. The case manager must explain case management and the role of the case manager to the patient/family. Patients and their families often assume that a nurse case manager will provide services similar to nurses that they have experienced, so roles and responsibilities need to be clarified. The purpose and goals of case management are discussed with the patient and with the family.

BOX 2-3

Red Flags: Who Needs Case Management?

The overall principle in identifying who needs case management is to identify patients who are high risk, high cost, and/or high volume. Consider any of the following characteristics or problems.

- Fixed financial resources (e.g., Medicare, Medicaid)
- Comorbidities
- History of frequent hospital admissions
- Chronic illness
- Cognitive deficit
- Mental illness/substance abuse
- Frequent use of emergency services

- Need for multiple health care services (e.g., home care, rehabilitation, medical equipment)
- Inadequate caregiver support

Clinical Examples:

- Acquired immune deficiency syndrome (AIDS)
- Multibirth pregnancy
- Premature infant
- Cancer
- Schizophrenia
- Chronic obstructive lung disease
- Diabetes
- Asthma

From the very early stages, the patient plays an active role in the entire case management process. Effective case management is patient-centered. The depth of the assessment depends on the needs of the patient and case management services required. This assessment includes not only the patient, but also the family, the patient's health care providers (e.g., physicians, registered nurses, physical therapists), and past health care records as needed. The assessment needs to be comprehensive and include data related to:

- Demographics
- Health history
- Current medical status and chief complaint
- Medication
- Nutritional status and needs
- Psychological status and needs
- Social needs
- Functional status and needs
- Adjustment to illness and treatment
- Cultural and spiritual factors
- Health education needs
- Environment (home)
- Financial status and concerns

Planning done by case managers covers additional areas that are not part of a nursing care plan. Case managers must be knowledgeable about the benefits provided by the patient's health insurance policy in order to ensure that the care is cost effective. Claims assessment, for example, review of claims and bills, and review of the patient's health care benefits, is typically part of the assessment. Claims management has not been part of most nurses' education or experience, but an understanding of claims management is important. Additional information about claims management is found in Chapter 3.

The case management plan identifies appropriate treatment and setting. Outcomes are identified and reassessed throughout the process. Quality and cost are also assessed throughout the process. An interdisciplinary case management plan of care is developed, usually based on standard plan formats (e.g., protocols, clinical pathways). Using the assessment data the case manager identifies the actual and potential problems, identifies goals with the patient, and if necessary, with the family. Then the case manager identifies interventions and resources required to meet the goals. This leads to the development of the full case management plan. The plan should be interdisciplinary and address the following questions, with the critical terms in italics (Powell & Tahan, 2008, p. 185).

1. What are the patient's and family's *problems* that need to be addressed in this *episode of care?* Do the patient and family agree with the identified problems? What are the patient's and family's strengths and limitations? The focus should be on patient-centered care.
2. What are the *treatment goals* and *desired outcomes* the health care team must accomplish?
3. What are the necessary *interventions* (both diagnostic and therapeutic) that would address these problems and goals?
4. What *timeframe* should be established for meeting the goals and outcomes?
5. What are the *barriers*, including financial and reimbursement, to meeting the goals and the desired outcomes?

Case managers deal daily with making decisions and need to be effective decision makers.

Nurse case managers are familiar with all of these questions because they are also critical in the nursing process; however, many nurses often do not consider question 5. Case managers need to be aware of potential financial and reimbursement barriers. This is the most effective way to be prepared and plan to overcome these barriers. The case manager must then move to the next phase, implementation, which emphasizes coordination.

PHASE II: PATIENT AND ENVIRONMENTAL INTERVENTIONS. Implementation requires thoughtful use of the plan to ensure that the patient's outcomes are met. Coordination and monitoring are critical components of the **intervention phase.** The case manager does not provide direct care, but rather the case manager ensures that all patient needs are met in a timely manner by the appropriate provider. Utilization review/management (UR/UM), as discussed in Chapter 5, is important throughout the case management process. **Environmental interventions** are much more important in case management than in most areas of nursing. These interventions include such activities as linkage with community resources, consultation with families and caregivers, education, maintenance and expansion of social networks, collaboration with health care providers, and advocacy. In addition, some case managers may be involved in clinical interventions that are provided to patients, for example, telephone triage. The case manager focuses on ensuring that care is provided in a timely manner, is appropriate, and is delivered in the most cost-effective setting, all of which require collaboration and active coordination.

PHASE III: DISCHARGE PLANNING AND TRANSITIONAL PLANNING. Discharge planning and **transitional planning** are part of the case management process. Discharge planning is an older term and is different from transitional planning in one particular way. Discharge planning typically refers to the plans that are made to discharge a patient from acute care and is required by federal regulations and accreditors. Care managers can be very involved in this process to ensure that the patient receives the best follow-up care if it is required. Transitional planning "refers to care and services that promote the safe and timely transfer of patients form one **level of care** to another (e.g., acute to subacute, intensive/critical care unit in a hospital to a regular unit), or from one type of setting to another (e.g., hospital to home). It focuses on moving a patient from the most complex to less complex care settings, or in some cases the reverse, should the patient require more intense services" (Powell & Tahan, 2008, p. 196). Times of transition or handoffs are high-risk experiences when communication and coordination may be inadequate and may lead to errors and decrease quality of care (Stanton & Lammon, 2008). The Institute for Health Improvement (IHI) has examined this concern. See the chapter's Internet Links section to learn more about one example of transition: from hospital to home. During times of transition the role of the case manager is the same as other times: to assess, identify problems, identify barriers, plan interventions and consider required resources, consider reimbursement issues, implement the plan, and evaluate. Throughout the process the case manager must coordinate, collaborate, and communicate with an awareness of increased risk of errors and ineffective care. When errors occur, this can lead to additional problems and complications requiring longer treatment and increased costs.

PHASE IV: EVALUATION.   Throughout the case management process the case manager needs to be aware of health insurance plan benefits and reimbursement issue to ensure that care is covered. **Continuous reassessment** is required so that the case management plan is current, adjusted to the patient's treatment plan and needs, and outcomes are reassessed. Routinely asking for patient and family input is also critical because their views may change. Evaluation is ongoing. At some point the case manager may terminate or conclude the case management services. This requires a review of outcomes, a discussion with the patient to close the relationship and the case management services, and transition to next stage that would not include case management. This may mean that the patient no longer requires any medical care, or it could be the patient still requires medical care but case management is no longer required. Common reasons for termination are (CMSA, 2002):

- Targeted goals and outcomes are met.
- There is a required change in health care setting or level of care.
- There is loss of or a change in insurance benefits.
- The patient and/or family request that case management be terminated.
- The case manager is no longer able to provide case management services.
- The patient and family obtain the maximum benefit from case management.
- The patient and/or family exhibit nonadherent behaviors to case management plan of care.

Evaluation takes place in all phases of the process as outcomes are assessed. Outcomes must be clearly identified and changed as needed. The aspect of evaluation that is different from the typical nursing process phase of evaluation is the importance of cost–benefit analysis. Does the money spent on case management services save money? If it does not, then the case manager must reconsider the approach taken. Further discussion on outcomes and quality improvement is found in Chapter 5.

CASE MANAGEMENT PROGRAM CHARACTERISTICS

Case management programs can vary; however, there are basic characteristics that are found in most programs. The focus on a *targeted patient population* is a unique characteristic of case management programs. Rather than providing case management for all patients, case management focuses on specific types of patients or problems. Case management has frequently been *nurse-driven* because nurses have played an important role in its evolution, and an increasing number of nurses are in case manager positions.

Family-focused care is the third program characteristic. Families or significant others are included in all aspects of care throughout the continuum of care as well as during each episode of care. Family education about the illness and treatment is an integral component of case management. The fourth characteristic is the use of *protocols*, which are referred to by many different names, such as clinical pathways, guidelines, and CareMaps®. Though names may vary the general purpose is the same—to provide a description of the care that should be provided. It is generally accepted that these tools increase efficiency, improve decision making, decrease costs, eliminate inappropriate treatment, and provide consistent treatment approaches. The fifth characteristic is *outcome-driven* care, specifically outcomes that are defined and measurable. Outcomes are identified and monitored throughout the case management process. *Interdisciplinary* care is the sixth characteristic. Case managers must work with a variety of health care professionals depending on the needs of the patient. Because care is complex, *multiservice* care is required. The case manager ensures that care is appropriate and timely. *Service coordination* links patients to services and involves assessment of needs, planning, delegation, referrals, and monitoring. Multiservice care is interrelated care and requires the brokerage of services or getting the patient the services needed by making the arrangements and ensuring accessibility of services. The ninth characteristic of case management programs is *specialization,* and it is often a part of multiservice care; for example, case managers may specialize in care of the elderly, substance abuse, or disabilities. Another characteristic, *episode-based* care, focuses on care that is needed from all services provided from first contact to the last contact for a specific problem or treatment across a continuum of settings. *Continuum of care*, which is an important part of the entire case management process, has no end and includes **primary care,** care for high-risk patients, wellness care, and long-term care. An episode of care is one part of the continuum. Continuum of care emphasizes longitudinally-based care. Coordination and collaboration are essential characteristics for outcome-driven case management. Case management is used for patients with complex problems, requiring coordination of services and interdisciplinary care. The final characteristic is *research-based* care, as case management relies on research results to provide direction for care and development of protocols (**evidence-based practice, or EBP,** one of the critical IOM core health care professions competencies). Another characteristic could be added to most case management programs. As an increasing number of case managers are looking at the full continuum of health, with an increased *emphasis on wellness*. For example, disease management programs emphasizing wellness have been developed, as discussed in Chapter 6, and case managers usually implement them. Health promotion and prevention are becoming increasingly important in the case management process for all patients. Some of the factors that impact case management program design are identified in Box 2-4.

BOX 2-4

Case Management Program Design

- Targeted patient population
- Nurse-driven
- Family-focused
- Use of protocols
- Outcome-driven
- Interdisciplinary
- Multiservice
- Specialization
- Episode-based
- Continuum of care
- Coordination and collaboration
- Research-based

CASE MANAGEMENT MODELS AND SETTINGS

Why Do We Have Different Case Management Models?

Case management has general characteristics, and there are also different perspectives or models of case management. Regardless of the model, the following characteristics are found in each model (Powell & Tahan, 2008, p. 41).

1. **Outcomes-oriented care delivery** that focuses on monitoring and measurement of patient safety, continuity, and quality of care
2. Appropriate resource allocation and utilization that is justified by the patient's condition and the required treatment, with cost effectiveness as the ultimate outcome
3. Comprehensive care planning including early assessment, intervention, and linking patient's condition and the required treatment, with cost effectiveness as the ultimate outcome
4. Integration and coordination of care delivery to eliminate fragmentation and/or waste
5. Collaboration across care providers and care settings
6. Advocacy to ensure that needed services are obtained and expected outcomes are met
7. Use of licensed professional as the case manager
8. Compliance with the standards of accreditation and regulatory agencies
9. Open lines of communication and sharing of important information across care providers, care settings, and the patient/family
10. Consumer and staff satisfaction

Generally, models of case management can be classified as **"within the walls"** or **"beyond the walls"** (Cohen & Cesta, 2005). "Within the walls" case management models provide services within a hospital or acute care setting. "Beyond the walls" is a more expansive classification, and includes case management provided in the community, payer-based settings such as an MCO, Medicaid, or long-term care organizations. In all models, case management has a critical role to play in reducing errors and ensuring that quality care is provided, particularly during handoffs or transitions. This role is related to the need for collaboration and coordination in the highly complex health care system and numerous risk factors that can result in harm to the patient (IOM, 1999). Case managers understand this issue and the importance of getting the patient into and out of the health care system in and effective and efficient manner.

Nurses and social workers are frequently responsible for developing case management programs. Programs can best be designed by considering these questions.

- What is the setting or context (e.g., acute care, insurer, home care)?
- What is the scope and nature of the patient population? Are the patients acutely or chronically ill? Are the health problems single-episode, or will cyclic interventions be required? What is the patient population's socioeconomic profile? Who are the principal payers associated with the patients? What are the patients' health conditions and needs?
- Where is the case manager's role based—in the acute care setting, in the community, as a component of third-party payers, or within a social agency?
- Will the case managers also be involved in clinical decisions such as telephonic triage, or will they focus on the coordination of care that is provided by others?
- What are the primary goals of the case management program?
- What types of case management interventions might be provided? What resources are needed to accomplish this?

- What are the types of reimbursement that will be used (e.g., capitation, prospective payment system, managed care)?
- Who will be providing the care (e.g. types of health care professionals—primary care provider-physician, physical therapist, nurse, specialty physician, and so on)?

The answers to these questions will aid in the design of the case management program and the case management model that is developed for a specific setting.

Level of care is a concept that is important for the case manager as the patient is assisted and is a concept well known to nurses. Patients require different types of care that are provided in different settings based on their acuity level and care needs. The typical levels of care are: acute (hospital); subacute (requires high level of nursing, medical, and therapy services and can be provided in a hospital unit or a separate organization (may also be referred to as transitional care); skilled nursing facility (SNF) providing 24-hour nursing care and rehabilitation, social services, either short term or long term; home health; and hospice (Powell & Tahan, 2008).

Case Management Compared with Care Management

Two terms, *case management* and **care management,** can be found in the practice setting and literature. Both terms include the care coordinator element. There are different views as to what these two terms mean, and the difference between care management and case management can be confusing. One view is care management focuses on care for an entire patient population as opposed to specific patients. Some refer to this as disease management, though others see disease management as a tool used by case management. Disease management is discussed further in Chapter 6. In comparison, case management focuses on individual patients. Case management is a strategy that is often used in conjunction with care management for a specific patient population. Some patients within the care management patient population require more individualized assistance, which is then provided with case management. Powell and Tahan (2008) define the two terms. "Case management is the management of acute and rehabilitative health care services—delivered under a medical model, primarily by nurses" (p. 162). Whereas, care management is "the management of long-term health care, legal, and financial services by professionals serving social welfare, aging, and nonprofit care delivery systems—delivered under a psychosocial model" (Powell & Tahan, p. 162). The Internet Links section at the end of the chapter provides some websites that discuss care management. The conclusion that can be drawn from these two terms that often have the same definition or similar characteristics is that health care professionals are still not clear about what all this means. For the purposes of this content, care management refers to the management of care for an entire patient population, such as enrollees of a managed care organization, and case management is the coordination of care for individual patients. It is the latter that is the focus of this book.

Developing a case management model requires that thought be given to the critical players, elements, skills, and functions. Typically, the critical players are the patient/family, case manager, health care provider(s), and the third-party payer. The major elements of a case management model are the same as the elements of the nursing process: assessment, planning, implementation, and evaluation. Skills and functions are discussed in other sections of this chapter. Identifying one model or the ideal case management model has not been possible. Some factors that make it difficult to develop one acceptable universal model are the setting or the organization in which case management is used, external and internal factors affecting services, several case managers from different organizations assigned to the same patient who requires the use of case management, and the needs of patients and services required. This situation has led to the development of a variety of case management models.

Case management takes place in many settings and organizations. Typically, these are acute care hospitals, home health agencies, ambulatory care settings, psychiatry, behavioral health care services, substance abuse or occupational health services, and rehabilitation agencies. Case management is also found in MCOs and other types of third-party payer organizations. Case managers may be viewed as external or internal. External case managers provide case management services outside a health care provider setting, such as a hospital or long-term care. These case managers usually work for third-party payers, occupational health services, community agencies, or Workers' Compensation. Internal case managers provide these services within a health care provider setting, such as within a hospital, home health agency, or long-term care facility. Health maintenance organizations (HMOs) not only finance care but also provide care, and thus their case management would be considered internal. This would not be true of other types of MCOs, such as preferred provider organizations (PPOs), point-of-service (POS), and other types of third-party payers because they do not provide direct care. Case managers coordinate care within the health care system, with health care providers, and with HCOs, typically coordinating with several different providers and HCOs, assessing utilization of resources, and communicating with the patient, family, providers, and payer. As more health care agencies and organizations use case management, the problem of duplication will undoubtedly arise. In some situations, the patient's insurer may assign a case manager and then the patient's home care agency may decide to assign a case manager. When the patient enters the hospital, another case manager may become involved (Goodwin, 1994). Each of these case managers has a case management plan and outcomes, and conflicts are bound to occur. The problem of multiple case managers has yet to be resolved, but this can clearly impact coordination effectiveness.

Models may vary from setting to setting, but a key consistent characteristic is the emphasis on the continuum of care and coordination. Several examples of case management models that are used in different settings are highlighted in Box 2-5 and described in more detail below. This is not an inclusive list. New models are created as need arises.

- *Social case management* is a model that emphasizes comprehensive long-term community care services to delay hospitalization. The primary patient population for this model is the elderly. Both health and social needs are covered in this model.
- *Primary case management* operates within the medical model of care and provides gatekeeping, primarily to prevent hospitalization. The physician acts as the gatekeeper and thus might be called the case manager in this model. The focus is on treatment for a specific health problem. An advanced practice nurse who is a primary care provider could also function in this model as the case manager.

BOX 2-5

Examples of Some Case Management Models

• Social case management	• Population-based case management
• Primary case management	• Ambulatory care case management
• Medical/social case management	• Home health care case management
• Private case management	• Patient navigation
• Telephonic case management	

- *Medical/social case management* is the model in which nurses are frequently the case managers. The focus is on a long-term care patient population who are at risk for hospitalization and who require coordination, assessment of resource utilization, planning, outcomes, and so on.
- *Private case management* is found in companies that provide case management functions. These functions may be coordination of services (social, functional, financial), mental health assessment and counseling or referral, monitoring, and evaluation services. Examples of interventions that might be used are: placement in long-term care facilities, homemaker care, respite care, and transportation. These services are often not covered by third-party payers and require that the patient pay out-of-pocket for these services. An example of a program based on this model is the use of case managers for the elderly who live a distance from their family. Case managers who are in the geographic area of the elderly are hired by the family to represent them or act as their "eyes and ears." These case managers are usually social workers who assist with coordination of health care needs and services and social needs, such as long-term care placement, transportation, meals-on-wheels, and social activities (e.g., day care treatment programs). This type of program is growing due to the trend of adult children living in different geographic areas from their parents. These families have the choice of uprooting their parent from his or her own environment to live with them or supporting the parent in the parent's familiar environment. This case management helps the parent and also adult children as they cope with the many problems that frequently occur, often on a daily basis (Cohen & Cesta, 2005).
- *Population-based care management (PCM)* is becoming a more effective, more significant approach to case management. PCM is based on the idea that "persons must be cared for in the context of their health status; in consideration of the interplay between existing conditions, or risk for conditions" (Howe, 1998). Typically, case management has focused on patients with complex health problems, but PCM offers a different case management focus. According to PCM, there are three classifications of patients: (1) the well, (2) the at-risk, and (3) the unstable. PCM focuses on the middle classification or the at-risk persons. This allows these patients to move into and out of the other two classifications. The at-risk group either is at risk for a chronic illness or has an illness that is stable and controlled but at risk for complications. This group continues to need primary prevention as would be found in the well persons' group and care to prevent them from becoming unstable.

  Population-based care is the community focus that nurses have been advocating for some time. The goal is to improve care for a specific population that has common health needs. Why has this become more popular today? Cost control of health care for these groups is a major reason. In addition, focusing on outcomes and achieving them can be more successful with this approach. Effective delivery of services requires a thoughtful approach to address the needs of the population. The key aspects of population-based care are highly relevant to nursing care. These aspects are health assessment and planning, health promotion and disease prevention, focus on groups of patients, patient and family education emphasizing self-care management, and evaluation and interpretation of health care trends and needs. Case management can play a major role in the community. Case managers can work with segments of the population that need greater coordination such as the elderly, people with chronic illnesses, patients covered by Medicaid with complex issues, and children with special needs.
- *Telephonic case management* has grown over the years and includes more than use of the telephone to assist in delivering case management. With the growth of the Internet, telephonic case management now includes e-mail and other forms of electronic communication. MCOs use this model as a method for their case managers to

work with identified members. It is cost effective and proactive. This approach can provide triage services to help members determine the steps that they need to take to resolve a medical problem by determining if the problem is emergent, urgent, or non-urgent. The case manager uses standardized protocols to guide decision making. This service can be provided 24/7, but it may also be provided in more traditional timeframes. Through this approach case managers can assess, intervene, and evaluate care and patient needs and outcomes. This may decrease the patient's need to go to the emergency department or in for a physician appointment. Health education can be provided along with health promotion and prevention information. Insurer case managers can also use this approach to follow up on patients after hospitalization or following other treatment. Hospital case managers can do the same. Case managers may also explain the claim process, authorize services, and coordinate care with multiple health care providers.

- *Ambulatory care case management* is a type of community-based case management. Patients with chronic illness requiring disease management may benefit from case management focused on their ambulatory care. Typically, these patients have long-term care needs and may require care from multiple health care providers and specialists, increasing the need for coordination.
- *Acute care case management* is one of the major settings that use case management. Hospitals are concerned about quality and costs. A case management program is a method of controlling costs and quality. The case manager works with ambulatory care patients who are high risk for complications and longer hospital stays and high-cost care, thus controlling LOS and transition periods. The case manager collaborates with the care team, patient, family, and health care providers that will care for the patient after discharge. Family involvement is very important. In some cases this is now referred to as clinical resource management (CRM) with the activities "focused on the process of access, the nature and appropriateness of treatment, and alternatives for timely transition to a post-acute venue" (Powell & Tahan, 2008, p. 81). Disease management and outcomes management are types of CRM. (Chapter 6 discusses disease management and outcomes management.)

In clinical case management the case manager focuses on quality and safety and use of appropriate interventions. "Using EBP protocols is important as is working with physicians when orders are developed. Eighty percent of medical costs are initiated through physician orders" (Powell & Tahan, 2008, p. 87). Computerized physician order entry (CPOE) has become more common. CPOE has had an impact on decision making and monitoring quality and safety. Physician profiling is also used by case managers to describe typical care patterns for specific physicians and use of resources such as laboratory testing, medications, procedures, use of intensive care, and therapies such as respiratory and physical therapy. A typical method for categorizing this information is to focus on specific diagnostic-related groups (DRGs) discussed in Chapter 3, or the primary diagnosis. Then within the DRG or primary diagnosis, specific physicians are profiled who might have a patient with the specified diagnosis. Physicians can then be compared. Third-party payers use this information to monitor physician performance, and case managers are often involved in the monitoring process. This information also helps case managers to understand physician practices and provides alerts to potential problems such as a physician who might overprescribe or order unnecessary laboratory tests.

Hospital case managers are involved in the entire acute care continuum of care (Powell and Tahan, 2008). This continuum includes three common phases. Access or entry into the acute care setting is the first phase. The second phase is throughput or care management—"all the people, processes, and systems that work independently or dependently to deliver care, treatment or services to the patient" (Powell &

Tahan, 2008, p. 89). The third phase involves transition or handoffs from one level of care to anther. This could occur when the patient moves from one unit to another such as from intensive care to a less intense unit or from discharge to home or to rehabilitative facility. The case manager works with the health care team, patient, and family during all these phases to ensure the patient receives care needed that is covered by insurer, provided in a timely manner, and is safe, quality care so that outcomes can be met. Resource management plays a critical role. What does the patient need to meet needs and reach outcomes? Can the need be met in a timely manner? Examples of resources are equipment, supplies, medication, and laboratory testing. Case managers have to think ahead based on assessment of the patient's current and future needs and the case management plan, which is routinely updated as the patient's condition and needs change.

- *Home health care case management* has also increased as home health care has become more common across the United States, both in urban and rural areas. The goals of home health care management are similar to other areas of case management— to control costs and ensure that patient outcomes are met. The red flags are also similar—patients with chronic illnesses, complex illnesses, high risk for rehospitalisation, and the need for more intensive services. There is greater reimbursement today for home care. Case managers need to be concerned with home health care nursing services, rehabilitation services (physical, speech, and occupational therapies), durable equipment and supplies, and social services. Patients need to be followed by a physician providing physician orders. A case manager in a hospital may have identified a patient requiring home health care, and later home health care case management may be added on. The case manager makes sure that prescribed services are covered by the insurer and that the correct services are accessible, thus coordinating care for the patient. The case manager may be an employee of the home health care agency or an employee of the patient's insurer. In either case, the case manager needs to work closely with all relevant staff. The case manager helps the patient and the patient's family to understand home health care, the services prescribed, and insurer benefits or services covered. A top concern is continual assessment to determine if the patient requires the prescribed services and to provide assessment, control of costs, and avoid the use of unnecessary care.

Case management is used in a variety of health care settings, typically hospice settings and palliative care, rehabilitation and long-term care, telehealth and telemedicine, workers' compensation, disability, and occupational health. The use of case managers in reimbursement organizations is discussed in Chapter 3. Case management may also focus on a specialty area such as substance abuse, mental health or behavioral health care, maternal-child, and geriatric care. There are a great many different settings and models in which the nurse case manager may work. New models are developed as need arise; for example, a newer model is nurse navigation or **patient navigation.**

Patient Navigation

Nurses are working in other roles that have similarities to case management including "nurse navigator" and "clinical nurse leader." The concept of "navigation," introduced by Harold Freeman, M.D. at the Harlem Hospital Center (New York City) in 1990, was developed to eliminate barriers to breast cancer screening and diagnosis among the impoverished community (Freeman, 2006). Dr. Freeman's program used lay people to reach out into the community, provide appropriate education, and overcome numerous barriers to cancer screening (2006). Although there are still many lay navigators, nurses are moving into these "patient navigation" or "nurse navigation" roles, which are most often used in cancer care.

BOX 2-6

Navigation

Navigation is a barrier-focused intervention that has the following characteristics:

- Patient navigation is provided to individual patients for a defined episode of cancer-related care (e.g., evaluating an abnormal screening test).
- Although tracking patients over time is emphasized, patient navigation has a definite endpoint when the services provided are complete (e.g., the patient achieves diagnostic resolution after a screening abnormality).

- Patient navigation targets a defined set of health services that are required to complete an episode of cancer-related care.
- Patient navigation services focus on the identification of individual patient-level barriers to accessing cancer care.
- Patient navigation aims to reduce delays in accessing the continuum of cancer care services, with an emphasis on timeliness of diagnosis and treatment and a reduction in the number of patients lost to follow-up.

Source: Summary of information from Wells, K.J., Battaglia, T.A., Dudley, D.J., Garcia, R., Greene, A., Calhoun, E., et al. (2008). Patient navigation: State of the art or is it science? *Cancer, 113*(8), 1999–2010.

According to Battaglia, Roloff, Posner, and Freund (2007, p. 359), navigation is "a type of care management that encompasses a wide range of advocacy and coordination activities." The National Cancer Institute, which is currently studying this role through the Patient Navigator Research Program, reports that navigators provide a wide range of services to patients, including education, assistance with logistics and accessing the health care system, identification of resources, appropriate follow-up, and emotional support for the patient and family.

A very small number of studies on navigation have been published (Nguyen & Kagawa-Singer, 2008). There is no wide agreement regarding a definition of navigation or required education and qualifications for navigators (Wells et al., 2008). However, review of the published literature by Wells et al. (2008) finds some common ground about navigation, as highlighted in Box 2-6.

Although there still is much to learn about the ideal candidate to fill the navigator role and how to apply the new role in different settings, navigation is increasingly being embraced in health care settings. Nurses with a holistic view of patient care and broad-based education can have great impact in this role.

Another new nursing role may also function as a case manager or nurse navigator in some situations. The Clinical Nurse Leader (CNL) is a nursing role proposed by the American Association of Colleges of Nursing (AACN) to respond to recommendations made in a number of landmark reports including *To Err is Human: Building a Safer Health System* (IOM, 1999), *Crossing the Quality Chasm* (IOM, 2001), *Health Care at the Crossroads: Strategies for Addressing the Evolving Nursing Crisis* (Joint Commission on Accreditation of Healthcare Organizations), and *Health Care's Human Crisis: The American Nursing Shortage* (Robert Wood Johnson Foundation, 2002) among others. Fragmented care, use of resources, patient safety, health care quality, use of technology, evidence-based practice and workforce shortages are just some of the issues raised in these reports (AACN, 2007).

Educated at the master's level, CNLs are advanced generalists and clinical "integrators who provide centralized care coordination and put evidence-based practice into action to ensure that patients benefit from the latest innovations in nursing science" (Rosseter, 2009). Compared to air traffic controllers (Rosseter, 2009) and orchestra conductors (Tornabeni, Stanhope, & Wiggins, 2006), CNLs look at the big picture, working with all providers and components of the care continuum to influence patient care (Tornabeni et al., 2006). As described by the AACN on its website (http://www.aacn.nche.edu/CNC/index.htm), the CNL role is broad and encompasses duties and responsibilities necessary to work toward improvements in today's challenging health care environment.

When the CNL role was introduced, concern and confusion existed regarding this new role, especially about how it relates to nurse managers and Clinical Nurse Specialists (CNS). While some roles and responsibilities may, at times, overlap, the CNL should complement nursing roles already in place. As a generalist, the CNL does not conflict or compete with the specialized knowledge and role of the CNS. Further, according to the AACN (2007), the CNL does not act as the nurse manager, who is responsible for supervising staff (including the CNL) and the day-to-day management and oversight of a unit. However, the CNL does assume a leadership role, "working in tandem with nursing staff and the multidisciplinary team for the purpose of delivering effective and efficient quality care and to improve patient health status" (Tornabeni, Stanhope et al., 2006). Although the role was originally developed primarily for the acute care setting, CNLs today are expanding into other areas including outpatient settings, community health, long-term care, and home health (Harris & Roussel, 2010). Section II provides further information about nurse navigation.

Summary

This chapter focused on case manager functions, competencies, and the case management process. All are inter-related. Case management frequently assists in lowering costs and improving care; however, it is not effective for all patients. Identifying patients who can benefit the most from case management is critical. There are many different types or case management models, and it is used in a variety of health care settings. This all impacts the actual services offered and the focus of the case management process.

Chapter Highlights

1. Collaborative care and cooperative effort are central to effective, outcome-driven care. Case management emphasizes collaborative care.
2. The four main case manager functions are: assessor, planner, facilitator, and advocate. The case manager is the care coordinator.
3. Effective case management requires a number of competencies: critical thinking, collaboration and interdisciplinary relationships, coordination, communication, conflict and negotiation, leadership, delegation, evaluation, and entrepreneurship.
4. It is critical to identify the patients who obtain the most benefit from case management. The typical types of red flags are: most expensive care, high frequency admissions in a short time, and LOS. Patients at high risk for complications are important to identify.
5. The case management process is similar to the nursing process; however, it includes additional focus areas such as reimbursement issues. The phases are: assessment and problem identification, patient and environmental interventions, discharge planning and transitional planning, and evaluation.
6. Case management programs vary based on the populations served, purpose of the organization offering case management, and the setting in which it is offered. Various case management models have been developed. New models are developed as need arises.

References

Alfaro-LeFevre, R. (2006). *Applying nursing process: A tool for critical thinking*. Philadelphia: Lippincott Williams & Wilkins.

American Association of Colleges of Nursing. (2007). *White paper on the education and role of the Clinical Nurse Leader*. Retrieved from www.aacn.nche.edu/Publications/WhitePapers/ClinicalNurseLeader07.pdf on August 16, 2009.

American Nurses Association (ANA) and the National Council of State Boards of Nursing (NCSBN). (2006). *Joint statement on delegation*. Silver Springs, MD: American Nurses Association.

American Nurses Association. (ANA). (2003). *Nursing's social policy statement*. (2nd ed.). Silver Springs, MD: Author.

Battaglia, T.A., Roloff, K., Posner, M.A., & Freund, K.M. (2007). Improving follow-up to abnormal breast cancer screening in an urban population. *Cancer Supplement, 109*(2), 359–367.

Burke, M., Boal, & Mitchell, R. (2004). Communicating for better care. Improving nurse–physician communication. *American Journal of Nursing, 104*(12), 40–47.

Case Management Society of America. (CMSA). (2002). *Standards of practice for case management.* Little Rock, AR: Author.

Cohen, E. & Cesta, T. (2005). *Nursing case management: From essentials to advanced practice application.* (4th ed.). St. Louis, MO: Elsevier Mosby.

Commission for Case Manager Certification. (CCMC). (2005). *CCM certification guide.* Rolling Meadows, IL: Author.

Fabre, J. (2005). *Smart nursing.* NY: Springer Publishing Company.

Finkelman, A. & Kenner, C. (2010). *Professional nursing concepts.* Boston: Jones & Bartlett Publishers.

Finkelman, A. (2001, December). Problem-solving, decision-making, and critical thinking: How do they mix and why bother? *Home Care Provider*, 194–199.

Freeman, H. (2006). Patient navigation: A community based strategy to reduce cancer disparities. *Journal of Urban Health: Bulleting of the New York Academy of Medicine, 83*(2), 139–141.

Goodwin, D. (1994). Nursing case management activities: How they differ between employment settings. *Journal of Nursing Administration, 24*(2), 29–34.

Hansten, R. & Jackson, M. (2004). *Clinical delegation skills.* Boston: Jones and Bartlett Publishers.

Harris, J.L. & Roussel, L. (2010). *Initiating and sustaining the clinical nurse leader role: A practical guide.* Sudbury, MA: Jones and Bartlett Publishers.

Howe, R. (1998). Population care management emerging as a significant approach to case management. *Inside Case Management, 5*(3), 3–5.

Institute of Medicine. (1999). *To err is human.* Washington, DC: National Academies Press.

Institute of Medicine. (IOM). (2001). *Crossing the quality chasm.* Washington, DC: National Academies Press.

Institute of Medicine. (2003a). *Priority areas for national action.* Washington, DC: National Academies Press.

Institute of Medicine. (2003b). *Health professions education.* Washington, DC: National Academies Press.

Institute of Medicine. (IOM). (2008). *Retooling for an aging America: Building the healthcare workforce.* Washington, DC: National Academies Press.

Joint Commission. (2009). *Health care at the crossroads: Strategies for addressing the evolving nursing crisis.* Oakbrook Terrace, IL: Joint Commission on Accreditation of Healthcare Organizations.

Landro, L. (2004, 20 October). Disease management: Pro and con. *The Wall Street Journal*, p. D4.

Mullahy, C. & Boling, J. (2008). The case manager as change agent in a new and improved health care model. *Professional Case Management, 13*(5), 286–289.

Mullahy, C. (2001). Case management and managed care. In P. Kongstvedt, *Essentials of managed healthcare.* (4th ed.). Gaithersburg, MD: Aspen.

National Cancer Institute. (n.d.). *The patient navigator research program.* Retrieved from http://www.crchd.cancer.gov/news/press-kit.html on July 13, 2009.

National Council of State Boards of Nursing. (NCSBN). (1995). *Delegation: Understanding the concepts and decision-making process.* Retrieved from NCSBN at https://www.ncsbn.org/887.htm?search-text=delegation&select=%23&x=14&y=9 on January 9, 2008.

Nguyen, T.N. & Kagawa-Singer, M. (2008). Overcoming barriers to cancer care through health navigation problems. *Seminars in Oncology Nursing, 24*(4), 270–278.

Powell, S. & Tahan, H. (2008). *CMSA core curriculum for case management.* Philadelphia: Lippincott, Williams & Wilkins.

Robert Wood Johnson Foundation. (2002). *Health care's human crisis: The American nursing shortage.* Princeton, NJ: Author.

Rosseter, R. (2009). A new role for nurses: Making room for clinical nurse leaders. *The Joint Commission Perspectives on Patient Safety, 9*(8), 5–7.

Stanton, M. & Lammon, C. (2008). The "wins" of change. Evaluating the impact of predicted changes on case management practice. *Professional Case Management, 13*(3), 161–168.

Tappan, R., Weiss, S., & Whitehead, D. (2004). *Essentials of nursing leadership and management.* (3rd ed.). Philadelphia: F.A. Davis.

Thomas, M. (2008). The providers' coordination of care. A model of collaboration across the continuum of care. *Professional Case Management, 13*(4), 220–227.

Tornabeni, J., Stanhope, M. & Wiggins, M. (2006). The CNL vision. *Journal of Nursing Administration, 36*(3), 103–108.

Wells, K.J., Battaglia, T.A., Dudley, D.J., Garcia, R., Greene, A., Calhoun, E., et al. (2008). Patient navigation: State of the art or is it science? *Cancer, 113*(8), 1999–2010.

Questions and Activities for Thought

1. Describe how the nine critical case management competencies are interrelated? How do the five IOM core competencies relate to these nine competencies?
2. Describe two examples for each of the four major case manager functions.
3. Discuss how delegation is related to case management practice. Provide examples.
4. Compare and contrast case management and care management?

5. Select one of the case management models and research the model in the literature. What can you learn about the model and its application? Why did you select this model to learn more about?

6. Search the current literature for information about new case management models.

Case

You have been assigned to Mr. Jonesville because he met case management red flag criteria. You work as a case manager for a hospital. Mr. Jonesville is 60 years old and has experienced his second myocardial infarction (MI) in two years. He arrested with the second MI and is now in the cardiac care unit. The patient is employed and travels a lot for his job. Given the current economic instability he is worried about losing his job. He is 20 pounds overweight. His wife is frequently at the hospital, and his two adult children also visit. You learn that he has not been compliant with recommended treatment between the first and second MI. Using the case management process, apply each of the four phases to this patient to describe how you would provide case management services.

Internet Links

- Institute for Health Improvement: Transition Example; From Hospital to Home
  http://www.ihi.org/IHI/Programs/Conferences AndSeminars/HospitaltoHomeOptimizingthe TransitionOct08.htm
- Institute of Health Improvement: Handoffs
  http://www.ihi.org/ihi/search/searchresults.aspx? searchterm=handoffs&searchtype=basic
- Institute of Health Improvement: Case Management

  http://www.ihi.org/ihi/search/searchresults.aspx? searchterm=case+management&searchtype=basic
- Kaiser Permanente's Care Management Institute
  http://www.kpcmi.org/
- National Association of Geriatric Care Managers
  http://www.caremanager.org/
- Dorland Health Care Information
  http://dorlandhealth.com/

CHAPTER 3

Reimbursement: A Critical Case Management Issue

OBJECTIVES

After completing this chapter, the reader will be able to:

- Discuss the relationship of costs and coordination of benefits in case management.
- Compare and contrast the types of third-party payers, including indemnity insurance, service benefit plans, workers' compensation, government health benefit plans, and managed care organizations.
- Explain the reasons for the growing uninsured problem.
- Describe the financial relationship between the insurer and the enrollee, including benefits, eligibility, and co-sharing expenses.

KEY TERMS

Actuarial data, p. 80
Adverse selection, p. 80
Aid to Families with Dependent
   Children (AFDC), p. 73
Annual limits, p. 82
Authorization, p. 75
Benefits, p. 60
Capitation, p. 67
Case rate, p. 81
Claims processing, p. 87
Consolidated Omnibus Budget
   Reconciliation Act of 1985
   (COBRA), p. 68
Cost shifting, p. 63
Covered services, p. 82
Deductibles, p. 67
Diagnosis-related groups (DRGs), p. 69
Discounted fee-for-service, p. 81
Enrollees, p. 60
Exclusions, p. 61

Experience rating, p. 80
Fee-for-service (FFS), p. 65
Gatekeeper, p. 62
Government benefit plans, p. 65
Indemnity insurance, p. 63
Insurance, p. 60
Insurance commission, p. 66
Medicare Catastrophic Coverage Act
   of 1988, p. 68
Medicare Part A, p. 71
Medicare Part B, p. 71
Medicare Part C, p. 71
Medicare Part D, p. 71
Medigap plans, p. 72
Out-of-pocket expenses, p. 82
Per diem, p. 81
Preexisting conditions, p. 84
Premium rate setting, p. 80
Primary care, p. 65
Provider panel, p. 78

INTRODUCTION

Health care **reimbursement** in the United States is a pluralistic payment system with multiple payers from both the public and private sectors. It is a complex system, with many players, motivations, and a long history of change. The use of health **insurance** began in this country in 1847 with a medical care policy issued by the Massachusetts Health Insurance Company of Boston. By the end of the 1860s, there were 60 health insurance companies. In 1911, Montgomery Ward and Company offered a plan that provided **benefits** to employees who were unable to work due to illness or injury (Health Insurance Association of America, 1998). Employers began to offer insurance instead of increasing wages. By the 1920s, insurance companies experienced overexposure and excessive costs; however, in the 1940s, the insurance industry expanded again. Blue Cross/Blue Shield plans were created. An important stimulus for businesses to offer insurance was the tax benefit it provided to employers. Employers' contributions for insurance benefits are exempted from federal and state taxes, which is a very important saving for employers. An interesting point about insurance today is that not all workers are signing up for health care coverage. This is particularly true for those earning low wages and for employees in their 20s and early 30s. The latter group does not want to spend the money on health insurance, thinking that they currently do not need it. With the growing health care economic problem described earlier and the need for health care reform, health insurance will undoubtedly undergo more changes in the near future. Case managers will need to be aware of these changes, which will impact reimbursement and health care delivery.

Today, the health care purchasers, typically employers and governments, are in a very influential position because the purchaser usually is involved in the major decisions (e.g., what is reimbursed, provider choice, length-of-stay [LOS], length of treatment, quality). Case managers require a greater knowledge of reimbursement and the insurance industry in order to meet their position responsibilities. This chapter focuses on critical information that lays the foundation for understanding health care reimbursement. Just saying that "insurance pays" is not enough. The case manager needs to know what this means and how it works, and in some cases, the nurse case manager may actually work for the third-party payer organization.

This chapter addresses content related to health care reimbursement, a complex topic, and the development and organization of managed care organizations (MCOs). Managed care refers to a health care system that focuses on the delivery and financing of health care services that are appropriate for the needs of the **enrollees** or members of a health care reimbursement plan, with particular emphasis on cost control, quality, and access to care. There is great variation among MCOs and in how managed care strategies are applied within the health care delivery system. Managed care strategies have been integrated throughout the health insurance industry. How do patients find their way through the health insurance maze and gain a better understanding of their own health care reimbursement, whether this is a more traditional insurer, an MCO, or government insurance such as Medicare? There are many confusing models that may have similarities but also many differences. Box 3-1 highlights some facts about health insurance coverage.

BOX 3-1

Health Insurance Coverage: 2007 Highlights

Due to the changing economic situation in the United States, the number of persons without insurance and with inadequate insurance has changed since 2007. The box below describes current data published on August 26, 2008.

- Both the percentage and number of people without health insurance decreased in 2007. The percentage without health insurance was 15.3% in 2007, down from 15.8% in 2006, and the number of uninsured was 45.7 million, down from 47.0 million.[1]
- The number of people with health insurance increased to 253.4 million in 2007 (up from 249.8 million in 2006). The number of people covered by private health insurance (202.0 million) in 2007 was not statistically different from 2006, while the number of people covered by government health insurance increased to 83.0 million, up from 80.3 million in 2006.
- The percentage of people covered by private health insurance was 67.5%, down from 67.9% in 2006. The percentage of people covered by employment-based health insurance decreased to 59.3% in 2007 from 59.7% in 2006. The number of people covered by employment-based health insurance, 177.4 million, was not statistically different from 2006.

- The percentage of people covered by government health insurance programs increased to 27.8% in 2007, from 27.0% in 2006. The percentage and number of people covered by Medicaid increased to 13.2% and 39.6 million in 2007, up from 12.9% and 38.3 million in 2006.
- In 2007, the percentage and number of children under 18 years old without health insurance were 11.0% and 8.1 million, lower than they were in 2006—11.7% and 8.7 million. Although the uninsured rate for children in poverty decreased to 17.6% in 2007, from 19.3% in 2006, children in poverty were more likely to be uninsured than all children.[2]
- The uninsured rate and number of uninsured for non-Hispanic Whites decreased in 2007 to 10.4% and 20.5 million (from 10.8% and 21.2 million in 2006). The uninsured rate for Blacks decreased to 19.5% in 2007 from 20.5% in 2006. The number of uninsured Blacks in 2007 was not statistically different from 2006, at 7.4 million.
- The percentage and the number of uninsured Hispanics were 32.1% and 14.8 million in 2007, lower than 34.1% and 15.3 million in 2006.

[1]For a brief description of how the Census Bureau collects and reports on health insurance, see the text box "What is health insurance coverage?" For a discussion of the quality of ASEC health insurance coverage estimates, see Appendix C.

[2]The number of uninsured children in poverty in 2007 was not statistically different from the number in 2006.

Source: U.S. Census Bureau. Retrieved July 19, 2009, from http://www.census.gov/hhes/www/hlthins/hlthin07/hlth07asc.html

CASE MANAGEMENT: COSTS AND COORDINATION OF BENEFITS

Who has an interest in supporting the use of case management? All types of **third-party payers,** MCOs, public sector insurers such as Medicare and Medicaid, workers' compensation, and employers have a vested interest in keeping the cost of health care down, and case management can help to reduce these costs. In addition, health care **providers** such as hospitals find value in using case management. Cost-containment strategies that are commonly used by third-party payers are:

1. Assessing benefits (e.g., excluding high-risk individuals, discovering those with preexisting conditions, determining what benefits will be covered)
2. Coordinating the care of catastrophic claims or chronic patients to better ensure that care is provided when needed, not abused, and to prevent further complications that lead to the need for more care
3. Performing retrospective utilization review (UR) of unusual or high-dollar cases.

These strategies require that the case manager understand the patient's insurance coverage and policy **exclusions.** The case manager needs to know what resources are available for alternative funding for medical benefits. In addition, some patients may require creative management of their benefits and their health care dollars to better ensure that their needs are met. The case manager communicates and coordinates with many people and services in order to provide the most cost-effective care that meets the required outcomes.

Costs are not as simple as they may appear. There are several approaches to assessing costs. Hard savings are avoided costs (Powell & Tahan, 2008). Examples of these savings that can be facilitated by the case manager are change in level of care or change in LOS and negotiation of frequency or duration of services. Soft savings are potential savings (Powell & Tahan, 2008). When case management is not used, soft savings are reduced, and costs are increased. Examples of these savings are avoidance of readmission, emergency department visits, or number of home visits.

How does the case manager reduce costs and maintain quality? A major intervention is to prevent errors, problems, and anything that slows down the provision of care. Mistakes can lead to complications, the need to alter treatment, and may sidetrack care that needs to be provided to meet the outcomes. Another cost focus is resource allocation, or appropriate use of staff and equipment resources. If the wrong equipment is used, complications may occur or treatment may need to be repeated, and costs then increase. If more expensive equipment is used, then costs increase. Delays (e.g., in assessment, receipt of laboratory results, treatment procedures, receipt of medications, use of equipment, transportation to get the patient from one unit to another or from home to a medical appointment) also cause problems and increase costs. Case managers frequently ask, "Why are these problems occurring?" Solving these problems will usually decrease costs and improve quality. For example, patients who receive timely laboratory reports can obtain more timely treatment, thus decreasing costs and improving the quality of care. The case manager needs to monitor case management plans to ensure that outcomes are met in a timely, effective manner and to make adjustments as needs change.

Case management itself is not free of cost. The development and implementation of a case management program and the use of case managers is an expensive process. The case manager must consider this when cost effectiveness is evaluated as well as understand that case management should lower, not increase, the costs of care. Different case management models and settings and their characteristics can alter the costs of running a case management program. Examples of these characteristics are: patient characteristics, type and number of case management services, administrative functions of the case manager, and how much support the case manager gets to meet the administrative functions. A critical element is to determine whether a patient can benefit from case management as mentioned in Chapter 2 by the identification of red flags. Providing case management for patients who do not need it is not cost effective. The case manager must both ensure that the patient gets the care that is needed as a **gatekeeper** and ensure as a broker of services that the care is the least expensive possible. The assessment of cost–benefits becomes very important in this process. It is not easy to meet the joint goals of a gatekeeper and a broker. The savings that are usually gained are through the prevention of hospitalization or the reduction of inpatient days. As case management becomes more common, further savings will be identified in other areas (e.g., preventive care, coordination of care, resource management). As is true with any new program today, its costs and benefits must be analyzed. Were outcomes met and at what cost? Answers to these questions are critical to the survival of a case management program.

THE HEALTH CARE INSURER: THE THIRD-PARTY PAYER

What is insurance? Insurance is "a system of reducing a person's exposure to risk of loss by having another party (insurer, third-party payer, MCO) assume the risk. In health care, the risk the health care insurance company assumes is the unknown cost of health care for a person or group of persons" (Casto & Layman, 2009, p. 3). Another term that is often heard in relation to insurance is third-party payer. A third-party payer is the organization, private or public, that pays or underwrites coverage for health care for another entity, such as a business or individual. The third-party payer provides either group coverage or individual coverage. Most people who have insurance coverage receive it as an employee benefit or through membership in an organization, which is called group coverage. Most group insurers are commercial or for-profit insurers. Individual or personal insurance is more expensive for the purchaser or the enrollee. Common reasons individuals purchase personal insurance are to cover gaps in their employment insurance; their employer does not provide coverage; they are self-employed; or they are not employed and cannot get Medicaid coverage.

In the insurance schema, the patient is referred to as the first party; the provider as the second party; and the third party is the payer or insurance carrier, such as a commercial insurer, Blue Cross and Blue Shield or Humana, MCOs, and federal government programs such as Medicare and Medicaid. The third-party payer actually pays the bills; however, the process is not simple. The third-party payer or insurer invests its capital in order to have funds to pay for unexpected medical expenses in its member group. As the use of insurance has grown, there has been an increase in insurer financial risk. The insurer could lose the money it invests, or it could miscalculate the amount of money it needs to cover all of its expenses, both expected and unexpected. If the insurer is a for-profit organization, it must yield profits to pay its stockholders. Insurer's administrative costs can be very high. These costs typically include staff such as administrative staff, case managers, facilities, supplies, information systems, and other similar costs.

Types of Third-Party Payers

There are three types of traditional health insurance plans: indemnity, service, and managed care plans. The other two major types are workers' compensation and government plans. The type of third-party payer that has had the most influence on health care reimbursement in the past 20 years has been managed care. Managed care plans are discussed in more detail in Chapter 4. Most types of payers are now incorporating some managed care approaches into their plans.

Indemnity Insurance

Traditional **indemnity insurance,** a form of commercial insurance, is a type of third-party payer that is slowly disappearing as new forms of payers are developed and managed care becomes more prevalent. The indemnity plan pays for health care services by means of a contract with a business or individual. The employer, and usually the employee, pays for the coverage. The insurance plan carries the risk, not the employer or provider. The choice of health care provider is left up to the employee, though second opinions may be required for certain medical problems and treatments. The providers are paid the fee that they request, and few cost-containment controls are placed on the providers. Case management may be used for catastrophic cases to control costs. Over time, this arrangement has affected health care costs because there are no incentives to decrease costs. The health care system experienced an increase in the amount of services it provided, resources it used, and an increase in LOS or treatment. **Cost shifting** is a method used by providers to cope with the low reimbursement that they received from some patients. The organization or provider raises fees for self-pay and commercially insured patients to cover their losses. This increase in fees is then used to cover the expenses of those who cannot pay for all of their expenses. As per-employee costs for health care increase for indemnity insurance, employers and employees begin to change to less expensive types of plans, such as those using some form of managed care. The characteristics of traditional indemnity insurance are summarized in Box 3-2.

BOX 3-2

Characteristics of Traditional Indemnity Insurance

- Fee-for-service reimbursement for providers
- Insurer assumes all financial risk
- No restrictions on choice of provider
- Limited financial incentives to be cost-effective
- No organized interest in quality measurement
- No organized interest in appropriateness of services

Service Benefit Plan

A **service benefit plan** pays the provider directly. The insurer negotiates the prices. The patient pays a portion of the costs. Examples of service benefit plans are Blue Cross and Blue Shield. These plans offer discounts in their professional panels and hospital discounts. Some of these plans use diagnostic-related groups (DRGs) or some equivalent to determine reimbursement. DRGs are discussed later in this chapter. The plan reimburses providers directly, and the patient does not get directly involved in payment. Providers must accept the fees schedule and not charge the patient above the required deductible and coinsurance.

Workers' Compensation

Workers' compensation is a special type of insurance that focuses on a specific population. It is a very expensive type of insurance for employers to offer. This insurance is an important part of the national health care delivery system. Case managers do work in workers' compensation programs. Workers' compensation is a "form of social insurance provided through property–casualty insurers. Workers' compensation provides medical benefits and replacement of lost wages that result from injuries or illnesses that arise from the workplace; in turn, the employee cannot normally sue the employer unless true negligence exists" (Kongstvedt, 2009, p. 250). Typically, employees are provided workers' compensation coverage, which is mandated by state law, employee medical benefits, and often disability benefits.

Workers' compensation is not equivalent to employee medical benefits. Actually, workers' compensation was the first form of social insurance used in the United States. It is a social contract in that it is a form of mutual protection for the employee and the employer and is required by federal law and delegated to states. The employer must follow state requirements related to benefits and limits. The financial status of the employer is not a factor in determining the type of plan it offers. Each state's workers' compensation commission is the authority that supervises these health care services. States, however, do vary in the benefits they require.

Disability costs are an important part of workers' compensation costs. Disability management is critical for most employers, because it is used to control costs. Case management is used to manage disability claims. Utilization review is also an important aspect. This is not, strictly speaking, health coverage. Most employers offer short-term disability that usually provides a percentage of a worker's pay for a short period of time after an incapacitating accident or illness or in addition may offer long-term disability. Some of the costs of both or either of these benefits may also be covered by employee contributions. These policies often cover pregnancy and maternity leaves, usually for 10 weeks. Long-term disability becomes effective when short-term disability insurance coverage ends. Why is this insurance important? Paying for this care without any insurance can be a major financial crisis for most employees.

Diagnosis-specific protocols of expected lengths of disability are used to manage the disability. Many workers who experience a disability feel a sense of entitlement to the benefit, and some experience a secondary gain from receiving this coverage. The entitlement or the workers' feeling that this benefit is "a right" can lead to workers' demanding excessive medical care, and this in turn delays their return to work. Employer costs also increase. Case managers play a critical role in this process by managing the employee's expectations and responses.

Keeping workers' compensation separate from the traditional health care delivery system has not always proven to be the most cost-effective method of providing medical care for work-related injuries and illnesses. Workers' compensation is regulated under state laws. States vary in benefit levels, medical reimbursement schedules, and the amount of control that the employer has over employee medical choices. Occupational health nurses play an important role in prevention of work-related injuries and illnesses as well as providing on-site treatment and follow-up.

Managed care is also used in by worker' compensation programs and might also use case management, a provider network, utilization review, a toll-free number for reporting treatment, or a gatekeeper. A gatekeeper, usually the **primary care** provider, manages the patient's care and referrals to specialty care. Early attempts to move workers' compensation into the managed care environment met with some concern about labor–management relations, equity, access to care, and workers' rights. Despite these concerns, workers' compensation has incorporated an increasing number of managed care strategies.

Government Health Benefit Programs

The federal government is the major player in the health care arena because it covers a large portion of health care reimbursement in the United States. The federal **government benefit plans** are Medicare, Medicaid, the Federal Employees Health Benefit Program (FEHBP), TriCare, and the Civilian Health and Medical Program of the Uniform Services (CHAMPUS). In addition, states provide health care coverage for state employees. Case managers may be used with these programs, particularly for complex problems.

FEDERAL EMPLOYEES HEALTH BENEFIT PROGRAM (FEHBP).   The FEHBP is a special insurance in that the employer is the federal government providing health care insurance to its federal employees, retirees, and their dependents in same way that any other employer might provide coverage. Because of this, it is not technically a government plan but rather an employer plan. This coverage is mandated by law and administered by the federal government's Office of Personnel Management. Members or enrollees of the FEHBP choose from a wide variety of health care plans, including managed care plans, during the government's annual enrollment period. Minimum benefits are required for plans to contract with the FEHBP. The federal government pays part of the premium. The enrollee must pay other costs. Managed care plans are an employee option through the FEHBP. In fact, it was the federal government's success, although limited, with managed care in the 1970s that encouraged the federal government to develop and enact the Health Maintenance Act of 1973. In 1990, the Omnibus Budget Reconciliation Act (OBRA-90) mandated the use of certain managed care strategies in the government's **fee-for-service (FFS)** plans to reduce costs such using hospital precertification for nonemergency procedures and case management.

MILITARY HEALTH CARE.   Health care coverage for military personnel and their dependents is another major health care expenditure for the government. The military health services system is not only an insurer but also a provider through its health care facilities globally. It provides health benefits to all active-duty military personnel and through its CHAMPUS program to retirees, dependents, and survivors. Many of these beneficiaries are over 65 years of age, and this proportion is expected to increase with the aging of the baby boomers. CHAMPUS was an FFS insurance program for dependents; however, due to its increasing costs, the federal government also uses managed care such as HMOs, point-of-service (POS), and preferred provider plans. The Veterans Health Administration has also undergone recent changes (e.g., introducing primary care, regional centers and marketing, case management). This system provides ambulatory care, acute care, and in some cases long-term care, for military veterans.

STATE INSURANCE PROGRAMS.   States also offer insurance to their state employees. A state government is usually a state's largest employer and consequently its largest insurer. Usually, there is some degree of choice among plan options for state employees. The state or a contracted provider administrates these plans. State employees contribute to the payment of this coverage in the same way they would if they were employed in the private sector.

Each state has an **insurance commission** that is responsible for regulating both the solvency of all insurers doing business in the state and the marketing of insurance. The commission may also determine the type of insurance that may be sold in the state. A particularly important responsibility is the regulation of the level of reserves that the insurance companies must maintain. Reserves are the amount of funds the insurer holds in savings to ensure that it can pay future claims to better ensure the insurer's solvency. If the insurer does not have these funds and many claims are made, the insurer may not be able to pay its claims. Clearly, this would be a major issue for its enrollees. To further prevent this from occurring and to serve as a backup, each state has a fund to protect policyholders (enrollees) from an insurer that cannot pay its claims. The National Association of Insurance Commissioners (NAIC) assists state insurance regulators in the work that they do to ensure the public interest in the health care insurance industry.

MEDICARE.   The number of patients who are covered by Medicare and Medicaid make these two federal and state programs major sources of health care reimbursement in the United States. The number of people they cover is increasing. These programs have had a major effect on all aspects of health care, its delivery, reimbursement, accreditation, and quality. Every day, in all types of clinical settings, patients who are covered by Medicare and Medicaid receive care. Knowledge of these two programs is important in order to understand what services the patients can receive. As these two programs actively use managed care, it is also important to understand the changes that have been made in them due to managed care.

An Overview of Medicare.   Medicare is the federal health care insurance program that was established in 1965 by Title XVIII, Health Insurance for the Aged, as an amendment to the **Social Security Act of 1935.** Medicare is funded by the Medicare Trust Fund, which includes payroll tax contributions, and it is the largest single payer in the United States. For many years, Medicare has played a major role in health care delivery despite the fact that it is a complex program that is difficult to understand. President Johnson signed the Medicare legislation in 1965, but President Truman took the first steps toward this legislation. He envisioned this program as a critical step toward national health insurance (Daschle, 2008). Despite some efforts to make universal coverage available, it is still not available; however, Medicare has survived and changed. With the introduction of changes in reimbursement methods, such as DRGs, Medicare spending decreased. Interest in using managed care approaches to further decrease health care costs has increased over the years. As demonstrated in Figure 3-1, as a share of the federal budget, Medicare spending is expected to increase in the next 20 years, making the need for further cost reduction very important.

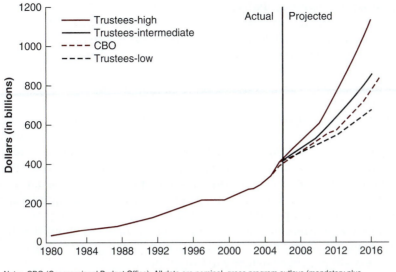

Note: CBO (Congressional Budget Office). All data are nominal, gross program outlays (mandatory plus
administrative expenses) by calendar year.

FIGURE 3-1   Overall Medicare Spending: 1980 Actual through 2016 Projected   *Source:* Medicare
Trustees Report 2007. CBO March 2007 baseline.

The elderly are living longer, thus requiring longer periods of health care services,
and medical prices are going up. These factors will have a major impact on the size of
the trust fund that will be available long term for this federal program. Case management for Medicare patients is not uncommon given the complexity of needs of this population. There has been considerable concern about the growth of Medicare. The "baby
boomers," people born between 1946 and 1964, are entering the Medicare beneficiary
age range. This greatly increases the number of Medicare beneficiaries.

Legislative and Regulatory Issues Related to Medicare.   The following discussion provides information about the legislation and regulations that have affected Medicare and
its move toward managed care approaches to control costs.

- *Social Security Act of 1935 and Amendments*   The Social Security Act of 1935
  with its subsequent amendments is the landmark legislation that established
  Medicare and Medicaid and made the federal government the major player in
  health care. The creation of Medicare and Medicaid not only allowed many who
  could not afford care to receive care but also gave the federal government power
  to dictate standards, reimbursement methods, and influence other aspects of care.
  Few hospitals can avoid treating patients covered by these two programs, and
  when they do treat these patients, they must meet federal requirements.
- *Tax Equity and Fiscal Responsibility Act of 1982*   The Tax Equity and Fiscal
  Responsibility Act of 1982 (TEFRA) introduced Medicare to managed care by promoting the use of health maintenance organizations (HMOs) with Medicare contracts. There are two types of Medicare contracts. *Risk-based* contracts require that
  the managed care organization accept a **capitation** payment for all Medicare services. *Cost-based* contracts provide reimbursement on an FFS basis. If the MCO provides services for less than the capitation, the MCO has two choices: It can return
  the unused portion of the Medicare payment to Medicare or provide additional
  benefits. Most MCOs choose the latter and also require limited or no copayments
  and **deductibles.** Adding benefits made these plans more attractive to Medicare
  beneficiaries.

- *Consolidated Omnibus Budget Reconciliation Act of 1985*   The **Consolidated Omnibus Budget Reconciliation Act of 1985 (COBRA)** affected most hospitals. It requires that all hospitals treating Medicare patients also treat all patients who request care in their emergency rooms, regardless of whether they are covered by Medicare or are able to pay. This law has had a major effect on emergency services, their inappropriate use, and escalating costs. Once a hospital receives federal funding, such as Medicare, this federal law applies to the hospital's emergency services.
- *Medicare Catastrophic Coverage Act of 1988*   The Medicare Catastrophic Coverage Act was signed into law in 1988. This law recognized the economic disparity that existed among the elderly. The decision was made that elderly people with greater personal funds should pay more for Medicare; however, this law did not last long. Two years later, it was repealed. This is an example of the power that the consumer's voice, even a minority of the more affluent elderly, can have on legislation. This group of beneficiaries did not like paying higher premiums. In addition, the pharmaceutical companies were concerned about the drug benefit that was included, and they feared this would lead to greater price controls. They had a very strong, effective lobby in Congress.
- *Balanced Budget Act of 1997 (BBA)*   BBA expanded the ability of Medicare to offer MCOs to its beneficiaries. This included Medicare beneficiaries who had been enrolled in HMOs since 1985. The law increased the options to not only include Medicare HMOs, but also Medicare preferred provider organizations (PPOs), Medicare POS plans, and several other MCO plans (Kongstvedt, 2009). Medicare contracts with nongovernmental insurers for these plans. (The types of MCOs are discussed in Chapter 4.)
- *Medicare Prescription Drug Improvement and Modernization Act of 2003 (MMA)*   This legislation created Medicare Part D, the newest Medicare benefit part. The focus of Part D is prescription coverage, a long-needed benefit for Medicare beneficiaries; however, this Medicare Part D is administered by private entities.

The Healthcare Financing Administration (HCFA) is the agency within the U.S. Department of Health and Human Services (DHHS) that administers the Medicare program and the federal portion of Medicaid. It develops regulations to implement relevant federal laws. The HCFA also grants all managed care contracts for Medicare beneficiaries, evaluates, and reports on MCO performance. Medicare is financed from four sources. The most important source is the mandatory contributions made by employees and employers to the trust fund, which is used to provide hospital care. Employees contribute to the fund during their employment years, as do employers; however, the money that they contribute is actually used to reimburse care for people who are currently covered by Medicare. It is not saved to cover care for the contributing employees in the future. This means that current Medicare beneficiaries are actually covered by current employer and employee contributions. The other fund sources are general tax revenues, premiums paid by beneficiaries, and deductibles and copayments.

Some initiatives that are used to decrease Medicare costs include efforts to reduce hospital, home health, and provider payments. In some cases, these savings have exceeded expectations. There are, however, some results that are troubling and that have had a ripple effect throughout the health care system. Today, patients are often sicker when they receive care, and thus need more intensive care at a time when nursing staff levels are reduced. Families are also greatly affected when they are left with the burden of caring for seriously ill family members at home with limited or no health care support such as home care. This all has implications for case management because more patients could benefit from this assistance.

BOX 3-3

Diagnosis-Related Groups

What Are DRGs?

Diagnosis-related groups (DRGs) are the basis of payment to hospitals under the Medicare prospective payment system (PPS). Each DRG represents a group of patients that are similar, both clinically and by use of resources. There is a specific payment rate for each DRG that is calculated by a formula. DRGs are the fixed payment amounts for each Medicare inpatient, regardless of length-of-stay (LOS). The location of the hospital, urban or rural, and wage levels are factored into this fixed price. Exceptions are those patients who are outliers or those with exceptional expenses.

How Are DRGs Assigned?

The patient's physician documents the patient's principal diagnosis by using classifications and terminology found in the *International Classification of Diseases, 9th Revision,* *Clinical Modification* (ICD-9). In addition to the principal diagnosis, the following are documented:

- Up to four secondary diagnoses
- Principal procedure and additional procedures
- Patient's age, sex, and discharge status

This information is reported to the hospital's Medicare fiscal intermediary. The information is used to classify the patient into one of 25 major diagnostic categories (MDCs). The principal diagnosis is the condition that caused the hospitalization. The patient is then assigned a DRG from within the MDC. Most MDCs are divided into surgical DRGs and medical DRGs. These DRGs may also be categorized by age, sex, and the presence or absence of complications or comorbidities.

What Is the Major Complaint about DRGs?

Severity of illness is not adequately considered.

MS-Diagnosis-Related Groups.   **Diagnosis-related groups (DRGs)** is a statistical system that classifies care into groups. These groups, which include inpatient care, are then used to identify payment rates. This is a per-stay reimbursement that focus on a single episode of care related to a diagnosis and includes all predetermined services delivered for that episode. The DRG system is a prospective payment system that is used as the payment system for Medicare reimbursement. Some third-party payers also use it. Box 3-3 summarizes some information about DRGs.

The DRG system considers the types of patients a hospital treats or its case mix and the costs for treatment. Resources used and LOS or bed days are important aspects of the incurred costs. Case mix characteristics include severity of illness and intensity of service as described in Table 3-1.

This system focuses not on the number of patients, but rather on the types of patients and the resources they use. The major diagnostic categories (MDCs) are based on

TABLE 3-1   DRG Criteria: Severity and Intensity

Severity of Illness	Intensity of Illness
Clinical findings	Physical evaluation
Chief complaint	
Working diagnosis	
Vital signs	Monitoring clinical elements
Imaging	Treatment/medications
Diagnostic radiology	
Ultrasound	
Nuclear medicine results	
Hematology, chemistry, and microbiology results	Scheduled procedures
Other clinical parameters	

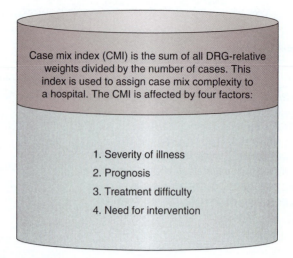

Case mix index (CMI) is the sum of all DRG-relative weights divided by the number of cases. This index is used to assign case mix complexity to a hospital. The CMI is affected by four factors:

1. Severity of illness
2. Prognosis
3. Treatment difficulty
4. Need for intervention

FIGURE 3-2   DRG: Case Mix Index

anatomical or pathophysiological groups and/or their clinical management. Within each MDC, there are a number of DRGs. The DRG rates are also affected by the:

- Location of the hospital (rural or urban)
- Wage index, which affects hospital costs
- Teaching hospital status and house staff training
- Recognition of outliers

Outliers are patients with cost of care or LOS that is outside the expected. If a patient's hospital stay is longer than expected, or total costs are greater than expected for the patient's DRG, then the patient is considered to be an outlier. Hospitals are very concerned when they have outliers because they need to investigate the reasons to ensure that costs are controlled. Figure 3-2 describes the case mix index, another important component of the DRG system.

DRGs have had and continue to have an impact on care. Coordination of all aspects of care becomes critical in order to meet LOS requirements for a specific DRG. Patients who stay longer incur more costs. Timely admissions and discharges are important components of cost-effective care. The nursing staff does most of the documentation, and it is this documentation that provides important information that is required to assign the DRG. The DRG is assigned after the patient is discharged, when it is too late to change the care or the documentation. The DRG system takes outliers into consideration. Changes in care and the coordination of that care may be required to decrease the number of outliers and thus decrease financial risk for the organization and risk of additional payment denials. There is no doubt that Medicare and DRGs have had a tremendous impact on health care. They have decreased lengths-of-stay in hospitals, but this has also increased the need for home health care, long-term care facilities, and ambulatory care. Costs have shifted to other settings, ones that were thought to be more cost effective.

Medicare Eligibility.   Eligibility requirements include the following (Medicare, 2009). A person can receive Part A benefits at age 65 without having to pay premiums if the person:

- Is eligible to get Social Security or Railroad benefits but has not yet filed for them,
- Or already receives retirement benefits from Social Security or the Railroad Retirement Board,
- Is the spouse of a Medicare-covered government employment.

If the person is under 65, the person can receive Part A benefits without having to pay premiums if the person has:

- Received Social Security or Railroad Retirement Board disability benefits for 24 months
- End-stage renal disease and meets certain requirements

Employers are prohibited from forcing employees who are between the ages of 65 and 69 to use Medicare instead of their employer's health coverage, which would be a financial benefit for employers. If employers could do this, then they would not have to provide coverage for older employees in this age group, reducing health care insurance costs for employers. There continue to be new proposals to change benefits, eligibility, and funding for the Medicare program. Medicare has not been immune to managed care since the federal government does offer managed care options in the Medicare program. Health care reform under the Obama administration will have an impact on Medicare.

Medicare Benefits.   The Medicare program is composed of four parts: Parts A, B, C, and D (Centers for Medicare and Medicaid Services [CMS], 2009).

- *Medicare Part A* is the hospital insurance plan, paying for inpatient treatment, skilled nursing facilities (not custodial or long-term care), home health care, and hospice care. Premiums are not paid if the beneficiary or spouse paid Medicare taxes while working. A person may purchase this coverage if the person does not meet past tax payment requirements but must meet citizenship or residency requirements and be 65 or older.
- *Medicare Part B* is the supplementary medical insurance program, which includes coverage for physician services, outpatient treatment, laboratory testing, and some preventive services. This part is voluntary and requires that the enrollee or beneficiary meet the requirements to be entitled to Part A and also be willing to pay Part B premiums. The Medicare beneficiary must also pay deductibles and copayments, which are not high. If the person also qualifies for Medicaid by meeting the requirement of limited financial resources, Medicaid pays the Medicare deductibles and copayments.

    Medicare Part B is very different from Part A. Part B resembles typical indemnity coverage and is supplemental medical insurance. Its benefits include physician services and outpatient hospital services, including emergency services, ambulatory surgery, diagnostic tests, laboratory services, durable equipment, and some preventive services. Though enrollment in Part B is voluntary, most beneficiaries enroll because it provides coverage at a reasonable cost. Part B benefits are funded by premiums paid by beneficiaries, annual deductibles, and copayments.
- *Medicare Part C* (Medicare Advantage Plans, such as an HMO or PPO) provides health coverage choice administered by private companies approved by Medicare. There are extra costs, which vary from plan to plan, and Part C includes benefits found in Part A and Part B and usually covers prescription drugs. Other services not typically covered by Medicare that might be covered are: long-term nursing care, custodial care, dental services, vision services, hearing aids, and other services. This part of Medicare will be reduced over time due to changes made by health care reform legislation in 2010.
- *Medicare Part D* is the Medicare prescription drug coverage. "The benefit is voluntary for regular Medicare beneficiaries, but dual eligible's (having both Medicare and Medicaid) are automatically in the program. It is primarily paid for by federal subsidies, with a portion of the voluntary benefit paid by beneficiaries in the form of premiums and cost sharing" (Kongstvedt, 2009, p. 158).

Medicare benefits do change. One example is use of telemedicine services. In 1997, it became possible to receive Medicare reimbursement for telemedicine services under Part B (Centers for Medicare and Medicaid Services, 2009). In 2008, this benefit was expanded to include nursing homes, allowing them to charge a fee for patients using telemedicine to reduce cost and need for travel to medical appointments. Telemedicine coverage was also expanded to community mental health centers and renal dialysis facilities.

Medigap Plans. **Medigap plans** are a special supplemental insurance plan for Medicare beneficiaries. These plans are not government plans but rather are offered by third-party payers but approved by the CMS. The benefits and costs of Medigap plans vary. Typically, the Medicare beneficiary must be enrolled in Medicare Part A and B, paying premiums for Part B, and then pay the premium to the Medigap insurer. As long as the premium is paid the plan is automatically renewed annually. The Medigap plan must meet Medicare's standard plan requirements and follow required policies. Consumers should compare plans because their costs vary. Spouses must buy separate plans; one plan does not cover both spouses. Why would a Medicare beneficiary buy a Medigap plan? The plan helps to pay some of the additional Medicare health care costs such as copayments, coinsurance, and deductibles and may cover services not covered by Medicare, thus filling the gaps. The plans do not cover long-term care, vision or dental care, hearing aids, eyeglasses, and private duty nursing.

Medicare+Choice: A Managed Care Approach. The Balanced Budget Act of 1997 Medicare+Choice was created to cope with the ever-increasing cost of the Medicare program and the financial drain on the Medicare trust fund, and it is hoped, to prevent future Medicare financial problems. This new change in Medicare did not terminate the indemnity program and its FFS component. Currently, beneficiaries have a choice as to whether they will participate in a managed care plan. They can choose from several managed care program options. These include PPOs, provider-sponsored organizations (PSOs), private fee-for-service (PFFS), and medical savings accounts (MSAs). Health plan participation in Medicare+Choice requires that its options meet Medicare standards related to enrollment, coverage and benefits, access, beneficiary protections, quality assurance, provider protections, and premiums. The HCFA must also publish comparative information about these plans for the consumer. After a review of the plan's proposed benefits, premiums, and other beneficiary out-of-pocket costs to ensure they are in compliance with Medicare regulations, contracts are approved annually by the HCFA.

Mixing Medicare and managed care has not always gone smoothly. Some of the critical issues that have arisen are disenrollment patterns, discontinuation of contracts by MCOs, and cherry picking (choosing healthier persons as enrollees to reduce costs). Issues related to choices that Medicare beneficiaries must make—more than they had prior to this change—and how the consumer copes with these options and changes have led to the need to better assist consumers.

Medicare allows enrollees to disenroll from their plans at any time. Disenrollment rates provide data about enrollee dissatisfaction. Beneficiaries or enrollees may disenroll for a number of reasons, but typically, beneficiaries are concerned about access to care, access to a health care provider of their choice, and dissatisfaction with the plan such as poor communication or poor customer relations. There are also the natural reasons such as change of residence. Disenrollment also affects treatment. Continuity of care is interrupted, and patients often must develop new relationships with providers. The following are some questions that case managers could use as a guide to determine if a Medicare patient was having problems with a Medicare HMO plan and dissatisfied with the plan:

- Did the doctor take complaints seriously?
- Did the patient get appropriate responses to medical problems (e.g., physician appointment, hospitalization, referral to specialist)?

- Was the patient's problem improving due to medical care or worsening?
- Did the patient feel that he or she had been denied care that was needed?

It is important to learn more about the dissatisfaction with the physician or plan in order to resolve problems and prevent disenrollment. Questions such as the ones identified might be helpful in preventing disenrollment. Consumers have had an impact on changes that have occurred in Medicare due to their complaints and feedback to the CMS. Complaints from providers have also had an impact.

MEDICAID.   Medicaid is the health plan for low-income individuals. The need for this program has grown owing to the higher costs of insurance, employer cutbacks on insurance coverage, greater number of unemployed persons, and many other factors that have resulted in people not being able to access health care. Despite this program, there are still many Americans who do not have health care coverage. Health care reform legislation of 2010 will lead to an increase of the number of people covered by Medicaid over the next 4 years, reducing the number of uninsured. About 22 million people will remain uninsured after all of the changes are implemented.

Medicaid Legislative and Regulatory Issues.

- *Social Security Act of 1965, Title XIX*   The Social Security Act of 1965, Title XIX, established the jointly funded Medicaid program. Each state and the federal government share the costs associated with Medicaid. The federal government develops the federal guidelines for the program, with the HCFA acting as the overall federal agency responsible for its implementation. This legislation was a major breakthrough in establishing a program to provide care for those who could not afford it. The regulations related to this program have grown more complex since 1965, and other laws have also affected the program.
- *Personal Responsibility and Work Opportunity Reconciliation Act of 1996*   In 1996, there were several attempts to make major changes in Medicaid, and most were not passed. However, the Personal Responsibility and Work Opportunity Reconciliation Act of 1996 (also known as the Welfare Reform Act) was signed into law (Casto & Layman, 2009). While the law eliminated **Aid to Families with Dependent Children (AFDC),** families who were eligible for AFDC are usually eligible for Temporary Assistance for Needy Families (TANF); these are usually low-income families with children. Prior to this law, Medicaid eligibility income thresholds were set by individual states, and there was thus great variation in eligibility. Now, poorer states receive a greater percentage of federal matching funds to provide greater parity in state programs. The goal of this legislation is to move people off welfare and into jobs; however, many lose their health benefits because they take jobs that do not offer benefits. This law provides 6 to 12 months of Medicaid coverage during the transition to work. There has been improvement with more people employed; however, there are now more uninsured because of this change and for other reasons such as the increased use of temporary staff who get no health coverage, increasing self-employment, and so on.
- *State Children's Health Insurance Program (SCHIP)*   This program, established by the Title XXI of the Social Security Act, was signed into law in 1997. It is a "state/federal partnership that targets the growing number of children not covered by health insurance" (Casto & Layman, 2009, p. 73). It covers children from families whose incomes are too high to receive Medicaid but too low for private insurance. There is state variation in SCHIP. These children may then get their coverage through Medicaid or through a separate state program. SCHIP has been successful, though it has had a rocky history. President Bush would not expand

SCHIP; however, President Obama signed legislation expanding SCHIP as one of his first acts as president in 2009. SCHIP covers inpatient services, outpatient services, physicians' medical and surgical services, laboratory and radiological services, and well-baby and immunization services.

Medicaid is not just a state program, but a program funded jointly by the federal government and individual states. Each state has its own Medicaid program that provides funding for health care and long-term care or nursing home care. What is the role of the federal government? The federal matching funds are designed so that poorer states receive a larger percentage of the federal Medicaid funds to ensure more equity among the state programs. The state programs must meet federal guidelines established by HCFA. Each state, however, determines its own benefits, eligibility requirements, and provider fee schedules. This is where problems and inequality occur. There is a difference in programs from state to state, particularly in eligibility requirements. All states, however, must include persons who qualify for AFDC, all needy children under the age of 21, Old-Age Assistance, Aid to the Blind, persons who are permanently and totally disabled, and the elderly over 65 years and on welfare. When states set eligibility standards below the federal poverty level, this can cause major problems for many people who need these health care services and cannot receive Medicaid reimbursement. Eligibility standards may have a major effect on providers that may provide care with no reimbursement to cover their costs.

The Medicaid program has also undergone many changes owing to the need for cost containment and the increasing use of managed care models and strategies. Medicaid is a program that has been troubled with bureaucracy and inadequate funding. Because of these factors, many providers are not willing to care for Medicaid beneficiaries. Medicaid managed care, however, has made it easier for some providers to participate in the program. Medicaid is a complex program with many regulations. As cost-containment strategies increase, there is concern that coverage for some people will be eliminated or reduced to a point that many Medicaid beneficiaries may not have their health needs met. Advocacy for these patients is very important.

Medicaid Eligibility.   Welfare reform changed Medicaid eligibility. States may modify their AFDC eligibility criteria, which continue to be the criteria used for TANF to establish eligibility for Medicaid services (Casto & Layman, 2009). A state may lower its income standard, but it may not be any lower than what it was in May 1998. This decreases the number of eligible persons. Second, a state may increase income or resource standards and expand eligibility. This increases the number of eligible persons. Welfare reform also established some specific provisions about eligibility. The most controversial provision is the refusal to work/transition. This gives states the option to discontinue Medicaid coverage for persons who refuse to work and lose TANF. Exceptions are children who are not heads of household and pregnant women. Legal immigrants are also included in these provisions.

Health care coverage for immigrants has been a longtime problem. "The passage of the Personal Responsibility and Work Opportunity Reconciliation Act (PRWORA) in 1996 changed the eligibility requirements for immigrants, making it more difficult for immigrants, especially those newly arrived in the U.S., to obtain Medicaid coverage. For the first time, the 1996 law tied legal immigrants' eligibility for Medicaid to their length of residency in the U.S. These restrictions also applied to SCHIP, which was established in 1997" (Henry J. Kaiser Family Foundation, April 2006, p. 1). The following information summarizes Medicaid and SCHIP eligibility rules for immigrants today. Legal permanent residents (immigrants with green cards) are not allowed to apply for Medicaid or SCHIP for the first five years that they are in the United States. Refugees do not fall under this rule. State Medicaid programs must cover the following groups (Casto & Layman, 2009, p. 71):

- Low-income families with children, including those who meet eligibility for TANF
- People who receive federal Supplemental Security Income (SSI) based on state criteria
- Infants born to Medicaid-eligible pregnant women
- Children under the age of 6 whose families meet income criteria
- Recipients of adoption assistance and foster care
- Medicare recipients who are elderly and disabled and meet income criteria
- Special protected groups (short-term), for example, persons who lose SSI assistance because of increased wages or Social Security payments

Eligibility is usually influenced by poverty criteria, which are established annually by federal poverty guidelines. These guidelines are based on prospective estimates for a given year. The federal poverty threshold is based on retrospective data for a given year and used by the Census Bureau for its reports.

Medicaid Benefits.   Due to the great variation in the types of Medicaid beneficiaries, Medicaid must provide services across the health care continuum, from preventive care to long-term care and across the lifespan of the enrollee. Medicaid required benefits include (CMS, 2009):

- Inpatient hospital care
- Outpatient hospital care
- Physician services
- Laboratory and radiological services
- Nursing facility services for beneficiaries 21 and older
- Home health care for individuals eligible for nursing facility services
- Medical and surgical dental services
- Family planning services and supplies
- Rural health clinic services
- Pediatric and family nurse practitioner services
- Federally-qualified health center services
- Pregnancy-related services and service for other conditions that might complicate pregnancy
- Sixty days of postpartum pregnancy-related services
- Nurse-midwifery services
- Early and periodic screening, diagnosis, and treatment services for individuals under 21

Optional benefits that states may offer are: prescription medications, prosthetic devices, hearing aids, and care for people who are mentally retarded. The number of people who are without insurance and unemployed has overtaxed the Medicaid program. This problem is only increasing and will also need to be addressed in health care reform initiatives. Patients who use Medicaid often have complex medical and socioeconomic issues and could benefit from case management.

Every state Medicaid program provides pharmaceutical services even though it is an optional service. It is provided in order to prevent the use of more costly services, such as surgery or extensive inpatient treatment. States do try to control pharmaceutical use by requiring prior **authorization,** prescription caps, and prospective utilization review. Other services that may be provided are: case management, transportation, hospice services, personal care services, inpatient psychiatric services, physical and occupational therapy for speech/language/hearing disorders, and respiratory services for children who are dependent on a ventilator. Home and community services may also be provided if the state receives a waiver to do so.

Medicaid Managed Care Risk.   Medicaid, as has been true with all areas of health care, has turned to managed care strategies to decrease its costs (Kongvedst, 2009). There is, however, concern that some of the managed care strategies, such as capitation, may result in underserving patients. In fact, some of these strategies, such as the use of copayments and deductibles, are prohibited in traditional fee-for-service Medicaid. Proponents of managed care strategies emphasize that managed care focuses on better coordination, prevention, decreased hospitalization, and methods to predict and control costs. Traditional Medicaid pays only for services provided to Medicaid beneficiaries; however, in the managed care model, Medicaid must pay a capitated amount to providers even though services may not be provided. States must ensure that contracts with MCOs meet the following provisions: enrollment, marketing, emergency care, access to care, grievance procedures, and quality of care.

Special Considerations for People with Chronic or Disabling Illnesses.   Medicaid managed care must include care needs for people with chronic and disabling conditions even though these care needs are often not as important for other groups of Medicaid recipients. These needs are individualized care with needs beyond traditional medical care, comprehensive service systems, and care without cure. The latter is most important, because the need for treatment is typically long term. States have taken various approaches to meeting the needs of these patients in Medicaid managed care.

The Uninsured.   The uninsured is a growing problem in the United States, as discussed in earlier chapters. There continues to be an increasing number of people without coverage, and this is a startling anomaly considering the country's excellent economy compared with that of many other countries. Children are at greater risk of having no insurance coverage. Sick people approaching 65 have the greater number of medical problems and higher costs. The people who are most likely to have insurance are those who are over 65, which is due to Medicare coverage. Adults who work for hourly wages often do not have insurance. Young adults also may decide not to pay for insurance, feeling that they have no need for it. People without insurance avoid preventive care and wait to receive medical treatment until it is an emergency, and thus the care frequently costs more.

One reason for this growth is the number of people who have lost Medicaid eligibility and thus health care coverage. Some people leave welfare for low-wage jobs, though this is difficult in a time of high unemployment. Low-wage jobs typically do not offer health care coverage. Another group is people who are hired for temporary or contract positions. Many of these people had health insurance coverage in their full-time positions, which may have even been in high-level or professional positions. As more companies outsource, they hire people to fulfill only specific needs temporarily. These positions come without any benefits. In 2008, the most current numbers, the number of people without health insurance is 45 million, and this number continues to increase (Cover the Uninsured, 2009). Health care reform legislation of 2010 will gradually increase coverage and thus decrease the number of uninsured, increasing the insured by estimated 32 million.

HOW DOES HEALTH INSURANCE WORK?

An individual experiences uncertainty about health care needs and treatment costs. Without consumer uncertainty, there would be less need for insurance and less financial risk associated with health care. Given this uncertainty, there is a need to share the financial risk with other consumers to decrease individual financial risk.

When individuals decide to join an insurance plan, they put a specific amount of money into the pool or the insurance fund. The pool consists of the group of people that the insurer is covering for health care services. This could be done without the insurer, which acts at the intermediary between the consumer and the health care providers, but it is not typical. The insurer takes on the role of managing or administering the pool of money. Plan members really do not want to do this for themselves. For example, a large manufacturing company offers several health care coverage options to its employees. This company does not want to use its own resources to administer employee health care coverage, so it contracts with insurers. The insurer or third-party payer typically provides the following administrative services (Casto & Layman, 2009; Kongvedst, 2009).

- Administrative structure and staff
- Enrollment of new members and re-enrollment of current members
- Claims and benefit administration (billing, collecting premiums, verifying claims and making claim decisions, paying providers, preventing fraud, establishing rates)
- Management of pended or appealed claims and adjustments
- Maintenance of records
- Marketing the plan
- Communication with providers
- Communication with members
- Quality improvement (handling complaints and grievances, collecting satisfaction data)

The insurer will be better served, as will the purchaser of the health care plan and the enrollees, if there are a large number of members/enrollees. This decreases the financial risk and the administrative costs and usually means that there is greater diversification in the health status of members, with some healthier than others, and premiums are usually lower. There will be a greater chance of a mix of needs: some requiring no care, others limited care, and some with major medical care needs.

Reimbursement and the role of the third-party payer is a complex process. What is the source of the money that is used for payment? Who decides what services will be covered and for what price? What is the relationship between the patient and the insurer? How does reimbursement affect the delivery of care? The first step in understanding reimbursement is to describe the many different types of third-party payers.

Key Players in Reimbursement Strategies and Risk Taking

The key players in reimbursement strategies are the insurer, provider, and the patient/enrollee, as described in Figure 3-3. Each of these key players may experience various levels of financial risk.

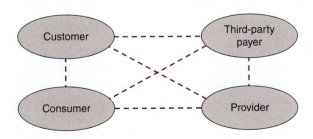

FIGURE 3-3   Key Players in the Health Care Environment

INSURER.   With the development of managed care, the insurer, third-party payer, or the MCO no longer carries all of the financial risk for health care. Reimbursement strategies used by MCOs are primarily aimed at reducing insurer financial risk. The insurer may use any of the managed care models and may be a national or regional insurer. With the advent of managed care, the insurer has increased power to influence care and reimbursement and has been more successful in decreasing its financial risk by using reimbursement and service strategies.

PROVIDER.   Who is the provider? Provider is a generic term. Any of the following may be considered a provider: physician, advanced practice nurse or nurse practitioner, nurse-midwife, registered nurse, physician assistant, nurse anesthetist, pharmacist, dentist, optometrist, chiropractor, podiatrist, hospital, home health agency, hospice, long-term care facility, psychiatric hospital, skilled nursing home, infusion therapy agency, and so on. In short, a provider is any person or organization that provides health care. An insurer **provider panel** includes a mixture of these providers, individuals, and organizations. The provider is carrying more and more of the financial risk. Providers, particularly physicians and hospitals, have had to reformulate their view of health care delivery, and this has increased stress in the health care delivery environment.

PHYSICIAN.   How are physicians reacting to greater use of managed health care reimbursement? Some are satisfied, but an increasing number complain about it. They are concerned about the increased time required to complete paperwork, telephone communication with the insurer, and meetings related to clinical reporting requirements. Physicians work longer hours and must see more patients for shorter times for less payment. Independent physician decision-making is frequently challenged by insurer requirements. In some communities, there is increasing competition for patients, and physician–physician relationships have been strained as physicians fight for patients and decrease their referrals. Advanced practice nurses who enter primary care experience similar problems.

HOSPITALS.   As hospitals try to cope with the health care changes, they began to restructure, reengineer, and merge in order to survive and compete. Health care changes have stimulated hospitals to recognize the need for more ambulatory services. They have developed or expanded these services, for example, ambulatory surgery, clinics, diagnostic services, and home health care. At the same time, they cope with more acutely ill admissions that require high staff levels and expertise. Administrative costs have always been a concern, but with the organizational changes in hospitals and the need to decrease their costs, administrative costs have become more important. Do health care administrative costs provide important information about overall health spending or cost efficiency? What is being sacrificed to reach a higher margin of profit or to cut costs? Has the hospital's efficiency improved? Has its quality decreased? How much charity care and community benefits and services have been reduced? Should the approach be more than looking at only dollar amounts, but rather the effect of the reduction in costs on the hospital and its services? These are difficult questions to answer and easy ones to avoid.

PATIENT/ENROLLEE.   Clearly, the patient or enrollee is a key player in the health care system. If patients did not exist, there would be no need for insurers or health care providers. When a person chooses a managed care plan, the person is no longer referred to as a policyholder, as was true with indemnity plans, but rather a plan member or enrollee. Managed care has also found ways to shift more financial risk to the patient by greater use of copayments, deductibles, and other payment requirements when the patient chooses to receive care from a provider not approved by the patient's insurer.

The goal is to increase the patient's recognition of costs and the patient's role in determining those costs by making choices, preferably choosing the less costly route. Costs play a critical role in insurance coverage decisions that people make.

MCOs expect their providers to effectively ration care to patients. Changes in the requirement that patients pay deductibles and copayments altered patient responsibility. Managed care's goals are to change patient behavior, increase patient financial risk sharing, and, hopefully, decrease costs. All types of insurers are using methods to increase patient responsibility in self-management of care and to reduce costs of care.

Financial Factors and Third-Party Payers

In the past few years, health care reimbursement methods have changed radically. Cost reimbursement was the method that was used for many years. With this method, assignment of benefits was usually made directly to the provider. The enrollee signed a form authorizing the third-party payer to pay the provider directly. This took the enrollee out of the payment process. If the third-party payer reimbursement is not timely in paying for services, the enrollee was still responsible the payment. The cost reimbursement system paid providers on the basis of reasonable historical costs. The following discussion describes some of the major financial factors that are important in understanding the past reimbursement methods, the changes that have occurred, and their application in the current reimbursement environment.

Fee-for-Service (FFS)

FFS or billed charges (fees, prices) is the traditional method used for payment of health care services. It is the price charged by the provider, and it is paid in three ways: (1) premiums, (2) deductibles, and (3) copayments. The provider establishes the fee-for-service, and the patient pays, usually through a third-party payer or the provider submitting a claim to the insurer. Historically, indemnity insurers used this type of payment. FFS payment typically did not put many limitations on the provider, and the insurer accepted the charges identified by the provider. There was little incentive to be cost effective when the provider knew the charge it requested would be paid in full.

Prospective versus Retrospective Payment

Typically, when a customer considers purchasing a product, the price is known before the purchase. This is prospective price setting. The seller sets the price (episode of care reimbursement), and then the purchaser decides to buy or not to buy the product, usually considering need, price, quality, and the like. The health care industry has had a different experience with setting prices. Third-party purchasers of health care services devised a **retrospective payment system** (FFS reimbursement). In this system, the provider spent money while providing the care for a patient (enrollee in an insurance plan), requested payment for these expenses, and then was paid. Providers liked this because they knew they would be paid for their services when they submitted their bills. Third-party payers thought this was a good approach, but after a time, this became an expensive way to do business. Then, third-party payers began to put some limits on what they would reimburse. There was no longer a blanket acceptance of all charges. The federal government via its Medicare and Medicaid programs was the first purchaser or third-party payer to develop a comprehensive prospective payment system (PPS), which resulted in the development of the DRG payment system. The purpose of this type of payment system was to decrease hospital costs. This system is not based on actual charges but rather on predetermined prices, based on average levels of use of resources, made by the payer, not the provider. The provider knows before the care is provided what the payer will pay for the service; usually, additional resources such as specialty care that may be used are not figured into this amount. These additional charges need to be negotiated and may not be paid.

Relative Based Value Units (RBVU)

The relative based value unit system (RBVU) is a payment system in which health care reimbursement is based on the relative value of a specific procedure (Kongvedst, 2009; Casto & Layman, 2009). RBVU is "based on CPT coding. Each CPT (Current Procedural Terminology) code has been assigned a relative value unit (RVU). An RVU is a unit of measure designed to permit comparison of the amount to resources required to perform various provider services by assigning weights to such factors as personnel time, level of skill, and sophistication of equipment required to render service" (Casto & Layman, 2009, p. 158). Unit values are assigned to over 4,000 specific procedures representing 85% of Medicare services based on their complexity or physician work (WORK) (i.e., time, skill required), physician practice expenses (PE), and malpractice costs. Geographic area is also important since costs vary across the country. This system has lowered reimbursement for procedures.

Premium Rate Setting

Premium rate setting is one of the most important decisions that a third-party payer can make. Rating is pricing. The third-party payer determines the premiums (prices or rate) for its products or services that are paid by the insurance member or enrollee. Premiums are usually calculated as an amount per member per month (PMPM). If the third-party payer miscalculates, it can mean that the insurer loses money and may become financially unstable. How does the third-party payer determine the amount to charge? **Underwriting** is the process of determining the risk of illness and need for treatment for specific employers and their employees and the identification of the premium rates. **Actuarial data** or assumptions with statistical relevance are used to help the third-party payer arrive at the premium rate. These assumptions might include utilization rates, age and gender mix of enrollees, cost of medical services, and so on. The third-party payer uses either community rating or **experience rating** to identify their premium rate.

Community Rating by Class (CRC) is a method in which everyone pays the same premium. When using CRC to set insurance premiums, the insurer ignores any differences in expected costs among insured groups or people. This type of approach can lead to an insurer having sicker enrollees or enrollees with higher risk in their coverage pool. Underwriting is the way in which insurance companies project what the expected covered health costs will be for a particular person or group. Medical underwriting includes assessment of the health or chronic illness of a person or group. The issue of whether health insurance premiums should be based on CRC or experience rating is a complex one involving social concerns, **adverse selection,** and privacy issues. CRC is less common today. One result is that higher cost groups (and individuals) are charged higher premiums. Some employers may not hire people with chronically ill dependents for fear that it will increase their health care premiums. This is referred to as selection bias. CRC has disadvantages. If the standard CRC method is used, all employer groups receive the same rates. No consideration is given for such factors as the type of industry or employer, the enrolled population or the size of the group. Why would these factors make a difference in the risk and thus the rate that needs to be charged? Is it an industry that has a high risk of injuries, stress-related disorders, cancer, and so forth? These factors may indicate that the employees have greater health problems, and this increases health care expenses. If it is a large business, the risk is spread over a greater number of employees, so if some employees need more care, there is a greater pool of funds to cover care. There is also a greater chance that some enrollees will be healthier than others. Older employees and women in their childbearing years usually require more medical care. Using CRC to make adjustments in rates can help the third-party payer to reduce potential financial problems.

As premiums rise, healthier individuals may refuse to pay increased premiums, or in difficult economic times people may not have the extra funds to pay. They drop out of the plan. Third-party payers then have a smaller number of healthier enrollees, and they must continue to increase premiums to cover a sicker pool of enrollees.

The second method used to determine rates or premiums is experience rating. Experience rating considers the actual medical claims history or utilization history of the employees as well as anticipated care based on such factors as age and gender. As historical data are used to determine the rate, a larger data pool provides more credible data. Consequently, experience rating works best with larger employee groups. If a business's employees have a high claims rate, then premiums will be higher with the employer and the employee paying more for their medical care.

Discounted Fee-for-Service

Discounted fee-for-service is a payment method that offers to pay the provider a specific percentage of the provider's usual charge or a reduced rate. The percentage can be a straight one in which only a certain percentage is taken off the charge, or it can be a sliding scale with the percentage changing based on specified criteria. Discounted services are part of a contractual arrangement with a third-party payer and are used by all traditional indemnity plans as well as some MCOs. An insurer may contract with a health care facility or any type of provider to receive a discount for services provided. For example, an insurer's enrollees who receive care at that facility receive a 20% discount or rather are only charged 80% of the usual charge for the services. Sliding scales are reflective of the volume of services provided. If the insurer requires a specific level of service, the fee scale will be adjusted or decreased. Most health care facilities, such as hospitals, have many contracts with insurers that have different discounts. If all care is not reimbursed at 100% of the cost, this leaves the health care provider with expenses that are not covered. This can have serious ramifications for the provider over the long term if the provider cannot cover these unpaid expenses. Providers, such as hospitals, outpatient clinics, physician practices, and home health care agencies, must be careful about the amount of care that is discounted and consider how the unpaid portion will be covered.

Per Diem Rates

A **per diem** rate is reimbursement that is fixed, based on each day in a health care facility (e.g., $600 per day). Services that may be covered, as well as expected LOS and intensity of services, may be included in the agreed-upon per diem rate. This rate may also be discounted by the contract between the third-party payer and the provider. The per diem rate is an estimate of what the charges would be; however, this is all that is paid even if the actual expenses are greater. This is a prospectively determined, pre-established rate. Usually, per diem rates vary for specialty areas, for example, different daily rates for critical care, psychiatric care, medical care, surgical care, or obstetrical care. Per diem reimbursement is the negotiated rate per day times the number of days of care. Home health is usually reimbursed on a per-hour or per-visit basis.

Case Rates

The **case rate,** which is a prospective, pre-established rate, is based on the type of case (e.g., a flat fee is paid for a vaginal delivery). This is similar to DRGs; however, case rating

BOX 3-4

Out-of-Pocket Expenses: More Than You Think—An Example

Physician's bill for office visit: Bronchitis	$120	Patient's total out-of-pocket	
Insurer's reasonable and customary charge		expenses_Copayment ($30) +	
for this visit	$100	uncovered portion ($20) =	$ 50
Patient's copayment of 30% ($100 ×.30) =	$ 30		
Uncovered part of bill to be paid by patient		**The $50 represents 41.6% of the total charge of $120.**	
($120 − $100) =	$ 20		

is a less complex rating system. It is a negotiated fixed rate for specific treatment for a specific problem or diagnosis. Case rates can be adjusted for patients requiring more services.

Copayments/Coinsurance

A copayment/coinsurance is the fixed payment that the employee must pay per physician visit, procedure/treatment, or prescription. This is payment sharing between the insurer and the enrollee/patient. The payment typically is required at the time of the service and usually is an established amount, such as $5 or $10, or it can be a percentage. What is the true copay? Copayments may be found in all types of coverage, including HMOs. Box 3-4 describes an example of a patient's **out-of-pocket expenses** for a commercial insurance plan. Employers are increasing their efforts to contain costs and are using more cost-shifting strategies. This increases the out-of-pocket expenses for employees.

Enrollee and Eligibility

When an employee joins a health plan or when an individual purchases insurance, the person becomes an enrollee/member/subscriber in the plan. The enrollee's family is not usually referred to as the enrollee. They are dependents that may be included in the plan's coverage, if this is an option available to the enrollee. The contract or **covered services** plan describes the eligibility criteria, benefits, and payments. These criteria identify when the enrollee and dependents are eligible for the services and when they are not eligible. For instance, a dependent child typically is not covered after a specific age or when no longer considered a dependent of the parent.

Coverage renewability is particularly important with individual health insurance policies and long-term care contracts. Until the Health Insurance Portability and Accountability Act (HIPAA) was passed in 1996, this was a major problem for enrollees or dependents with major or chronic health problems. This legislation provides guaranteed renewability, with exceptions for enrollee fraud and nonpayment of premiums.

Annual Limits

Annual limits are very important, particularly for employees and their families who experience major medical expenses in a year. All plans have some type of limit on the amount that the employee is required to pay annually. For example, coverage for an individual employee might have an annual limit of $1,000 and for the employee's family coverage $2,000. After this is paid, the health care services are covered 100%. In addition, some plans have lifetime limits on benefits such as number of psychotherapy sessions, which mean that after the employee's total expenditures for health care reach a specific amount, the plan will not pay for any more services. Plans may have a lifetime limit as high as $1 million; however, for some major illnesses, such as prematurity, major mental illness, or severe injuries with disability, this amount can quickly be spent.

This may seem like an attractive benefit, but in reality it may not cover the costs. Not all plans have lifetime limits. Health care reform legislation of 2010 will eliminate annual and lifetime limits beginning with some changes by September, 2010.

Covered Services/Benefits

Benefits are a very important part of any health care plan, and a major concern for case managers. Important factors are the covered services, exclusions (services not covered), and limitations. There is great variability among plans in their benefit description and what is included or excluded. For an employee makes decisions about coverage, benefits can be a critical issue to consider, depending on the health and financial needs of the employee and the employee's family. In some cases, when there are major or chronic health problems, paying higher premiums to obtain maximum benefits may be the wisest choice. Some plans offer a cafeteria-style option, with employees choosing the benefits that are most important for them. Examples of benefit categories that are typically included in a cafeteria-style plan are health benefits, pension and savings, childcare benefits, other types of insurance, and time off from work. Plan benefits are also important to the provider because medical decisions are often based on the benefits that will be covered, not necessarily what the patient needs. What does the employee need to consider when reviewing covered services, exclusions, and limitations?

Covered services are the health care services that the plan will cover or reimburse; however, the care or services must be medically necessary. What are the criteria used to determine if care is medically necessary? The key question the insurer asks is: Is the service, equipment or supply (drug or device) actually necessary to protect or preserve the health of a person (member, enrollee) based on evidence-based medical knowledge or practice (Kongstvedt, 2009)? This is not always easy to determine. The insurer determines medical necessity with input from the provider. Clearly, this is an area that creates conflict. Typical benefits included in health care plans are:

- Hospital room and board
- Outpatient and inpatient surgery
- Office and inpatient physician visits
- Nursing services
- Diagnostic and radiological laboratory tests
- Ambulance services
- Medical equipment for home use

Some plans include more specialized care, such as home health care, extended care, hospice care, inpatient and outpatient mental health care, and alcohol and substance abuse treatment. When plans cover these services, specific descriptions are included in the covered services document or plan. Typically, home health care is used when skilled nursing care is required and usually covers supplies and equipment required for the delivery of the skilled care. Hospice care is provided for the terminally ill and may include a specific time period for expected death, such as within six months of admission to hospice care. Extended care is provided for patients who need less intensive care than hospital care and require skilled nursing care, rehabilitation, and/or convalescent services. Mental health services and alcohol and substance abuse treatment services usually have more stringent limitations. The insurer identifies not only the benefits that are offered but often who may provide these services, a requirement that must be met for the insurer to cover or pay for the health care service.

Special health care needs are always a concern for the insurer because these needs increase costs. Dental and vision coverage are services that receive special attention. If an employer offers these services, it usually covers only one of them. Employers are beginning to pay a smaller portion of the premiums for these services. Some are offering only the option of dental HMOs. In addition, the use of medical technology has become an increased concern for insurers and for consumers. The development of new medical technologies is a major step forward for health care delivery, but they cost money to develop and to use. Insurers must evaluate new technologies carefully before agreeing to cover these new therapies.

Health promotion and disease prevention have become more important to insurers, particularly in the managed care environment and are included in health care reform of 2010. In the past, traditional indemnity plans usually did not cover or provide limited coverage for these services, but even traditional insurers are more concerned about enrollees' health in general. Examples of preventive care that might be included in benefits are annual physical exams, childhood immunizations, and mammograms, usually within a specified age range. Health promotion examples are health education classes, wellness centers, and smoking cessation groups.

Prior to the passage of HIPAA in 1996, insurers used preexisting conditions to control some of their costs. Preexisting conditions are health conditions that exist prior to the date that insurance becomes effective. This was a problem for enrollees who had chronic illnesses, such as rheumatoid arthritis or renal disease. HIPAA requires that a group insurer may only refuse or limit coverage of a new employee with a preexisting condition treated or diagnosed in the six-month period prior to enrollment for 12 months. This 12-month period is reduced by the period of continuous coverage before enrollment in the new policy and is for one time only. For example, a person with renal disease who was diagnosed with the illness maintains continuous coverage for five months. Upon changing jobs, the person's coverage can be limited or denied for seven months. At the conclusion of the seven-month waiting period, the person becomes eligible for the same insurance coverage offered to all employees. Having once met the 12-month waiting period, a person cannot be denied coverage when changing jobs as long as the person has had continuous coverage. The issue of **preexisting conditions** has long been a concern of members or beneficiaries; however, the health care reform of 2010 has eliminated the ability of insurers to limit care coverage based on preexisting conditions.

What happens with health insurance coverage when an employee leaves a job, either for another job or unemployment? Two federal laws address this concern. The Consolidated Omnibus Budget Reconciliation Act of 1985 (COBRA) provides protection for employees from businesses of 20 or more employees and their dependents. These employees have the opportunity to continue group insurance for up to 18 months. This option is much less expensive than purchasing individual insurance, though COBRA is not inexpensive. The individual must continue to pay the full premium and continue to obtain the group rates, but the individual must also pay a fee. If the individual misses a premium payment, COBRA eligibility is lost. If the worker does not want COBRA, family members may still use it. This is particularly helpful if a family member has a preexisting condition that is not covered by the worker's new employer.

In addition to the extension of coverage, COBRA established a federal requirement that all hospitals that participate in Medicare and offer emergency services must treat all patients requiring emergency treatment or who are in labor. It would be rare for a hospital with an emergency service not to participate in Medicare. Inability to pay cannot be used to deny treatment to patients who need emergency services. This is a major protection for the patient; however, the critical issue is the definition of an emergency and who defines it. Some patients use the local emergency department as their physician office. Insurers are concerned about this use, but the patients for whom this law is addressed often have no insurance. If hospitals meet these COBRA criteria, they cannot deny patients emergency services. How does this affect emergency service expenses? What is the hospital's moral obligation? Neither of these questions can be ignored, nor are they simple to answer.

Employee Contributions to Coverage: Deductibles and Copayments

The employee pays some parts of the insurance coverage, representing member cost sharing. The amount an employee pays, the premium, varies from plan to plan depending on the amount paid by the employer, the insurer's contract, and the amount of health care services used and how they are used. These costs continue to increase, which has led to major health care costs for individuals over the past few years. The employee contribution to medical coverage usually includes some form of deductible, copayment, coinsurance, and annual limits. These methods decrease the insurer's costs of covering small claims, which are expensive to administer. Insurance plans are highly variable, and these methods may not be included in all plans and can vary in how they are applied. Deductibles and copayments/coinsurance represent the employee's out-of-pocket health care expenses and are used by the insurer to control its costs.

A deductible is the amount the employee must pay before the third-party payer will pay for health care services. There are two ways that the deductible is handled. Some plans require that the employee pay a single deductible for the employee and also for family members, which is applied to all services in the plan. The deductible for family members is often higher. The second method is the use of separate deductibles for categories of services, such as hospitalization, ambulatory care, mental health care, and so on. Deductibles may also be required if the employee uses a provider outside the plan's list of approved providers. Usually, when employers and employees pay high premiums, the employee pays a lower deductible. Some plans may have deductibles for only some services, such as pharmaceuticals. Deductibles are usually not used by HMOs. Most major medical plans start with a deductible of $100, $250, or higher.

This payment keeps the cost of the plan down because the enrollee is accepting responsibility for the most frequent charges, those under the deductible limit. After the deductible is paid, the enrollee also shares the expenses by paying the copayment or coinsurance. Typically, this is shared with the insurer on an 80/20 basis. Each dollar above the deductible is paid in this manner—insurer 80 cents and enrollee 20 cents. If the medical bill is large, 20% can be a sizable amount. A patient example illustrating how this is implemented is found in Box 3-5.

In 2010, President Obama signed into law the Patient Protection and Affordable Care Act (P.L. 111-148) and the Health Care and Education Reconciliation Act (P.L. 111-152). This new laws will have a major impact on health care reimbursement, though many aspects

---

BOX 3-5

Deductibles and Copayments: A Patient Example

Hospital bill	$20,000	Deductible must be paid before the insurer will pay its portion. Patient must pay deductible and copayment.
Patient deductible	−$ 200	
	$19,800 Medical charges after deductible paid	Deductible $ 200
		Copayment +$ 3,960
Medical charges after deductible paid	$19,800	**$ 4,160 Total amount to be paid by patient**
Patient share/copayment	× .20	Despite insurance coverage, the patient must still pay $4,160, which is not a small amount.
	$ 3,960 Amount of medical expenses to be paid by patient/copayment	

of these laws do not take effect immediately. Rules and regulations that cover these laws also have an impact on their implementation. Case managers need to keep current with changes that will occur in health care delivery. Box 3-6 provides an overview of examples of reimbursement changes that will take effect over the next few years.

BOX 3-6

Examples of Reimbursement Provisions in Patient Protection and Affordable Care Act of 2010 (P.L. 111-148) and the Health Care and Education Reconciliation Act of 2010 (P.L. 111-152)

On March 30, 2010, President Obama signed into law health care reform legislation. This information only represents some examples of the provisions, not all of the law's provisions.

Effective 2010
Provision

Lifetime limits on benefits and restrictive annual limits will be prohibited.

Seniors will get a $250 rebate to help fill the "doughnut hole" in Medicare prescription drug coverage, which falls between the $2,700 initial limit and when catastrophic coverage kicks in at $6,154.

Insurers will be barred from imposing exclusions on children with preexisting conditions. Pools will cover those with preexisting health conditions until health care coverage exchanges are operational.

New plans must provide coverage for preventive services without copays. All plans must comply by 2018.

Young adults will be able to stay on their parents' insurance until their 27th birthday.

Businesses with fewer than 50 employees will get tax credits covering 35% of their health care premiums, increasing to 50% by 2014.

Improve care coordination for dual eligible's (Medicare and Medicaid) to improve access and quality.

Medicaid to cover tobacco cessation programs for pregnant women.

Qualified health plans must cover a minimum coverage without cost-sharing for preventive services rated A or B by the U.S. Preventive Services Task Force, recommended immunizations, preventive care for infants, children, and adolescents, and additional preventive care and screenings for women. (See http://www.ahrq.gov/clinic/uspstfix.htm for information on the task force.)

Provide new options for home and community-based services through Medicaid.

Temporary funding ($5 billion) for national high-risk insurance pool for coverage of individuals with preexisting medical conditions who have been uninsured for at least six months.

Insurance plans may not place lifetime limits on benefits and restrictive annual limits.

Insurers may not rescind policies to avoid paying medical bills when a person becomes ill.

People receiving coverage from large employers are not expected to experience major changes in premium costs or coverage.

Effective 2011
Provision

A 50% discount will be provided on brand-name drugs for Prescription Drug Plan or Medicare Advantage enrollees. Additional discounts on brand-name and generic drugs will be phased in to completely close the "doughnut hole" by 2020.

Cover only proven preventive services and eliminate cost-sharing for preventive services in Medicare and Medicaid.

The Medicare payroll tax will increase from 1.45% to 2.35% for individuals earning more than $200,000 and married filing jointly above $250,000.

States can offer home- and community-based services to the disabled through Medicaid rather than institutional care beginning October 1.

Medicare will provide free annual wellness visits and personalized prevention plans. New plans will be required to cover preventive services with no copay.

Pharmaceutical companies will provide a 50% discount on brand-name prescription drugs for seniors; additional discounts phased in over the next ten years.

A plan to provide a vehicle for small businesses to offer tax-free benefits will be created. This would ease the small employer's administrative burden of sponsoring a cafeteria plan.

Community Living Assistance Services and Supports (CLASS), a voluntary long-term care program, will be created. When employees contribute to the program for five years they will be entitled to a $50 per day cost benefit to pay for long-term care. CLASS does not cover all long-term care expenses. This is the first national government-run long-term care insurance program, primarily offered through employers.

Develop a Medicaid plan option for enrollees with at least two chronic illnesses, one condition, and risk of developing another, or at least one serious and persistent mental health condition, to designate a provider as a health home.

Provide access to comprehensive health risk assessment and a personalized prevention plan for Medicare beneficiaries. Health risk assessment model to be developed with 18 months after law's effective date.

Provide incentives to Medicare and Medicaid beneficiaries to complete behavior modification programs (criteria need to be developed).

Community First Choice Option for Medicaid beneficiaries with disabilities to receive community-based attendant services and supports rather than institutional care.

Provides incentives to reduce Medicare readmissions due to infections or other preventable causes.

2012
Provision

Create the Independence in Home demonstration program; providing primary care services in the home for high-need Medicare beneficiaries with goal of reducing preventable hospitalization, readmissions, improve health outcomes, improve efficiency of care, reduce costs, and achieve patient satisfaction.

Required mental health parity, which means deductibles, copayments, and limits on the number of visits or days of coverage for mental health and substance abuse treatment must be no more restrictive then for medical and surgical needs.

Establish more training for behavioral health professionals.

Develop nongovernmental research centers to investigate effective treatment for mental illness.

Effective 2013
Provision

Health plans must implement uniform standards for electronic exchange of health information to reduce paperwork and administrative costs.

Increase Medicaid payments for fee-for-service and managed care primary care services provided by primary care physicians (family medicine, general internal medicine, or pediatric medicine).

2014
Provision

Citizens will be required to have acceptable coverage or pay a penalty of $95 in 2014, $325 in 2015, $695 (or up to 2.5% of their income) in 2016. Families will pay half the amount for children, up to a cap of $2,250 per family. After 2016, penalties are indexed to the Consumer Price Index.

Companies with 50 or more employees must offer coverage to employees or pay a $2,000 penalty per employee after their first 30 if at least one of their employees receives a tax credit. Waiting periods before insurance takes effect is limited to 90 days. Employers who offer coverage but whose employees receive tax credits will pay $3,000 for each worker receiving a tax credit.

Insurers can no longer refuse to sell or renew policies because of an individual's health status. Health plans can no longer exclude coverage for preexisting conditions. Insurers can't charge higher rates because of heath status, gender, or other factors.

Health insurance exchanges will open in each state to individuals and small employers to comparison shop for standardized health packages.

Medicaid eligibility will increase to 133% of poverty for all nonelderly individuals to ensure that people obtain affordable health care in the most efficient and appropriate manner. States will receive increased federal funding to cover these new populations.

Adapted from Patient Protection and Affordable Care Act of 2010 (P.L. 111-148)

Health Care and Education Reconciliation Act of 2010 (P.L. 111-152); Health Reform http://www.healthreform.gov/; White House Health Reform http://www.whitehouse.gov/healthreform; The Henry Kaiser Family Foundation http://www.kff.org; "How People Will Be Affected by the Overhaul" by R. Wolf and A. Young, *New York Times*, March 24, 2010, p. A18; "Bill Spreads Pain, Benefits," *USA Today*, March 23, 2010, pp. 4A–3A; "Options Expand for Affordable Long-Term Care" by P. Span, *New York Times*, March 30, 2010, p. D5; "For Consumers, Clarity on Health Care Changes" by T. Bernard, March 21, 2010, retrieved from http://www.nytimes.com; Finkelman, A. (forthcoming). *Leadership and management*. Upper Saddle River, NJ: Pearson Education.

Claims Processing

Claim adjudication or **claims processing** is the process of determining whether a claim meets all the covered services requirements. The third-party payer claims department is responsible for paying claims in a timely manner. Claims data provide important information about enrollees, their health status, utilization of services, provider practice patterns, provider billing patterns, and risk factors (Kongvedst, 2009; Casto & Layman, 2009). The payer, the purchaser of insurance, and the employer use these data. These data are critical to health insurer success.

Claims processing is a costly process but a necessary one. The claims department is responsible for the following tasks.

- Processing and paying claims (capture the claim to enter it into the system; ensure that the member has coverage required to pay the claim at time claim was incurred; determine amount to be paid and to whom; pay the claim)
- Handling claim inquiries from members, providers, and employers
- Correcting claims payment errors
- Collecting reimbursement from third parties
- Identifying fraudulent and inappropriate billing practices
- Analyzing and tracking data
- Maintaining records of transactions

Complete and accurate information is critical in this process. The insurer must determine if the claim is to be paid, denied, or pended for further review. Generally, claims are paid within 30 days. Typical reasons a claim may be denied or pended include the following (Kongvedst, 2009; Casto & Layman, 2009):

- Incomplete information
- Inadequate authorization
- Service not covered
- Patient not a member of the plan
- Provider not part of the plan provider network

Encounter data describe claims for services provided in a capitated payment system. Each patient encounter is entered into the database as if it were a claim. Why is this important if services are paid by a capitated amount and not per service? If the third-party payer does not track these data, it will not know what services were actually provided, the volume and type of services, or the utilization rates. These data are important historical data that the third-party payer uses to determine the prices for its products and its capitated rates. There is also an increasing need to use these data in the assessment of the care provided and in provider performance evaluation. Claims data are also important to case managers because this data can track patient needs, interventions, and outcomes.

Summary

Health care reimbursement is a complex process that is highly relevant to health care delivery. Case managers need to understand how this process works and the players in the process. Reimbursement and managed care are inseparable. Medicare and Medicaid are clearly the most important health care delivery and reimbursement programs in the United States. For many years, these programs have tried to meet the critical health care needs of several groups of the population. These two programs are not without their limitations and problems. Just as managed care has affected other types of delivery and reimbursement, it has also affected Medicare and Medicaid. Both programs are incorporating managed care into their programs. Patients enrolled in these programs have complex needs, are often vulnerable, and require expertise and advocacy and benefit from case management. Health care reform legislation of 2010 will have a significant, long-term impact on health care reimbursement.

Chapter Highlights

1. Insurers use a number of strategies that focus on service and reimbursement to control their costs and provide quality care.

2. Primary care plays a major role in the heath care system and has substantially changed the practice of medicine and the health care environment. The PCP

is the gatekeeper for the health care system; however, patients complain about this approach when it limits their choices. It is not clear what changes will be made in the future about the PCP, but it is clear that there will be changes.

3. Specialty care has suffered from the primary care approach, particularly when patients must obtain approval from their PCP or MCO prior to seeing a specialist.

4. Insurers use utilization management and authorization. These are important service strategies that assist in controlling costs and ensuring that appropriate treatment is provided in a timely manner.

5. Insurers have been developing different types of service strategies to assist patients who have chronic health care needs and to provide health promotion and disease and illness prevention. Some examples of these strategies are disease management and demand management. Case management is often an integral part of these programs.

6. Because diagnostic and ancillary services can be very costly, they are monitored carefully by insurers.

7. The key players in the health care environment are the purchaser, insurer, providers, and the patient/enrollee. The employer selection of health insurers also affects the care provided. The role and power of the insurer has definitely increased in the past decade.

8. Managed care introduced the concept of performance-based reimbursement. All types of providers are evaluated prior to contract and at the time of contract renewal. This alone increases insurer's power.

9. Many of the reimbursement strategies that have been used by MCOs have received criticism (e.g., capitation, withholds, bonuses, authorization, formularies). Criticism has come from providers and patients. Some of these strategies have undergone change or they are no longer used in some areas. One of the concerns about some of the strategies (e.g., withholds, bonuses) has been that they encourage providers to undertreat.

10. Provider panels offer insurers more control over providers than traditional third-party payer insurance had over providers.

11. The common managed care models are HMOs and PPOs. There are several types of HMOs, for example, staff, group, network, and IPA. The PPO has become very popular because it offers more provider choice to the enrollee/patient.

12. Outcomes are more important today and are an integral part of the managed care requirements.

13. Carve-outs are used by insurers to control costs for high-cost services.

14. Data management and information systems are more important today to ensure performance monitoring and sharing of information across systems and providers.

15. Insurers may contract with providers for their services. These contracts define responsibilities and are time limited. Provider performance data are used to make decisions about contract renewal.

16. The health care reimbursement system is a pluralistic system with multiple payers, both public and private. It is a complex system that is rapidly changing.

17. The government—both state and federal—is a major player in the reimbursement system. States regulate insurance within their own states; however, the federal government is a major influence due to the size of the population that it covers for health care, for example, Medicare, Medicaid, federal employees, military personnel and their dependents, and veterans.

18. Prospective and retrospective payment systems are two approaches to reimbursement; however, prospective payment has become more popular since the introduction of the PPS and DRGs.

19. FFS was the primary method used in traditional insurance. Capitation, which is a prospective approach, has primarily replaced it.

20. Community rating and experience rating have been used to determine capitation rates; however, experience rating considers actual health care utilization and may provide more credible data.

21. Employees are contributing to more of their health care coverage through their premiums, deductibles, copayments, coinsurance, and annual limits. Out-of-pocket expenses are increasing.

22. Eligibility, covered services, benefits, exclusions, and limitations are all very important components for an insurance plan. There is great variability from one plan to another.

23. Claims processing is used by the insurer to control costs and ensure payment for services rendered and appropriate treatment for the problem.

24. The Healthcare Financing Administration is the administrator for the Medicare program, and the Medicare Payment Advisory Commission evaluates Medicare and advises Congress on the status of Medicare.

25. Medicare is composed of Part A (hospital services, continued treatment or rehabilitation in skilled nursing facility, hospice care); Part B (physician services and ambulatory care services); Part C (Medicare Advantage Plans); and Part D (prescription coverage). Each of these parts is reimbursed differently.

26. There is increasing concern about the growth of Medicare and the ability of country to fund the program, particularly with the expectation of a surge in the number of people who will be eligible in the future. Managed care approaches are important in decreasing Medicare costs.

27. Medicaid is a joint health care program shared between the states and the federal government.

28. The number of uninsured is increasing. Many of the uninsured are children who qualify for Medicaid but whose parents are not enrolled in Medicaid. The uninsured is a serious problem and needs resolution.

References

Casto, A. & Layman, E. (2009). *Principles of health care reimbursement*. Chicago: American Health Information Management Association.

Centers for Medicare and Medicaid Services. (CMS). (2009). Medicare and Medicaid Programs. Retrieved from http://www.cms.hhs.gov/MedicaidGenInfo/ on June 11, 2009.

Cover the Uninsured: Number of uninsured, 2008. Retrieved from http://covertheuninsured.org/content/overview on November 22, 2009.

Daschle, T. (2008). *Critical. What we can do about the healthcare crisis*. New York: St. Martin's Press.

Health Insurance Association of America. (1998). *Source book of health insurance data*. Washington, DC: Author.

Health Insurance. Info. (2009). Retrieved from http://www.healthinsurance.info/HICOMM.HTM on February 28, 2009.

Henry J. Kaiser Family Foundation. (KFF). (April, 2006). *Kaiser commission on key facts: Medicaid and the uninsured.* Retrieved from http://www.kff.org/medicaid/upload/7492.pdf on June 10, 2009.

Henry J. Kaiser Family Foundation. (KFF). (2009). More than half of Americans say family skimped on medical care because of cost in past year; worries about affordability and availability of care rise. Retrieved from http://www.kff.org/kaiserpolls022509nr.dfm on February 28, 2009.

Institute of Medicine. (IOM). (2008). *Knowing what works in healthcare: A roadmap for the nation*. Washington, DC: National Academies Press.

Kongstvedt, P. (2009). *Managed care: What it is and how it works*. Boston: Jones and Bartlett Publishers.

Powell, S. & Tahan, H. (2008). *Core curriculum for case management*. (2nd ed.). Philadelphia: Lippincott Williams & Wilkins.

Powell, S. (2000). *Advanced case management: Outocmes and beyond*. Philadelphia: Lippincott Williams & Wilkins.

Questions and Activities for Thought

1. Interview a case manager in your community. Discuss the implications of reimbursement on the case management process and outcomes.
2. Explain the relationship between risk taking and reimbursement.
3. Review your own health insurance policy. What does it say about eligibility, covered services, benefits, exclusions, and limitations? What are your financial obligations? Do you have provider choice? What is the grievance procedure? How does your policy compare to classmates' policies?
4. Describe the major differences between Medicare and Medicaid from a federal and state perspective.
5. Discuss the role of the federal government in health insurance coverage.
6. What is the importance of the difference in prospective and retrospective payment from the perspective of the provider?
7. What impact will health are reform legislation of 2010 have on reimbursement? (May have to research current information about the implementation of the legislation.)

Case

As a hospital case manager, you encounter many patients who are covered by Medicare. A new case manager has been hired to help you as the patient load has increased. The hospital is concerned about complications that this population experiences, and this impacts costs and reimbursement. How would you explain Medicare reimbursement to the new case manager who is new to case management and reimbursement?

Internet Links

1. http://www.nachc.com
   This is the site for the National Association of Community Health Centers. What information is available about prospective payment and other reimbursement?
2. http://www.ahrq.gov/consumer/
   Visit this site and select "Choosing Quality Care."
3. http://www.ahrq.gov/research/mar07/307RA4.htm
   What does the site tell you about managed care as a method to control costs?
4. http://www.health-mart.net
   This is an interactive site that allows you to compare hospital performance data, such as LOS, cost of stay,

and the like. Select a diagnosis; the site will assign it to a DRG. Then, select a place (state, city, specific hospital). What can you learn about performance related to a diagnosis? Compare and contrast data.

5. http://www.os.dhhs.gov/
What is the role of the HCFA? What are some of the initiatives that the HCFA is working on at this time? What statistics and data are available on the site related to managed care and reimbursement?

6. http://www.ahcpr.gov
Visit this site and click on "Data." What data provided by Nationwide Inpatient Sample (NIS) might be used by a managed care organization? By providers? What information is available about the distribution of projected health care expenditures? What information is available about trends in personal health care spending?

7. http://www.familiesusa.org
What can you learn about Medicare and Medicaid from this site? Who sponsors this site?

8. http://www.medicare.gov
Visit the site and click on "Medicare Compare." This activity can be done individually or in a small group. It is an interactive site that provides a Medicare health plan comparison database. You will be able to retrieve information about local Medicare plans.

9. http://www.medicare.gov/MPPF/Include/DataSection/Questions/

Visit the site and compare Medigap policies. You will be able to retrieve information about local Medigap plans. What tips are provided? What are the Medicare beneficiary rights and protections?

10. http://www.medicare.gov/NHCompare/
Visit the site and click on "Nursing Home Compare." This activity can be done individually or in a small group. It is an interactive site with a nursing home comparison database. You will be able to retrieve information about local nursing homes. Review the guides on choosing a nursing home. How do they compare? Review the family survival guide.

11. http://www.medicare.gov/health
What are the new Medicare preventive services? How are these reimbursed? Visit some of the specific diagnoses or procedures to learn more about the preventive services that are provided.

12. http://www.odphp.osophs.dhhs.gov
Who sponsors this site? Review the Prevention Reports. What are some of the topics? Select one to read and summarize.

13. http://www.ahcpr.gov
Review the types of insurance, such as HMOs and PPOs. What are the typical questions that are asked about them? What does the site tell you about disability insurance and long-term care insurance?

CHAPTER 4

Reimbursement and Managed Care

OBJECTIVES

After completing this chapter, the reader will be able to:

▪ Describe the types of reimbursement strategies.

▪ Describe the types of service strategies.

▪ Compare and contrast managed care coverage with other types of health care coverage.

KEY TERMS

Bonuses, p. 96
Capitation, p. 95
Carve-outs, p. 96
Formulary, p. 96
Gatekeeper, p. 102
Group model HMOs, p. 94
Health Maintenance Organization
   Act of 1973, p. 94
Health maintenance organizations
   (HMOs), p. 94

Open-access HMOs, p. 95
Preferred provider organization
   (PPO), p. 95
Primary care, p. 101
Provider panel, p. 93
Providers, p. 93
Reimbursement strategies, p. 96
Service strategies, p. 92
Staff model HMOs, p. 95
Withholds, p. 96

INTRODUCTION

This chapter continues the content on health care reimbursement. It focuses on managed care. Several managed care models are described, and the reimbursement and **service strategies** used to control costs and improve care are discussed. Many types of third-party payers now use these strategies, too.

MANAGED CARE MODELS AND THEIR CHARACTERISTICS

The HMO was the first managed care model; however, many others have been developed. Why did this happen? Consumers were not always happy with HMOs. The problem of increasing health care costs became a serious issue in the 1980s. Insurers, which were in competition with HMOs, began to develop new models for health care management, and employers were interested in these other options. Today, health care professionals and consumers must navigate a maze of different managed care organization (MCO) models. Trying to compare and contrast their characteristics can be an overwhelming task; at the same time, it is getting harder to distinguish among the managed care models. In the earlier period of managed care development, it was easier to see the major differences in the MCO models and other types of third-party payers. But first, before we discuss these differences, it is helpful to review a definition of managed health care, which has been described as "a regrettably nebulous term. At the very least, managed care can be described as a system of health care delivery that tries to manage the cost of health care, the quality of that health care, and the access to that care. Common denominators seen in MCOs include a panel of contracted **providers,** who are mostly physicians but may include other health care professionals such as advanced practice nurses, that is less than the entire universe of available providers, some type of limitations on benefits to subscribers who use non-contracted providers (unless authorized to do so), and some type of authorization system" (Kongstvedt, 2009, p. 230).

The most important difference in the managed care models is the relationship between the MCO and the participating providers, particularly physicians. The role of traditional indemnity insurance has been to process and pay medical bills. MCOs have a more comprehensive approach that has affected how they are organized. MCOs continue to process and pay medical bills, but they have become more involved in the management of their members' health care, focusing on appropriate care, when it is needed, and illness and disease prevention and even more health promotion.

Provider Panels

The managed care **provider panel** is a key managed care concept. It is a group of providers that are contracted to provide service to enrollees in the MCO. Providers can be direct care providers, for example, physicians, advanced practice nurses, nurse midwives, hospitals, clinics, long-term care facilities, home health agencies, laboratories, durable equipment suppliers, pharmacies, and so on. Provider panels are selected and organized in a variety of ways. These differences are found in the descriptions of each MCO model. Providers are accepted or rejected based on the MCO's criteria. Clearly, this has serious consequences for providers, for example, physicians who may not be accepted for a provider panel. It can even cause providers to lose patients who have to select another provider when their insurer no longer includes the original provider in its panel. If the person continues with the provider who is not in the panel, then the person must pay out-of-pocket for the care.

Control is a major issue with MCOs. Physician providers may be selected as individual physicians or as groups of physicians. Medical groups contract with an MCO as a group, but the MCO still evaluates individual physicians within the group. A medical or practice group is typically two or more physicians who work together to provide medical services to patients. Nurse practitioners and nurse midwives may be part of a medical group and in some cases have formed their own groups. Usually, these provider groups share a single office or may have satellite offices to expand their geographic coverage. There is one medical record for each patient that is shared among all the providers in the medical group. This facilitates coordination of care for the practice and for the patient.

Types of Managed Care Models

The following section describes the organization and characteristics of typical managed care models: HMOs, exclusive provider organizations, preferred provider organizations, independent practice associations, physician–hospital organizations, the integrated delivery system, and point-of-service (POS). The common characteristics found in the different managed care models are (Kongstvedt, 2009, p. 28):

- Tighter elements of control over health care delivery
- Addition of new elements of control
- More direct interaction with providers
- Increased overhead cost and complexity
- Greater control over utilization
- New reduction in rate of rise of medical costs

Kongstvedt (2009) describes a continuum of managed care models. The first example focuses on the least amount of cost and quality control, and the sixth example provides the most control of costs and quality (p. 27).

1. Indemnity with precertification, mandatory second opinion, and case management
2. Service plan with precertification, mandatory second opinion, and case management
3. Preferred provider organization (PPO)
4. POS health plan
5. "Open-access" HMO
6. Traditional HMO (open-panel with subtypes of independent practice association [IPA] and direct contract HMO; network model; closed-panel HMO with subtypes of group model and staff model)

HEALTH MAINTENANCE ORGANIZATIONS (HMOs). Health maintenance organizations have changed since their creation in the 1920s. The HMO pays the bills for its members' health services, but it also manages and provides care to its members. The **Health Maintenance Organization Act of 1973** describes an HMO as:

- An organized entity that ensures health care service delivery in a specific geographic area
- Provides basic and optional benefits
- Enrollees join voluntarily

HMOs integrate the delivery of service with reimbursement for those services. The HMO is the original model or prototype of managed care. It develops incentives to encourage its providers to provide the lowest-cost care to the HMO members. An HMO contracts with providers for health care services required to meet the comprehensive health care needs of the HMO members and often are considered HMO employees. This is done on a prepaid basis. Employers pay the HMO to provide these services via premiums, and the HMO agrees to provide specific services. Typically, HMOs have focused on comprehensive care, illness and disease prevention, and health promotion. Patient volume and risk for illness and disease are important factors when an HMO seeks contracts with employers. The four major types of HMO models are staff, group, network, and independent practice association HMOs. An HMO's control over its providers decreases with each of these models.

OPEN-PANEL HMOs. In an open-panel HMO, the MCO contracts directly with a provider or indirectly to provide services to HMO members. The providers work in their own offices, where HMO members come to receive care (Kongstvedt, 2009).

GROUP MODEL HMOs (CLOSED-PANEL HMOs). Group model HMOs contract with one or more medical practice groups, usually multispecialty, to deliver care for their members. Depending on the contractual arrangement, the physician groups may provide care exclusively to the HMO members or may also provide care to other patients who are not members of the HMO. Some group model HMOs also provide their providers with office space and may assist with administrative and laboratory support services. Reimbursement is by **capitation.** A specific amount is paid to the provider monthly or annually per member to provide all the care each member requires. If the member does not require care, the provider does not have to return the payment, but if the member's health care requirements incur more expenses than are covered by the payment, the provider receives no additional payment.

STAFF MODEL HMOs (CLOSED-PANEL HMOs). **Staff model HMOs** hire physicians as full-time employees, and the physicians are paid a salary. All premiums and revenues go to the HMO. In comparison with physicians working with other types of HMOs, these physicians have less opportunity to receive financial rewards for decreasing costs and less decision-making autonomy. They are HMO employees. Most of these HMOs actually own their own clinics, and some own hospitals. Clearly, members of this type of HMO have less provider choice. They typically go to one site for all of their care and see physicians who are salaried. In this type of HMO, the HMO has much more control over physicians and other providers (e.g., nurse practitioners, nurse midwives, other health care professionals, hospitals). Staff and group models are the most restrictive form of the managed care models.

Over time, owing to consumer complaints there has been a movement to provide greater provider choice for members and yet focus on cost and quality. **Open-access HMOs** allow a member to see a specialist in the provider network without first seeing a primary care provider (PCP), but they require that the member pay an additional copayment. Some offer a self-referral option that can be used when the member needs it. This is not like a POS model in that members do not receive reimbursement coverage if they choose a provider who is outside the HMO's provider network.

PREFERRED PROVIDER ORGANIZATIONS (PPOs). A **preferred provider organization** is a delivery network of providers, physicians, advanced practice nurses, hospitals, and other providers. The PPO does not assume any financial risk or receive premiums, but it does charge an access fee to the MCOs for use of the PPO provider network. The PPO itself is not directly involved in the delivery of health care services; rather, it acts as an intermediary to negotiate and manage the managed care contracts on behalf of the individual providers. Capitation is not common with a PPO. Reimbursement is usually based on the fee schedule identified by the PPO. The PPO has access to a large volume of patients through its contracts, and this is an incentive for providers to join a PPO and accept discounted fees. Typically, members pay lower deductibles and coinsurance when they use providers in the PPO. Utilization management (UM) and quality assurance are not a focus of PPOs as they are with other MCO models. Purchasers of the plans must also use other organizations to provide utilization management and case management services—services that are typically done by MCOs to ensure that enrollees' needs are met and control costs. Some PPOs do not meet the accepted criteria to be classified as an MCO. PPOs have become very common today and are used by different types of insurers.

There are other types of MCOs such as integrated delivery system, exclusive provider organization, IPA, and physician–hospital organization. Case managers may work for or have association with all of these models; however, the major models are the HMO and the PPO.

REIMBURSEMENT STRATEGIES

Reimbursement strategies probably receive the brunt of the criticisms directed at managed care. Strategies that may be used are: actuarial cost models, capitation, payer mix, diagnosis-related groups (DRGs), discounts, **withholds**, bonus, length-of-stay (LOS) management, authorization, formularies, and **carve-outs**. Understanding the definitions of reimbursement strategies, the purpose of these strategies, and the key players who use them is important for the case manager.

Definition and Purpose of Reimbursement Strategies

Reimbursement strategies require an understanding of the incentives that are important to health insurers and buyers of health care (e.g., employers, the government). The incentive for the health insurer is profit, which requires reduced costs. The incentive for the buyer, who is usually the employer, is reduced costs. The situation becomes complicated when one considers that the goal of the provider, especially the physician, advanced practice nurses, other health care professionals, and hospitals, is to provide quality care. Clearly, there are conflicting goals, and this affects the outcomes. The choice of reimbursement strategies has caused more conflict than service strategies. Financial loss is an important consideration. Compared to traditional insurers, managed care focuses more on shifting that risk to the provider. This section discusses how this shifting of financial risk is operationalized and its effect on health care. An important factor related to reimbursement is the key players and their roles.

Performance-Based Reimbursement Evaluation

Provider performance has never been more important. It was not as important in the traditional fee-for-service (FFS) arrangement when, with few exceptions, the provider was paid regardless of the expense or quality of the care. Today, when MCOs contract with new providers for their provider panels or renewed contracts, the MCOs base their provider selection on specific criteria. Why is this so important? The MCO wants providers who offer cost-effective, quality care that meets the MCO criteria. As managed care developed through the 1980s and 1990s, cost effectiveness became more important than quality. Today, quality issues are slowly becoming more important as demonstrating by greater emphasis on the Institute of Medicine (IOM) quality reports and their recommendations to improve care.

How does an MCO gather data about provider performance and then use this information to determine provider reimbursement? The common approach emphasizes on process, or how the service is provided. MCOs are interested in the type and frequency of treatments, laboratory tests, the use of radiology and other ancillary services, hospitalization rates, LOS rates, referrals to specialists, and the use of the MCO **formulary** and how these affect patient outcomes. All types of third-party payers have adopted this approach.

The goal of performance-based reimbursement evaluation is behavior modification. How the MCO goes about reaching this goal can vary and can mean the difference in success or failure. Rewards work better than sanctions, but both have been used. The MCO may financially reward providers who meet the MCO's criteria for cost-effective care by offering **bonuses** or close the provider off from receiving new enrollees. The goal is to discourage the use of inappropriate and costly services. MCOs typically use continuing education, data and feedback, practice guidelines, and protocols to encourage the provider to change behavior. As is true for all types of behavior modification, feedback is more effective if given frequently rather than in an annual review.

Typically, objective data collected are utilization rates, overall medical costs or medical costs per member per month, and productivity, such as number of patient visits per day. Some insurers use financial incentives to encourage providers (hospitals and physicians) to improve care provided and outcomes. This is called pay for performance (Kongstvedt, 2009). This requires the insurer to collect data on providers' quality, accessibility, and satisfaction of care provided.

Types of Reimbursement Strategies

ACTUARIAL COST MODELS.   Actuarial cost models are very important in the financial decision process and to rate setting. Plans identify medical expenses on estimated costs for each service on a per-member, per-month basis. Because actuarial cost is a component of many of the reimbursement strategies used by the insurers, it is critical that this be done well. Factors such as age, gender, mix of enrollees, disability level, distribution of the population, health services utilization rates, and cost for medical services are used to determine estimated medical expenses.

CAPITATION.   The growth of managed care introduced capitation is one of the major changes that has occurred in health care reimbursement. Capitation is a prepayment to a provider to deliver health care services to enrollees of a health plan. This is usually a monthly payment, but it can also be paid on an annual basis. The provider agrees to provide all care for the enrollee's health care needs that the PCP is qualified to provide. If the enrollee requires no services in the allotted time period, the provider is still paid the capitated amount. If the enrollee's care incurs additional expenses, the provider receives no extra payment. The capitation method is dependent on a contract between the provider and a third-party payer. The focus is on covered lives or the total number of persons who are enrolled in a health plan instead of focusing on individuals. Services that are included are defined in the contractual arrangement. What happens to financial risk with capitation? It shifts to the provider, which must cover all services as defined by the payer for the capitated amount, regardless of the frequency of those services. This should influence the types and amount of services provided; however, this has been one of the areas that have received frequent provider and consumer complaints. Capitation can be used with an individual provider or a group of providers, such as a multispecialty group that agrees to provide all services to the insurer's enrollees.

What are some of the pros and cons of capitation? The major advantage is that it transfers financial risk to the provider. It also provides the insurer with a clearer picture of budgetary needs. The insurer knows that for each enrollee in a specific plan it will pay a specific amount of money to providers to cover all identified health services. There are no surprises if a patient develops an illness that requires more services than originally expected, at least not from the perspective of the insurer because the insurer does not cover these services. The provider, however, will have major problems if the monthly capitated amount does not cover the actual expenses, and this is a disadvantage of capitation for the provider. Thus, the financial risk has been shifted. A difficulty of capitation is the calculation of the capitation amount. It must be an amount that is acceptable to the purchaser, which is usually an employer or the government, and must reasonably cover the expenses. If the insurer is for-profit with stockholders, the insurer must also consider these stockholders and their financial expectations.

PAYER MIX.   Payer mix is an important consideration for the provider. It is the proportion of total revenues that the provider expects from different payers. It is very important for the provider to understand its payer mix in order to manage its internal resources and finances. The important issue is that all payers do not pay the same amount.

DISCOUNTS.   Discounts or discounted FFS is still a very common reimbursement strategy. How is this type of payment determined? The insurer decides the percentage of the provider's usual fee schedule or billed charges it will pay. The percentage and all other decisions related to the discounted payment are described in the provider contract. There are two types of discounts: a flat or straight discount and a sliding scale that varies with volume. Specific procedures or services may also be assigned different discount rates. How does this actually work? An insurer contracts with a hospital to provide health care services to its enrollees. For example, the insurer may decide to take a 20% discount off all patient charges, 30% off laboratory testing, and so forth. The contract may also stipulate that there is a fee maximum before the discount is taken. For example, the insurer will give a discount of 20% for laboratory testing, but the maximum payment is limited to $400, even if the bill is actually more than this. The insurer does not want to pay more than what is customary. The sliding scale discount is linked to the volume of services actually provided. When volume increases for the specified service, the discount rate decreases. The provider is rewarded, then, for providing services to more enrollees. The insurer, however, expects that these services meet medical necessity criteria and monitors the provider. Use of discounts is a reimbursement strategy that decreases the amount that the insurer actually pays for services. Providers must be careful that the overall loss that is incurred with discounts is not so low that their expenses cannot be covered.

WITHHOLDS.   Withholds are used to shift utilization and financial risk to the provider. Under the capitation system, the provider is paid a specific amount per member per month (PMPM) to provide health care services that are identified in the contract with the insurer. When withholds are used, the insurer holds back a percentage of the monthly payment. For example, if the provider is to be paid $10 PMPM, $2 may be withheld by the insurer. What happens to this money? Why is this done? The provider may be paid this withdrawn amount at the end of year. The final decision to pay it at the end of the year is based on the provider's performance profile. The insurer evaluates the provider's utilization rates and compares them with other providers. Some insurers make their decisions based on the utilization rates of all of their providers and then determine if the withhold will be paid to all providers. Other insurers evaluate providers individually. The important fact is the provider cannot depend on getting this money at the end of the year. The insurer may decide to use the money that was withheld for other purposes. Withholds are also used with hospitals, but the withhold is taken out of the per diem rate. The hospital, as the provider, may or may not receive the withheld amount at the end of the year. Generally, the amount of payment withheld varies from 5% to 20%. Plan contracts may also have a clause stating that if their costs are higher than expected, the plan may increase the withhold. So, not only does the provider contend with the withhold, but the provider must also recognize that the amount of the withhold may increase at any time. Withholds are used to influence provider behavior, to change provider behavior to more cost-effective, quality care.

LENGTH-OF-STAY MANAGEMENT.   Hospital occupancy rates and LOS for all types of patients have been decreasing, as described in Chapter 2. Managed care supports this decrease. This change has increased the utilization of ambulatory care services, home care services, subacute services, and other types of services that replace inpatient treatment. Nursing has been concerned about the decrease because it has affected patient care and the needs of the patients. Hospitals have more acute patients because patients are kept out of the hospital until it is absolutely necessary to admit them. This has increased care needs. There is also increased pressure to provide rapid patient and family education, with little time to provide it. Productivity is a major concern, and it is also related to

LOS. Is money actually saved when LOS is shortened? At what point does the decreased LOS actually increase nursing costs? These are critical questions. Case managers are directly involved in LOS management.

FORMULARIES.   Advances in pharmaceuticals have helped patients to live normal lives and have decreased health care costs, but at the same time these advances have increased medical costs. This may seem contradictory; however, both have occurred. For example, new AIDS medications have decreased the number of hospitals days, but these drugs are also very expensive. Antibiotics prevent patients from becoming sick or sicker; however, some antibiotics are very expensive. Careful cost–benefit analysis is required. The federal government is more concerned about the increasing costs of drugs. To cope with these increasing pharmaceutical costs, the use of formularies is a critical reimbursement strategy that is used to control the ever-increasing costs of drugs. The formulary is the insurer's list of drugs or classes of drugs that the insurer prefers that providers use. There are three types of formularies: open, incentive, and closed. An *open formulary* means that the enrollee pays extra fees for using nonformulary drugs. With the *incentive formulary*, the insurer reimburses for drugs outside the formulary, but the enrollee is responsible for an additional copayment. This type of formulary is designed to encourage the enrollee not to use nonformulary medications. When a *closed formulary* is used, there is no reimbursement for drugs that are not in the formulary.

How does an insurer determine which drugs to include in its formulary? Most insurers use safety, effectiveness, cost, and cost effectiveness as their criteria. No insurer formulary includes all of the drugs approved by the Food and Drug Administration (FDA). The formulary typically focuses on generic drugs because these tend to be less expensive than the brand-name products, though usually chemically equivalent. Many drugs are the same, but their therapeutic effect or their side effects may vary. For some patients, excluding drugs that they have found helpful may be a serious problem. This is particularly important for patients with chronic illnesses for whom a specific drug is more effective. When the insurer's formulary changes and the drug is not included, or if the patient changes third-party payers and the new insurer formulary does not include the drug, the patient may suffer. Insurers must also consider the value of adding new drugs that are expensive, including biotechnology products. These drugs and products tend to be very expensive. Clearly, an insurer must weigh the costs and benefits of using these therapies. It needs data that demonstrate significant clinical advantages, but these advantages still may not be enough to support the decision to cover their use. Insurer protocols and authorization procedures are established for these highly expensive drugs. Another treatment issue is that most of the new biotech treatments are injectable, and insurers typically do not cover injectables under the category of pharmacy but rather as medical expenses. As these drugs become more common, this medical expense classification will require reconsideration. The pharmacy coverage may be different from other benefits, often more limited, and thus there may be some advantage in reclassifying biotech drugs as pharmacy expenses. Case managers are involved in prescriptions and the most effective use of drugs for their patients.

Providers are inundated with drug information via the mail, Internet, and the ever-growing pharmaceutical sales force. Drug companies are also marketing directly to the consumer/patient, which has increased the number of patients going to providers requesting specific medications through all types of media. All of this increases drug costs and the pressure that providers feel to prescribe drugs and, sometimes, specific drugs. The formulary presents other problems for the prescribing provider. Some providers have found that certain drugs work better than others or have fewer side effects, but the patient's insurer formulary does not reimburse for these drugs. This presents a conflict for the provider. In addition, most providers have contracts with many insurers. Each one has a formulary, and some are quite different from others. The provider, which is already inundated with paperwork and administration, is confronted with more information and differences. Many providers will choose the path of least resistance and use the least restrictive formularies, but these formularies may offer limited drug options. Authorization may also be required to receive reimbursement for nonformulary drugs.

POINT-OF-SERVICE (POS). The POS model provides more choice for the enrollee/patient, but at a price to the enrollee. At the time the enrollee needs a specific health care service, the enrollee may decide whether to use a provider in the panel or one outside the panel. If the enrollee chooses a provider outside the panel for care, then the enrollee pays higher copayments and deductibles. When the enrollee goes outside the panel, the provider is paid on an FFS basis. The insurer hopes that over time the enrollee will choose not to use the POS option and use the provider panel instead. A POS option may be found in HMOs, PPOs, and in indemnity plans. The POS supports patient choice while still providing for cost controls.

CARVE-OUTS. Carve-outs are used by some insurers to control reimbursement costs. Specific medical services are separated from other services for reimbursement services. How is a carve-out benefit reimbursed? There are several ways in which this is done. Under capitation, the insurer may designate that some services are not covered in the capitated amount and will be reimbursed on a fee schedule. Carve-outs are usually used for services that are not subject to discretionary utilization (Kongstvedt, 2009). In this situation, the insurer has clear guidelines that must be followed to use these services. For example, immunizations might be paid on a fee schedule, but the insurer would develop guidelines that direct their use. Some insurers approach carve-outs by using a separate provider network and organization for these services, which may be paid on a capitated reimbursement. A disease management approach may be used for some carve-out programs. Examples include mental health, substance abuse, oncology, and cardiology carve-outs. Mental health and substance abuse are the most common carve-outs. A disease management carve-out allows for better assessment of utilization and usually is used for diseases with a risk of high costs.

Why do carve-outs control reimbursement costs? The insurer requires greater control over the utilization of these services. If an enrollee is a member of a PPO, the plan usually uses an outside utilization review organization to better ensure that services are as cost effective as possible. Carve-out services may have different requirements for their use than other services, and the insurer may charge differently for them. For example, the plan may require that the enrollee obtain a referral from the primary care physician for the use of mental health services. The plan may require contact with different insurer staff for carve-out services than staff used for other services. These services may actually come under an entirely different plan. The provider panel may also be different, particularly since many of the services that are carved out require different types of professionals, such as psychiatrists, social workers, counselors, optometrists, and dentists.

SERVICE STRATEGIES TO CONTROL COSTS AND QUALITY

There is now more flexibility in consumer choice because consumers demanded more, and this has and will continue to make it more difficult for MCOs and other types of insurers to control costs. After a period of relative quiet when MCOs grew, consumers began to complain about their lack of choice, and eventually this had an impact—driving change to increase patient/enrollee choice of providers. MCOs also are now confronted with more powerful providers than in the early years of managed care.

Physicians and hospitals, as well as other types of providers, are joining together to gain more negotiating power with MCOs. External forces have become more important, with increased legislation and regulation that further constrain MCO efforts to control costs. Strategies that MCOs and insurers use to manage increasing costs and control quality have become increasingly important.

How do insurers cut health care expenses and yet still ensure quality care? Service strategies are used to manage the health care services provided. It is important for all health care providers to understand the strategies that are used and their purposes. Case managers play a major role in the use of choice and implementation of these strategies. In addition to using reimbursement strategies, service strategies are also used to reduce costs and improve care.

Service Strategies: Definition and Purpose

Service strategies are methods used by MCOs and insurers to manage delivery of care in all types of health care settings. The purpose of these strategies is to decrease costs and provide quality care. The goal is to find better, more cost-effective treatments; however, this is a strategy that has not been fully utilized. It is quite clear by now that as MCOs have been trying to decrease health care costs, provider roles, and responsibilities, provider–insurer/MCO relationships, patient needs, and societal health care needs have undergone major changes and will continue to do so. There is no doubt that health care delivery has been affected by managed care service strategies, but it is not always clear if costs have been better controlled with these strategies or if the quality of care has changed, positively or negatively.

Efficiency is a critical component of deciding on service strategies, minimizing costs, and choosing services with the maximum excess of benefits over costs. Just focusing cost-containment efforts on decreasing costs will not be enough in the long run. Achieving the desired outcome has become more important over the past few years, and this definitely relates to achieving greater benefits over costs.

Types of Service Strategies

There are many different service strategies that an insurer may choose to use. Examples of service strategies include changing practice patterns, **primary care,** specialty care, resource management, utilization management, disease management, health promotion and disease and illness prevention, and management of ancillary services. Case management is also a service strategy, and case management may choose to use some of the other service strategies. Some of these strategies directly affect health care delivery and all health care professionals. The strategies are described briefly here, and some of them are discussed in more detail in Chapter 7 as case management tools or methods to manage care.

CHANGING PRACTICE PATTERNS AND PRIMARY CARE.   There is no doubt that managed care has affected how physicians, registered nurses (RNs), and all other types of providers deliver their care and services today. The greatest change in practice patterns has been the move from the acute care setting to the home and community. Today, many providers focus more on ambulatory care, but at the same time patients in the hospital are more acutely ill and have shorter lengths-of-stay requiring more resources. Patients are then sent home not fully recovered and thus require more care at home. In addition, and in conjunction with this change, there is an increased emphasis on primary care, though there is much that needs to be done to continue the development of primary care.

The delivery of care, both diagnostic testing and treatment choice, has changed. Providers are now more concerned with what treatment is really necessary and how to get the job done quickly. Much of this is driven by reimbursement with a greater emphasis on evidence-based practice (EBP) (Institute of Medicine, 2008). Hospitals have changed the way that they deliver care and are more interested in shortening LOS, the utilization of resources, and the development of ambulatory services (e.g., clinics, wellness centers, ambulatory surgery, home care). Hospitals are moving more to integrating EBP, though there is a long way to go to reach success.

Why have practice patterns changed, and why do they continue to change? Owing to the increasing costs, buyers of health care have become increasingly interested in efficient care or evidence-based best practice. It is important to remember that the majority of buyers are employers and the government. In order to be competitive, insurers need to identify strategies that reduce costs, and these strategies usually affect practice patterns. As managed care has evolved, it is recognized that reducing costs is not the complete answer. Efficient care must also consider outcomes. For example, a third-party payer may decide to pay $1,000 to a specific provider to set a fracture because that provider can do it more cheaply. If the patient does not have a positive outcome and recovery, however, it does not matter if the provider held down costs. One thousand dollars were wasted. Cost cannot be isolated from service and the quality of that service.

Trust has been an important element in the physician–patient relationship, but there is now some concern about the effect that managed care and practice changes have had on this trust relationship. Some MCOs recognize that they are not only the payers of health care services but in some cases may also be providers (e.g., HMOs). Thus, the issue of trust becomes even more important to them. Trust is not only important in the physician–patient relationship, but also in the relationship between the insurer and the patient/enrollee. Most U.S. citizens do not speak highly of the health care insurance system and see the insurer as the adversary. This is critical for the case manager to understand because the case manager is often seen as representing the insurer, and in some cases the case manager is the insurer representative as an employee of the insurer. It is important that the insurer provide coverage as required by the plan contract when it is needed and that it is competent in its administrative tasks and the services it provides, such as selection of provider panels, quality assessment program, and utilization review.

The issue of advocacy is important in a trust relationship, and it continues to be more important in the provider–patient relationship than in the relationship between the enrollee and the insurer. In Chapter 5, the issue of advocacy and the case manager is discussed further. As discussed in Chapter 1, ethical issues related to reimbursement are important and frequently discussed in professional and lay literature. To whom the physician is responsible is a major concern. With financial incentives driving many physician decisions, can the patient trust the physician to be completely honest about treatment options, even the expensive ones? This is one reason why it is important for health care providers to understand incentives, other services, and reimbursement strategies used by insurers. These strategies affect how care is delivered; treatment patients receive or do not receive; (LOS) and length of treatment; communication with providers; and trust in all health care providers. Consumers also need to be aware of these strategies. In some cases, consumers (patients, enrollees) will turn to the case manager for guidance and information.

The PCP plays a major role in the managed care environment. "Primary care is a process of assessing, planning, coordinating, and providing health care from a consistent practitioner who serves as the central point of contact for all practitioners" the patient may be seeing (Powell & Tahan, 2008, p. 9). The major responsibility of this role is to coordinate comprehensive care and serve as a **gatekeeper.** Most PCPs are physicians (MDs) (internists, pediatricians, family physicians, and general physicians) or doctors of osteopathy (DO). All insurers classify obstetrician/gynecologist (OB/GYN) specialists as PCPs, meaning patients do not have to request a referral to see these specialists. Some states have laws requiring this service (Kongstvedst, 2009). Not all insurers require that every enrollee have a PCP. The MCO or insurer identifies the PCP qualifications, and these qualifications may vary among MCOs and insurers. In addition, pressures from consumers and physicians have also changed how MCOs describe PCPs. The traditional view is that the PCP is a family practice physician. Another important characteristic of a PCP is the patient does not need a referral from a provider to see the PCP.

The purpose of gatekeeping is to control overutilization of specialists and other medical costs. In the traditional FFS system, patients were free to see any physician they wanted when they thought they needed care, and this is still true in some plans, for example PPO, as long as the enrollee chooses from the insurer's list of providers. If the provider is not on the list, then the enrollee incurs additional costs. Providers that serve as gatekeepers are free to order laboratory testing, radiological examinations, procedures, drugs, and treatment. Gradually, third-party payers have developed a variety of methods to control overutilization. The critical concerns about utilization continue to be unnecessary testing and prescription of expensive treatment.

The insurer does not think that the patient is always the most qualified person to make the decision to consult with a specialist or whom to consult. The PCP, in the role of the gatekeeper, does this for the patient. In addition, the PCP coordinates the patient's care, which should improve the outcomes. Concerns about cost and appropriate treatment utilization are not illegitimate; however, consumers have generally disliked the idea of having to go through a physician or another provider in order to see a specialist. The PCP is typically paid on a capitated basis to provide the contracted services identified by the MCO. This strategy provides additional cost control. In addition, insurer performance profiles provide descriptive data on the provider's utilization of services, such as laboratory testing, referrals to specialists, use of formularies, and the like. This is used to control costs.

What does the PCP role mean for the enrollee? Choice is the critical issue for the enrollees and has become more of an issue in the managed care reimbursement environment. Usually the enrollee can see the PCP without a referral from any other provider. In the traditional HMO, the enrollee has limited primary care choice. Of course, the enrollee can ask to have a change in PCP, but this requires some effort on the part of the enrollee. Other MCO models vary in their use of PCPs and their effect on the enrollees' health care decisions. The PCP makes treatment decisions and specialty referrals with the patient and, in some cases, chooses the hospital. Patient participation in these decisions is influenced greatly by the health plan contract and the MCO.

SPECIALTY CARE.   In the early years of the managed care environment, the PCP and the authorization process began to influence how specialty care was used. The rigid approach to specialty care used in the early 1990s, however, has been loosening up. This has occurred primarily because consumers dislike limitations on physician choice and have spoken out against this approach. Specialty physicians also found the rigid process associated with gatekeeping and authorization a major deterrent to practice survival. Open access, allowing for greater direct access to specialists, has become more common. Usually, the patient must pay an additional copayment to have a choice of specialists, but some MCOs are not charging for the option of choice but are still requiring authorization from the PCP. MCOs are providing more information to enrollees about the use of specialists and access to them. This information is often found on the insurer's website. There was concern about increased utilization and continuity of care; however, some MCOs have found that these concerns have not played out the way they expected. Usually, these MCOs have developed systems to keep PCPs informed about their specialty usage.

Reliability of data is very important in assessing services provided and the health care delivery and planning decisions that are based on this data. Case managers help collect some of the data and also use databases in their practice of case management.

Specialty care is frequently capitated, unless it is part of a traditional HMO or other types of third-party payer plans. An HMO usually has all the necessary specialists included in its organization. Administration of a capitated system is expensive, so the MCO would not want to use capitation for low-volume specialties or for specialties that are not frequently used, such as neurosurgery compared to pathology or radiology, which have high-volume utilization rates. It is important for the MCO to monitor all PCP specialty referrals.

Hospitalists and intensivists have become more common in the past five years. These roles are typically filled by physicians, though some hospitals are now using nurse practitioners and clinical nurse specialists to fill these rolls. Hospitalists provide the overall medical coverage for patients rather than having the patient's PCP meet these responsibilities. This allows the PCP more time to care for patients in the outpatient setting. The patient returns to the care of his or her PCP after hospitalization. The intensivist is similar to the hospitalist but focuses on intensive care. It is important that both communicate with the primary provider. Patients may not like this arrangement because they do not get regular access to their usual physician. Both the hospitalist and the intensivist are hospital staff, paid by the hospital. PCPs are not often as current in inpatient treatment whereas the hospitalist and intensivist are. This arrangement can improve care, reduce lengths-of-stay, and ensure that outcomes are met.

RESOURCE MANAGEMENT. Resource management is important in any health insurance program and is a critical part of case management. The goal is cost-effective, efficient, quality care. Resources need to be used wisely. Resource management is interconnected with utilization and authorization. These resources must be managed better than they were in the past. It is now more important to identify clear outcomes, use scientifically determined best practices to achieve outcomes, measure progress, and when required, to reinvent the processes through which care is delivered. The drive to use EBP has influenced this need. An IOM report on EBP concludes that "the nation must significantly expand its capacity to use scientific evidence to assess 'what works' in health care" (Institute of Medicine, 2008, p. 1). The report notes that a significant proportion of health care costs are associated with care that has not been shown to be effective. This care consumes resources.

MANAGEMENT OF ANCILLARY SERVICES. Diagnostic and therapeutic services are ancillary services. Typical diagnostic services are radiology, laboratory testing, electrocardiography, invasive imaging, and cardiac testing. Examples of ancillary therapeutic services are physical therapy, occupational therapy, speech therapy, and cardiac rehabilitation. Pharmacy service is also considered to be an ancillary service and is discussed in more detail in this chapter's section on formularies. Why are ancillary services included in service strategies? These services are different from other services in that they require an order from a provider. Patients cannot just request a specific laboratory test or the like. In addition to this factor, these services have been identified as high-cost services with potential for overutilization. Their overuse or inappropriate use has often increased health care costs. How does the insurer control the utilization of these services? Case managers play a critical role in coordinating care to ensure that the patient gets the care needed when needed and to prevent overuse of ancillary services. Collection of utilization data about ancillary services is very important. These data are collected so that individual providers can be evaluated. Standards of care and protocols are developed to educate and guide the provider when decisions are made to use ancillary services. Another method employed to control usage is the authorization process and limiting who can authorize services, which provides more rigid control. Case managers may be directly involved in this process. Some insurers also limit how many times the enrollee can receive the service before reauthorization is required. For example, how many physical therapy sessions can a stroke patient receive before reauthorization is required? This control of usage has been a problem for some patients and providers. Case managers hear about these complaints and must explain to patients the reasons for these decisions.

Some insurers consider emergency service to be an ancillary service, and it is a service that has caused problems. In most cases, a patient goes to the emergency room because he or she feels there is an emergency. Use of emergency services tends to increase when people do not have insurance or have insufficient coverage for regular care. Use of the emergency room for any reason is expensive. Third-party payers have experienced inappropriate use of emergency services and know that it increases their costs. Hospitals have incurred an increasing amount of bad debt from patients who cannot pay and never will pay for their emergency services. Consequently, insurers want to avoid the excessive costs of emergency services. From the perspective of a service strategy, what does the insurer do? Clearly, the insurer wants the emergency service used when there is medical necessity. If a patient does not use the emergency services when there is an appropriate medical necessity, the patient may require more intensive care. For example, if a patient is experiencing symptoms of a cardiovascular accident and avoids going to the emergency room, the patient may experience a severe stroke that requires long-term hospitalization and rehabilitation. This is not what the insurer wants because this would only increase the patient's treatment needs and costs. The insurer does, however, want to control the use of emergency services when an alternative, less costly service can meet the medical needs of the patient. What can the insurer do to encourage appropriate use of emergency services? Some insurers ask that their enrollees use the insurer's nurse advice lines for assessment of the need for emergency services. The enrollee or patient calls the advice line, which may be covered by case managers, to discuss the need for emergency care. The nurse case manager uses established insurer protocols to determine the best approach for the patient. This is a form of authorization, but the patient may choose not to follow the advice. If the care is not authorized and the patient chooses to use emergency care, the insurance plan needs to be clear about the costs to the patient. Some insurers require prior approval from the PCP for emergency care. Others offer more flexible clinic hours so that patients can use a clinic if there is a suspected emergency. Urgent care centers may be used, but some are not less expensive than emergency rooms. To better control costs, insurers may have contracts with emergency services that include discounted services. One of the major issues with emergency services is that the MCO or insurer loses control over treatment decisions, particularly if the emergency department physician decides to admit the patient and the physician is not a member of the insurer provider panel. This is one reason why third-party payers have increasingly required insurer notification when enrollees use these services. Another problem area is the use of emergency services when the enrollee travels away from home, particularly when hospitalization is required. In these situations, the enrollee may have little choice about using a provider who is not a member of the provider panel. Some plans try to transfer the patient to a participating hospital as soon as possible, but this requirement needs to be included in the plan description. The Emergency Medical Treatment and Active Labor Act of 1986 (EMTALA) requires that all patients who come into an emergency department (ED) receive a medical screening, and this cannot be delayed due to insurance reasons. The insurer may try to deny payment even though the ED had to provide care, but hospitals will challenge this response (Kongstvedst, 2009). When a patient is admitted from the ED to hospital inpatient care, the ED charge may be incorporated into the hospital charge.

Summary

As discussed in this chapter, there are many MCO models with complex health care reimbursement. There are increasing problems with the models and reimbursement. As managed care has experienced less profit, there has been a drive to increase members; however, costs have increased faster than income. Managed care has used two approaches to improve the financial status. The first is to increase control over use of services and costs. The second is to gain more market power over hospitals, physicians, and payers through consolidation and acquisitions. Something, however, has happened that interfered with the success of these two approaches. Consumer and regulatory backlash have increased and will continue to increase, and both had an important impact on managed care.

Chapter Highlights

1. Insurers use a number of strategies that focus on service and reimbursement to control their costs and provide quality care.
2. Primary care plays a major role in the heath care system and has substantially changed the practice of medicine and the health care environment. The PCP is the gatekeeper for the health care system; however, patients complain about this approach when it limits their choices. It is not clear what changes will be made in the future about the PCP, but it is clear that there will be changes.
3. Specialty care has suffered from the primary care approach, particularly when patients must obtain approval from their PCP or MCO prior to seeing a specialist.
4. Insurers use utilization management and authorization. These are important service strategies that assist in controlling costs and ensuring that appropriate treatment is provided in a timely manner.
5. Insurers have been developing different types of service strategies to assist patients who have chronic health care needs and provide health promotion and disease and illness prevention. Case management is often an integral part of services strategies.
6. Because diagnostic and ancillary services can be very costly, insurers monitor them carefully.
7. Managed care introduced the concept of performance-based reimbursement. All types of providers are evaluated prior to contract and at the time of contract renewal. This alone increases insurer's power.
8. Many of the reimbursement strategies that have been used by MCOs have received criticism (e.g., capitation, withholds, bonuses, authorization, formularies). Criticism has come from providers and patients. Some of these strategies have undergone change, or they are no longer used in some areas. One of the concerns about some of the strategies (e.g., withholds, bonuses) has been that they encourage providers to undertreat.
9. Provider panels offer insurers more control over providers than traditional third-party payer insurance had over providers.
10. The common managed care models are HMOs and PPOs. There are several types of HMOs, for example, staff, group, network, and IPA. The PPO has become very popular because it offers more provider choice to the enrollee/patient.
11. Outcomes are more important today and are an integral part of the managed care requirements.
12. Insurers use carve-outs to control costs for high-cost services.

References

Institute of Medicine. (IOM). (2008). *Knowing what works in healthcare. A roadmap for the nation*. Washington, DC: National Academies Press.

Kongstvedt, P. (2009). *Managed care. What it is and how it works*. Boston: Jones and Bartlett Publishers.

Questions and Activities for Thought

1. What types of managed care models are used in your community?
2. Which of the service strategies discussed in this chapter are used in your geographic area? Have advantages for their use been identified? What criticisms have been made about them?
3. What is the major difference between a service and a reimbursement strategy?
4. What is your personal view of provider withholds and discounts?
5. Why is it important for a nurse case manager to understand service and reimbursement strategies?

Case

You are working on a patient and family education program to explain your employer's use of reimbursement and service strategies. As a case manager who works for a MCO, it is important for you to include this information in the initial phase of the case management process. You have found that when you do not do this, you get frequent calls from patients and they are less involved in their care. What would you include in this program, and how would you present it?

Internet Links

- Use the links provided at the end of Chapter 3.
- American Association of Managed Care Nurses
  http://www.aamcn.org/

CHAPTER 5

Quality Improvement and Case Management

OBJECTIVES

After completing this chapter, the reader will be able to:

- Critique critical issues related to defining quality.
- Discuss the influences of the Institute of Medicine's *Quality Chasm* series on quality improvement (QI).
- Compare and contrast a blame culture and a culture of safety.
- Discuss the relevance of quality improvement to case management.
- Describe the safety initiative.
- Describe how the following are used by health care organizations (HCOs) and insurers to better ensure quality care: policies and procedures, licensure and credentialing, standards of care, credentialing, utilization review/management (UR/UM), clinical guidelines, clinical pathways, benchmarking, evidence-based practice (EBP), provider performance evaluation, outcomes management, and risk management (RM).
- Analyze the relevance of case management certification to quality care.
- Explain the use of quality report cards by employers, consumers, and insurers.
- Discuss the reasons purchasers and consumers are interested in accreditation and its data.
- Describe the process for accreditation provided by the National Committee for Quality Assurance (NCQA) and Utilization Review Accreditation Commission (URAC).
- Discuss the importance of Joint Commission accreditation.
- Explain why case management program evaluation is important.

KEY TERMS

Access, p. 111
Accreditation, p. 118
Benchmarking, p. 120
Clinical guideline, p. 120
Clinical pathways, p. 115
Credentialing, p. 119

Evidence-based practice (EBP), p. 111
Health Plan Employer Data and
 Information Set (HEDIS), p. 128
Indicators, p. 124
National Committee for Quality
 Assurance (NCQA), p. 127

INTRODUCTION

This chapter discusses **quality** in the health care delivery system, health care reimbursement, and case management. It addresses some of the critical issues related to quality care and provides information about quality care and methods used to monitor care and the relationship of quality to reimbursement Case managers need to be knowledgeable about **quality improvement (QI)** and its impact on the case management process and outcomes.

WHAT IS QUALITY IMPROVEMENT?

The Institute of Medicine's (IOM) fourth health care profession core competency is to apply QI. The IOM describes this core competency as "identify errors and hazards in care; understand and implement basic safety design principles, such as standardization and simplification; continually understand and measure quality of care in terms of **structure, process**, and **outcomes** in relation to patient and community needs; and design and test interventions to change processes and systems of care, with the objective of improving quality" (2003, p. 4). As noted in this report and also in the IOM report *To Err Is Human* (1999), the U.S. health care system is dysfunctional and has problems with safety, quality, and inefficiency. Case managers encounter these issues as they try to ensure that the patients receive quality and timely care. The health care system is the focus of QI. The system is fragmented and in need of improvement. A system "can be defined by the coming together of parts, interconnections, and purpose. While systems can be broken down into parts, which are interesting in and of themselves, the real power lies in the way the parts come together and are interconnected to fulfill some purpose" (Plsek, 2001, p. 309). The health care system is composed of a continuum of services (e.g., clinics, hospitals, physician offices, long-term care facilities, home care, pharmacies, laboratories, etc.). Ideally, this system should be interconnected and be a functioning, effective system (Plsek, 2001). This does not mean that individual patient's needs and improvement of individual patient care is not important. Each patient's care is part of this overall emphasis on health care improvement. The ultimate goal is that each patient's outcomes will be met. QI now emphasizes improvement and describes problem identification as an opportunity to improve. The older term for QI is quality assessment or assurance. QI should be a continuous, active process. How can this be applied to the health care system that is rapidly changing?

Definition of Quality Health Care

Can quality be defined? This has long been a recurring question in health care. There is no universally accepted definition of health care quality, and this has made it difficult to assess quality. The IOM defines health care quality as the "degree to which health services for individuals and populations increase the likelihood of desired health outcomes and are consistent with current professional knowledge" (1990, p. 4). It is a complex concept. The view of quality can vary depending on who is defining it; for example, a physician, patient, nurse, case manager, or insurer will most likely define the term differently.

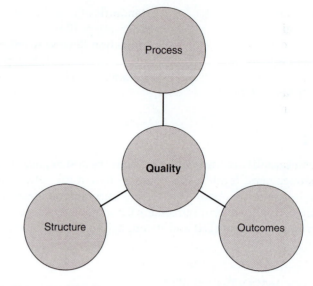

FIGURE 5-1   Three Elements of Quality

Can quality be measured, or are there some aspects that cannot be measured? Measuring the quality of the nurse–patient or physician–patient relationship quantitatively is difficult, and in many cases it is difficult to evaluate patient outcomes, though more is being done to evaluate outcomes. If knowledge about a specific illness is incomplete, it is difficult to measure quality care accurately. More research is required before standards and guidelines can be developed to describe the best treatment. There are three elements to quality that are usually included in a discussion about quality care and monitoring care, which relate to the IOM definition of quality (Donabedian, 1980). The three accepted elements of quality are *structure,* the environment in which services are provided; *process,* the manner in which services are provided; and *outcome,* the result of services. These elements serve as the framework for the assessment of care. Figure 5.1 describes these elements.

Increased Interest in Quality Care

In the past 10 years there has been increasing interest in the quality of health care, particularly since the publication of the IOM report *To Err Is Human* (1999). This report signaled that the system was experiencing frequent and important errors. This result led to the IOM initiative to examine the health care system in more detail.

CROSSING THE QUALITY CHASM: IMPACT ON QUALITY CARE.   *Crossing the Quality Chasm* (Institute of Medicine, 2001a) is the IOM report that followed *To Err Is Human* (Institute of Medicine, 1999) as part of the quality series. This report states that the U.S. health care system needs fundamental improvement. The report identifies six aims or goals for improvement, concluding that care should be (Institute of Medicine, 2001a, pp. 5–6):

1. *Safe:*   Avoiding injuries to patients from the care that is intended to help them.
2. *Effective:*   Providing services based on scientific knowledge (EBP) to all who could benefit and refraining from providing services to those not likely to benefit (avoiding underuse and overuse).
3. *Patient-centered:*   Providing care that is respectful and responsive to individual patient preferences, needs, and values and ensuring that patient values guide all clinical decisions.

4. *Timely:*   Reducing waits and sometimes harmful delays for those who receive and those who give care.
5. *Efficient:*   Avoiding waste, including waste of equipment, supplies, ideas, and energy.
6. *Equitable:*   Providing care that does not vary in quality because of personal characteristics such as gender, ethnicity, geographic location, and socioeconomic status (disparity concern).

The IOM developed new rules for the 21st century to guide care delivery and improve the health care system (Institute of Medicine, 2001a, p. 8). Consider how each of the rules might apply to case management.

- *Care based on continuous healing relationships.*   Patients should receive care whenever they need it—**access** is critical. *How does the case manager assist in ensuring that the patient gets care when needed from the most effective provider?*
- *Customization based on patient needs and values.*   This rule relates directly to patient-centered care. Patient needs and values are sources of evidence for **evidence-based practice**. *How can individual patient needs and values be included in the case management plan?*
- *The patient as the source of control.*   Patients need information to make decisions about their own care—patient-centered care. Health care systems and professionals need to share information with patients and bring patients into the decision-making process. *How can the case manager include the patient and patient's family/significant others in the decision-making process?*
- *Shared knowledge and the free flow of information.*   Patients need access to their medical information, and clinicians need access. *What should the case manager do when the patient asks to have access to medical information?*
- *Evidence-based decision making.*   Clinicians need timely access to patient information, so that care decisions are based on the best possible evidence available. Patients also need timely information. *How can the case manager ensure that care does not vary illogically from clinician to clinician or from place to place? How does health care informatics better ensure accurate, timely information for those who need it?*
- *Safety is a system property.*   Patients need to be safe from harm that may occur within the health care system. There needs to be more attention placed on system errors rather than individual errors. *How does the case manager prevent errors that might impact the patient's care?*
- *The need for transparency.*   The health care system should make information available to patients and their families that allow them to make informed decisions when selecting a health plan, hospital, or clinical practice, or choosing among alternative treatments. *How does the case manager effectively include information describing the system's performance on safety, EBP, and patient satisfaction in the case management process?*
- *Anticipation of needs.*   Health care providers and the health system should not just react to events that may occur with patients but should anticipate patient needs and provide care needed. *How are needs anticipated in the case management plan?*
- *Continuous decrease in waste.*   Resources should not be wasted—including patient time. *How does the case manager incorporate effective use of resources in the case management process?*
- *Cooperation among clinicians.*   Collaboration and communication are critical among health care professionals and systems (interdisciplinary teamwork). *How are collaboration and communication critical parts of the case management process and care coordination?*

ENVISIONING THE NATIONAL HEALTH CARE QUALITY REPORT. Following the development of the *Quality Chasm* report, which laid out the problem and critical concerns, the next question was, how do we learn more and how do we monitor the quality of care so that the interventions can be taken to improve care? *Envisioning the National Health Care Quality Report* (Institute of Medicine, 2001b) describes a framework that is now used to collect and organize annual data about health care quality, focusing on how the health care delivery system performs in providing personal health care. The framework for the annual report uses a matrix. "The matrix is a tool to visualize possible combinations of the two dimensions (consumer perspectives and components of health care quality) of the framework and better understand how various aspects of framework relate to one another" (Institute of Medicine, 2001b, p. 8). The IOM uses two dimensions in the quality matrix to describe quality. *The first dimension focuses on safety, effectiveness, patient-centeredness, and timeliness* (Institute of Medicine, 2001b, p. 41).

1. *Safety* refers to the avoidance of injury or harm when providing care that is intended to help a person. Subcategories are (1) diagnosis, (2) treatment (e.g., medication, follow-up), and (3) health care environment.
2. *Effectiveness* focuses on providing care that is based on scientific knowledge and avoids overuse and underuse. Subcategories are: (1) preventive care, (2) acute, (3) chronic, (4) end-of-life care, and (5) appropriateness of procedures.
3. *Patient-centeredness* focuses on the partnership between the patient (and also as appropriate with families and caregivers) and health care providers. Subcategories are (1) experience of care and (2) effective partnership. This process emphasizes the role of the patients in decision making about their own care.
4. *Timeliness* or receiving care when it is needed with the least amount of delay is part of this dimension. Subcategories are (1) access to the system of care, (2) timeliness in getting to care for a particular problem, and (3) timeliness within and across episodes of care.

The second dimension of quality care focuses on the consumer perspectives on health care needs and includes (Institute of Medicine, 2001b, pp. 56–57):

1. *Staying healthy* means that the individual needs to get health care to stay well and avoid illness.
2. *Getting better* requires care to reach recovery.
3. *Living with illness or disability* acknowledges that some health problems cannot be cured, and then the individual needs assistance in learning how to manage and cope long term.
4. *Coping with the palliative or end-of-life* requires that the individuals need support and care during terminal stages of illness. Families and caregivers are also involved in each of these consumer components of health care.

These components are considered to be key issues for individuals, affected by the individual's age. Across the life span, individuals view these components differently. This matrix could be used by case managers to evaluate individual patient's care and outcomes. Particularly important and somewhat different is the second dimension in the matrix. This dimension expands on the patient or consumer of health care services and personal health issues and perspectives, reinforcing patient-centered care.

The Agency for Health Resources and Quality (AHRQ), part of the U.S. Department of Health and Human Services (HHS), is mandated to collect data using this quality framework. AHRQ then publishes an annual report describing the results, which are available on the Internet. This health care quality report should "serve as a yardstick or the barometer by which to gauge progress in improving the performance of the health care delivery system in consistently providing high-quality care" (Institute of

Medicine, 2001b, p. 2). This report serves as the country's annual national report card; however, it does not replace the need for individual HCOs to monitor their own organization's quality. The information from the national annual report is used by HCOs in developing services, insurers, health policymakers, and health professions educators. It is also an information that case managers can use to increase their awareness of current quality concerns and a specific HCO's services.

Quality Improvement: A Growing, Complex Process

The IOM frequently comments on health care complexity and views this as a barrier to understanding safety and quality and to improving health care delivery. Implementing IOM QI approaches "requires that health professionals be clear about what they are trying to accomplish, what changes they can make that will result in an improvement, and how they will know that the improvement occurred" (Institute of Medicine, 2003a, p. 59). Why is health care so complex? Health care is different from other businesses that might have one product or a series of highly related products, such as manufacturing. Health care products are determined by the medical problem, the consumer/patient, patient prognosis, the setting, clinical staff expertise, treatment options, reimbursement, health policy, and legislation. Even geographic location can make a difference because there are practice pattern variations from one part of the country to another or rural access compared to urban areas. Specialty areas such as obstetrics, psychiatry, emergency care, intensive care, home care, and long-term care offer varied services that are influenced by their interventions, roles of the patient and family, patient education needs, prognosis and outcomes, and so on. Patients are very diverse in their needs, diagnoses, ethnic and cultural backgrounds, and overall health status and are influenced by genetic background, socioeconomic factors, patient preferences for health care, community differences, and health care coverage and reimbursement concerns. The latter is particularly important with the development of major economic problems when people lose their jobs and health care coverage. If patients put off elective surgery, then there is less surgery to schedule. This leads to financial issues for hospitals that may lead to a change in services or elimination of services that are too expensive to offer.

It is expensive to develop and maintain an effective QI program, but QI programs can lead to improved safety and quality and in the long run save money when complications or extended treatment is avoided. This is a concern of case managers who want to reduce costs and ensure effective treatment to meet patient outcomes. Developing a QI program that addresses monitoring and improving health care safety and quality is in itself a complex process and should consider the IOM matrix describing the two dimensions of quality. Health care can be improved moving to using best practice (EBP) and finding new approaches that are better than current care interventions. An effective QI program includes the following elements that are relevant to case management (Berwick, Enthoven, & Bunker, 1992; Donabedian, 1980; Institute of Medicine, 2001a; Institute of Medicine, 2003b, p. 59):

- Continually understand and measure quality of care in terms of structure or the inputs into the system, such as patients, staff, and environments; process, or the interactions between clinicians and patients; and outcomes, or evidence about changes in patients' health status in relation to patient and community needs
- Assess current practices and compare them with relevant better practices elsewhere as a means of identifying opportunities for improvement
- Design and test interventions to change the process of care, with the objective of improving quality
- Identify errors and hazards in care; understand and implement basic safety design principles, such as standardization and simplification and human factors training

- Both act as an effective member of an interdisciplinary team and improve the quality of one's own performance through self-assessment and personal change

Quality is difficult to understand and to monitor. The following are examples of issues identified by Bodenheimer in 1999 that arise when assessing quality and have been reemphasized in the IOM reports.

- Health care is not a single product.
- Different interventions require different measurements.
- Different groups focus on different issues when considering quality.
- Overuse, underuse, and misuse are critical in determining quality.
- Organizations need a culture of quality to improve.
- Assessment of quality is expensive, and this cost is shifted to purchasers and consumers.
- Patient satisfaction is a questionable measure of the quality of care.

Key questions on quality in the health care reimbursement environment should focus on the needs of the customer or purchaser of the care and the consumer/patient. The customer, typically the employer or government that purchases insurance for employees, wants the best value, affordable care, healthy employees, and no hassle. The consumer or patient wants services, access, choice, and affordability. Sometimes the customer's and the consumer's viewpoints collide.

Insurers are concerned about value or function of both quality and cost of health care. Both are critical to an insurer's survival. A recommended model for improvement suggested by Berwick and Nolan (1998) focuses on several questions: What are you trying to accomplish? How will you know whether a change is an improvement? What change can you try that you believe will result in improvement? Each of these questions could be asked daily by a case manager in planning, implementing, and evaluating. Berwick continues to push for health care improvement through the organization that he leads, the Institute for Healthcare Improvement (IHI). This organization's Internet site listed in the end-of-chapter link provides important information about QI in HCOs.

Placing Blame or Supporting a Culture of Safety

HCOs have typically handled errors by identifying the staff member who made the error or asking staff to report their errors by completing incident reports describing the error. Over time, this has become a more punitive approach and has not been effective. Most errors are much more complex than just an error made by an individual, a viewpoint supported by the IOM reports (Institute of Medicine, 1999). When an error occurs, the question should not be one of "Who is at fault?" but rather, "Why did our defenses fail?" (Reason, 2000). There are too many people involved in health care and the health care system is too complex to think that one individual is always the reason for an error. As case managers work with multiple health care providers and teams, it becomes important to understand that errors are more commonly due to system issues. The IOM reported that the health care system was focusing on the "blame game" rather than examining causes to improve. Staff are anxious or afraid to report errors, which may prevent them from doing so. Near misses or errors that are caught before they occur are also important to monitor. There is greater movement to change to a culture of safety instead of a blame culture. This approach sets the stage for greater communication about errors and near misses to improve care more. "A fundamental principle of the systems approach to error reduction is the recognition that all humans make mistakes and that errors are to be expected, even in the best organizations" (Reason, 2000, p. 768). Case managers encounter errors that impact their patients and may also be directly involved in making errors.

A CASE MANAGEMENT PERSPECTIVE OF QUALITY IMPROVEMENT

When reviewing case management, it is difficult to separate the effects of cost containment on the quality of care. Factors identified by Bower in 1992 are still relevant today and can be seen in the IOM's work on health care quality.

- Enhanced communication with, and education of, patients and their families, enabling them to better plan for, and make more fully informed decisions about care
- Earlier identification of discharge needs (often before an inpatient admission), resulting in the development of plans to address potential or real barriers
- Identification of patient problems and barriers to care within a time frame that allows the problems to be addressed proactively or concurrently, rather than retrospectively
- More effective and efficient communication among the disciplines involved in patient care, as well as with patients and their families
- Reduction or elimination of duplicate or overlapping care, tests, and treatments through improved sequencing and coordination of care activities
- Minimized or eliminated delays in required tests, treatments, or care
- Enhanced knowledge among clinicians regarding the financial aspects of care
- Attention to the needs of patients and the issues and problems encountered in providing efficient, effective care at both the individual and aggregate patient levels

Case management and its tools as discussed in Chapter 6 (e.g., **clinical pathways**) help to define quality care and outcomes and monitor care. Because these tools often include timelines and identified lengths-of-stay, the tools assist in clarifying when outcomes should be met. Data from research (EBP), standards, and experts are incorporated into the content and provide a sound basis for the plan of care and identified outcomes. Third-party payers are interested in providers that use case management because they want to see:

- Length-of-stay (LOS) reduction
- Cost-per-case reduction
- Patient outcomes met
- Increased patient satisfaction
- Increased physician/HCO provider satisfaction
- Decreased admission/readmission rates
- Decreased complications
- Appropriate, timely treatment decisions

In order to accomplish these outcomes, successful case management programs typically use the following:

- Identification of target populations based on specific plan to meet needs of identified population
- Accurate assessment of needs
- Formal written case management plans with involvement of the physician, other care providers, the patient, and family
- Consideration of needs across the continuum of care
- Use of information systems to monitor patient status and outcomes
- Recognition of the need to meet cost containment needs and patient care needs, ensuring quality care

The health care delivery system is complex and difficult to navigate, particularly for individuals with chronic illness who often use multiple services. Case management, however, is provided within the health care delivery system, and this can make it easier to be successful. The following are characteristics of the health care delivery system that are frequently barriers to success:

- There is confusion over access to services and information on available insurer services.
- Patients are not guaranteed that they will see the same physician at every visit, thus jeopardizing continuity of care.
- The choice of specialists may be limited.
- Data systems are typically disparate.
- Benefits may be limited and difficult to interpret.
- Physicians often have contractual arrangements with several MCOs or insurers, which differ in the benefits they cover.

The case manager can help patients and their families to cope, but case managers must also learn to cope with the complex delivery system to ensure that quality, cost-effective care is provided.

MEDICARE AND QUALITY

The Quality Improvement Organization (QIO) is the federal program that monitors medical necessity and quality for Medicare and Medicaid and the prospective payment system. What do QIOs do? "By law, the mission of the QIO Program is to improve the effectiveness, efficiency, economy, and quality of services delivered to Medicare beneficiaries" (Centers for Medicare and Medicaid Services, 2009). Based on this statutory charge, and Centers for Medicare and Medicaid Services (CMS) Program experience, CMS identifies the core functions of the QIO Program as:

- Improving quality of care for beneficiaries;
- Protecting the integrity of the Medicare Trust Fund by ensuring that Medicare pays only for services and goods that are reasonable and necessary and that are provided in the most appropriate setting; and
- Protecting beneficiaries by expeditiously addressing individual complaints, such as beneficiary complaints; provider-based notice appeals; violations of the Emergency Medical Treatment and Labor Act (EMTALA); and other related responsibilities as articulated in QIO-related law.

The CMS relies on QIOs to improve the quality of health care for all Medicare beneficiaries. The CMS views the QIO Program, which is required by law, as an important resource in its effort to improve quality and efficiency of care for Medicare beneficiaries. Throughout its history, the Medicare program has been instrumental in advancing national efforts to motivate providers in improving quality, and in measuring and improving outcomes of quality (Centers for Medicare and Medicaid Services, 2009).

In the fall of 2007, the CMS made a major change in the Medicare program. The CMS no longer pays for specific complications or what it terms as reasonably preventable medical errors that result in serious consequences for patients that occur in the hospital and could be prevented. These events are referred to as "Never Events." To be included on the list of "Never Events," an event must be characterized as (Centers for Medicare and Medicaid, 2007):

- Unambiguous—clearly identifiable and measurable, and thus feasible to include in a reporting system
- Usually preventable—recognizing that some events are not always avoidable, given the complexity of health care

BOX 5-1

Centers for Medicare and Medicaid: Never Events (2008)

The 10 categories of Hospital-Acquired Conditions (HACs) include:

1. Foreign Object Retained After Surgery
2. Air Embolism
3. Blood Incompatibility
4. Stage III and IV Pressure Ulcers
5. Falls and Trauma
   - Fractures
   - Dislocations
   - Intracranial Injuries
   - Crushing Injuries
   - Burns
   - Electric Shock
6. Manifestations of Poor Glycemic Control
   - Diabetic Ketoacidosis
   - Nonketotic Hyperosmolar Coma
   - Hypoglycemic Coma
   - Secondary Diabetes with Ketoacidosis
   - Secondary Diabetes with Hyperosmolarity
7. Catheter-Associated Urinary Tract Infection (UTI)
8. Vascular Catheter-Associated Infection
9. Surgical Site Infection Following:
   - Coronary Artery Bypass Graft (CABG) – Mediastinitis
   - Bariatric Surgery
     - Laparoscopic Gastric Bypass
     - Gastroenterostomy
     - Laparoscopic Gastric Restrictive Surgery
   - Orthopedic Procedures
     - Spine
     - Neck
     - Shoulder
     - Elbow
10. Deep Vein Thrombosis (DVT)/Pulmonary Embolism (PE)
    - Total Knee Replacement
    - Hip Replacement

Source: Centers for Medicare and Medicaid (CMS), (2009). Retrieved from http://www.cms.hhs.gov/HospitalAcqCond/06_Hospital-Acquired_Conditions.asp#TopOfPage on August 31, 2009.

- Serious—resulting in death or loss of a body part, disability, or more than transient loss of a body function
- Any of the following:
  - Adverse
  - Indicative of a problem in a health care facility's safety systems
  - Important for public credibility or public accountability

Never Events are highlighted in Box 5-1. This list will change as the CMS determines events that can be removed and events that need to be added. Current lists of events are available on the CMS website.

What does this change in reimbursement really mean? If a Medicare patient falls and injures himself or herself in the hospital, the CMS will not pay for the care needed to resolve the injury. The Never Event approach is of great concern to health care providers, who wonder if all of these incidents can be prevented. The second issue for health care providers is who will pay for the care if the CMS does not. Hospitals will have to cover the costs not paid by Medicare, and this will have a major impact on hospital budgets. Since there are limits on what the HCO can charge an individual Medicare patient, there would be no other source for payment. The purposes of this CMS change are to control Medicare costs and push for greater improvement in care. Since a large percentage of inpatients are Medicare patients, this change will have a major impact on the overall status of hospital budgets. With the growing economic problem, many hospitals are already having financial problems. This issue will only add to these problems. Following the CMS decision, some insurers have also issued their own lists of preventable medical errors by identifying what incidents they will not cover. This expands this type of payment policy to a greater number of patients. In the case of nongovernmental coverage, the patient could be billed for this care. Given the growing costs of health care to individuals, this will only make the problem worse. It is hoped that this approach will improve care, but there may be a heavy price to pay for it.

EXAMPLES OF SAFETY INITIATIVES

The IHI is described as "a reliable source of energy, knowledge, and support for a never-ending campaign to improve health care worldwide. It has helped to change health care by focusing on practical solutions that can be used by health care organizations, providers, and health care education" (Institute for Healthcare Improvement, 2009). Its projects and resources focus on safety, effectiveness, patient-centeredness, timeliness, efficiency, and equity, all of which are emphasized in the IOM *Quality Chasm* series. One of the IHI's collaborative projects with The Robert Wood Johnson Foundation (RWJF) is Transforming Care at the Bedside (TCAB). This is a "unique innovation initiative that aims to create, test, and implement changes that will dramatically improve care on medical/surgical units, and improve staff satisfaction as well" (Institute for Healthcare Improvement, 2009). Its website provides examples of TCAB pilots and results.

The Joint Commission's annual safety initiative goals, which began in 2003, identify annual safety goals that should be the focus of every HCO accredited by the Joint Commission (Joint Commission, 2009). The goals focus on the critical, current safety concerns. Joint Commission surveyors also emphasize the safety goals during **accreditation** visits. These goals have become important in staff education about safety and in efforts to monitor safety. The current goals are available on the Joint Commission website.

QUALITY IMPROVEMENT METHODS

HCOs use a variety of tools and methods to monitor safety and quality and ensure quality improvement. There are many methods used in the accreditation process of insurers and MCOs. Some are used to collect data, as sources of data, or to provide guidance about quality care. The following sections describe some of these methods.

Policies and Procedures

Policies and procedures set standards within an HCO or insurer that guide decisions and how care is provided and support greater consistency in how care is delivered. This can help to improve care. Policies and procedures should not conflict with regulatory issues in the state such as the Nurse Practice Act and should be in agreement with professional standards. Policies and procedures need to be readily available to staff for review when needed. Many HCOs have put their policies and procedures into their computer systems, reducing the need for hardcopy policy and procedure manuals and making it easier to access the information when needed. HCOs are beginning to recognize the need to use EBP when developing, reviewing, and updating policies and procedures. Case management policies and procedures should reflect similar characteristics, whether the case management is part of an HCO or part of an insurer's program.

Licensure, Credentialing, and Certification

Professional licensure verification is an important activity in all HCOs. It is important for case managers who also hold a professional license such as a registered nurse license. A license means the person has met expected minimal standards set by the state practice act. State laws require that certain health care providers have licenses. Allowing someone to practice without a license means the HCO and the individual are breaking the law. Some states require continuing education credits per licensure renewal cycle with the intent of improving practice. Nurses who are case managers should continue to maintain their registered nurse licensure. **Credentialing** is different from checking licensure. It is a more in-depth review process that includes evaluation of licenses, certification if required in a specialty area, evidence of malpractice insurance as required, history of involvement in malpractice suits, and education. Credentialing is primarily used for physicians that practice in a HCO. Nurse midwives and nurse practitioners may also require credentialing depending upon the services they provide. Licensure and credentialing information is kept on file and may be reviewed during Joint Commission surveys or by other accreditors. Certification has also become more important. Case management certification is available for case managers through the Commission for Case Management Certification (CCMC). See current information on certification at http://www.ccmcertification.org/pages/12frame_set.html.

Standards

A standard is an authoritative statement that provides a minimum description of accepted actions expected from an HCO or an individual health care provider such as a physician, nurse, case manager, and so on; and describes expectations about what should be done. Standards are developed by professional organizations, legal sources such as federal and state laws and nurse practice acts, regulatory agencies, and HCOs. Standards should be evidence-based and supported by scientific literature. The Joint Commission has standards that are used in its accreditation process, which are discussed later in this chapter.

Standards are important to health care professions and in health care in general, so it should be no surprise to learn that standards have also been developed for case managers. The CMSA has developed a set of standards for case managers that are patient-centered. The organization's **standards of care** focus on (CMSA, 2002):

- Assessment/case identification and selection
- Problem identification
- Planning
- Monitoring
- Evaluating
- Outcomes

The standards of performance focus on:

- Quality of care
- Qualifications
- Collaboration
- Legal
- Ethical
- Advocacy
- Resource management/stewardship
- Research utilization

These standards are under revision. Updates can be obtained from the CMSA website at http://www.cmsa.org. Many of focus areas of these standards are familiar to nurses because their content is similar to nursing standards.

The Joint Commission should not be ignored, because its standards are very influential in health care delivery systems. Case management standards include the major principles that are found in the Joint Commission standards, emphasizing appropriateness, timeliness, effectiveness, efficiency, continuity, efficacy, availability, safety, and attention to respect and caring (Joint Commission, 2009a). These principles are also employed in the IOM quality recommendations.

Clinical Guidelines

The IOM defines a **clinical guideline** as: "systematically developed statements to assist practitioner and patient decisions about appropriate health care for specific clinical circumstances" (Institute of Medicine, 1990, p. 38). The use of clinical guidelines is a method that focuses on improvement of care. The AHRQ is the most prominent agency in the development of clinical or practice guidelines. Guidelines identify outcomes and support best practice, and they can be useful in determining the quality and cost of health care. Professional organizations have also become very active in developing guidelines. How do guidelines enhance the quality of care? Data can help to identify quality problems, particularly problems related to underuse, overuse, or ineffective provision of care. Greater understanding of how patients respond to care for particular problems can help to prevent problems. Patient outcomes and patient satisfaction are important variables to consider as guidelines are implemented and data collected. This should all lead to a more complete view of care required for specific problems and improve guidelines. Chapter 7 discusses guidelines in more detail.

The Case Management Society of America (CMSA) (2009) first developed the Case Management Adherence Guidelines (CMAG) in 2004. The goal of the case management guidelines is to assist case managers with assessment, planning, facilitation, and advocacy of patient adherence. The CMAG offer a number of guidelines that focus on adherence, motivation, and knowledge. The disease-specific guidelines that have been published are: diabetes, deep vein thrombosis, depression, cardiometabolic risk, and a guideline devoted to medication nonadherence (Aliotta et al., 2007). These guidelines are accessible through the link provided at the end of the chapter.

Clinical Pathways

Clinical pathways are discussed in more detail in Chapter 7; however, it is important to recognize their use in the assessment of quality and cost of health care. Pathways focus on outcomes and the assessment of their achievement. They provide a **benchmarking** method for individual patients. The promotion of appropriate use of resources in a timely manner is an important component of each pathway, and this promotes cost-effectiveness. Box 5-2 provides a sample of quality rating items for cost-effectiveness analysis.

BOX 5-2

Sample Quality Rating Items for Cost-effectiveness Analyses

Framing
- Are the interventions and populations compared appropriate?
- Is the study conducted from the societal perspective?
- Is the time horizon clinically appropriate and relevant to the study question?

Effects
- Are all important drivers of effectiveness included?
- Are key harms included?
- Is the best available evidence used to estimate effectiveness?

- Are long-term outcomes used?
- Do effect measures capture preferences or utilities?

Costs
- Are all appropriate downstream medical costs included?
- Are charges converted to costs appropriately?
- Are the best available data used to estimate costs?

Results
- Are incremental cost-effectiveness ratios presented?
- Are appropriate sensitivity analyses performed?

Source: Agency for Healthcare Research and Quality. Developing the instrument and process for abstracting data. Retrieved from http://www.ahrq.gov/clinic/ajpmsuppl/saha2.htm#section9

Variances are analyzed when outcomes are not met to determine causes and actions that need to be taken to prevent further problems. This information also provides data that can be used to improve care for other patients. As many types of organizations and insurers develop pathways, how will organizations comply when each insurer may require a different pathway? Which pathway should be followed? Who is liable if the wrong one is followed? Case managers will need to reconcile differences and relate to individual patient case management plans.

Benchmarking

"The concept of discovering what is the best performance being achieved, whether in your company, by a competitor, or by an entirely different industry. Benchmarking is an improvement tool whereby a company measures its performance or process against other companies' best practices, determines how those companies achieved their performance levels, and uses the information to improve its own performance. Benchmarking is a continuous process whereby an enterprise measures and compares all its functions, systems and practices against strong competitors, identifying quality gaps in the organization, and striving to achieve competitive advantage locally and globally" (Six Sigma, 2008). Case managers find that many hospitals, other types of HCOs, and insurers use benchmarking today. One of the popular benchmarking approaches is Six Sigma, which is "a rigorous and a systematic methodology that utilizes information (management by facts) and statistical analysis to measure and improve a company's operational performance, practices and systems by identifying and preventing defects in manufacturing and service-related processes in order to anticipate and exceed expectations of all stakeholders to accomplish effectiveness" (Six Sigma, 2008).

Benchmarking is also a tool that links standards of care, guidelines, documentation, quality assurance programs, and clinical pathways. Benchmarking allows organizations to compare their performance both within the organization and with other organizations. The goal is to find new opportunities for cost and quality improvement.

Benchmarking focuses on using data to improve care and services and requires that staff use data-driven decision-making processes. It makes the organization and its staff aware of options. Benchmarking begins with the organization identifying the areas of greatest need that require monitoring and improvement and for which there is comparable performance data. Time should not be wasted on correcting problems that will not have an impact or for which it is difficult to obtain data.

A key component of benchmarking is sharing, and this has not always been easy for HCOs. If information is shared, it will benefit all, but this requires some trust. Any organization or insurer that participates in benchmarking will undoubtedly want its legal advisors to review policies and procedures related to this project. Competition has not disappeared—in fact, it has increased. Acknowledging competition and also participating in benchmarking can be a complex endeavor. The report card provided by the NCQA is an example of benchmarking, allowing for greater comparison and hopefully improvement of cost and quality of services as changes are made in insurers and with providers (National Committee for Quality Assurance, 2009). The link to this report is available in the Internet Links at the end of this chapter.

Evidence-Based Practice (EBP)

Evidence-Based Practice (EBP) helps to identify and assess high-quality, clinically relevant research that can be applied to clinical practice. It includes four elements that are described in Figure 5.2. The results are synthesized so that they can be used to improve care. EBP requires that information is available to answer specific questions (Institute of Medicine, 2008). The research literature is reviewed using explicit scientific methods

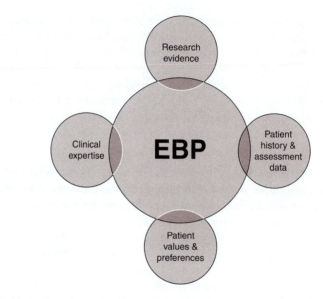

FIGURE 5-2 Evidence-Based Practice Elements

and includes all relevant research. This valuable information is then available to practitioners and should be helpful in directing their care decisions.

As seen in Figure 5.2, EBP is more than just research evidence. EBP can also be viewed as method to improve the quality of care because it entails basing decisions on several types of evidence to better ensure that the care needs are met in an effective manner. The AHRQ is the government agency that develops clinical guidelines based on EBP and provides a public Web-based repository of guidelines (National Guideline Clearinghouse, 2009). The AHRQ's goals are to: (1) support improvements in health outcomes, (2) promote patient safety and reduce medication errors, (3) advance the use of information technology for coordinating patient care and conducting quality and outcomes research, and (4) establish an Office of Priority Populations to ensure that they receive care—low-income groups, minorities, women, children, the elderly, and individuals with special needs. A key question one could ask is, does the lack of insurance impact access to high-quality, evidence-based care? According to the IOM (2004, pp. 42–43): "The difference health insurance makes is not just in increasing utilization but also in ensuring appropriate care. Although not all of the care that insured populations use is necessary and appropriate, overall, the care received by those with coverage contributes to health outcomes better than those experienced by otherwise comparable uninsured populations who on average receive many fewer and less appropriate services. People without health insurance are less likely to receive high-quality, evidence-based care that is recommended by professional groups. When appropriate care is not received, patients' health is placed at risk, conditions become more severe, and the effects can linger. Increased severity frequently demands more intense treatment (e.g., hospitalization)." Box 5-3 provides some examples of EBP literature that could impact case management for chronic illnesses.

Risk Management (RM)

The purpose of **risk management (RM)** is "to maintain a safe and effective health care environment and prevent or reduce loss to the health care organization" (Pike, Janssen, & Brooks, 2002, p. 3). RM interventions focus on decreasing financial loss for the HCO due to legal and malpractice issues by monitoring errors and incidents and decreasing

BOX 5-3

Evidence-Based Practice: Chronic Illnesses

Shafer, D. and Miller, M. (2009). Research on coordinating care for patients with chronic conditions. *Home Healthcare Nurse, 27*(7), 403–409. Read about four published articles that describe research about chronic disease care coordination. Give an example of EBP.

errors. When a medical error occurs, RM evaluates the risk for a lawsuit and takes actions as required. HCO attorneys are very involved in RM. Health care providers, particularly hospitals, insurers, and MCOs, retain legal services to assist them with RM. These preventive efforts are expensive; however, they are not as expensive as the cost of malpractice suits.

Assessment of Access to Care

Access to care is a critical issue in today's health care environment. Reduced access may result in poorer outcomes of care and can be costly when a patient's condition worsens because the patient was unable to access care when needed. How easy is it for the patient to receive care? Economic factors, transportation, and availability of appropriate health care providers may make it difficult for the patient to receive required care when it is needed. Access has been greatly affected by the diverse health care delivery and financial arrangements that are present in the health care environment today. There is also an ethical issue that is interwoven into any discussion of access. Is health care a right? This is an issue that has not been resolved. There is no state or federal law that says it is a right. The country spends more money on health care than any other service and yet not all citizens receive it. If barriers to coverage and proximity are removed, will we have equitable access? This is also an unknown. Access includes more than just initial entry into the health care system, but also includes how services are received within the system and the outcomes of that care. Case managers can have an impact on all of these factors.

- Ability to get to an appointment (e.g., hours of service for appointments, transportation, time off from work, childcare, and so forth)
- Ability to get specialty care or referral required
- Ability to pay for care
- Ability to know when care is needed and seek it
- Ability to understand health care information and utilize it
- Ability to access health care facility (e.g., disability access)
- Ability to choose health care providers
- Ability to get exams and tests in a timely manner
- Ability to better ensure patient-centered care
- Ability to implement EBP

A current concern is the effect of financial incentives on decisions that providers make about treatment after the patient enters the health care system. These incentives and decisions affect access. If a physician or another provider decides not to pursue further diagnostic testing based on the incentive arrangement in the provider's contract with an insurer, this affects the patient's accessibility to care. This potential medical underutilization is a major concern.

Other factors that are important in considering access are convenience, timeliness, handicap provisions, accommodations for language or sight, hours of operation, provider choice, waiting time for urgent and routine care, and timeliness of laboratory tests. Each of these can be used as **indicators** to determine accessibility of care. The IOM describes critical issues related to access of care and emphasizes that access should be timely so that patients receive personal health services when they need it (Institute of Medicine, 1993). Case managers work daily with access issues. How can case management impact these factors? The major focus today is on accessible primary care, particularly in relation to continuity, time, and provider type. Managed care emphasizes the use of the primary care provider as the gatekeeper or controller of access.

As the health care delivery system has changed, greater strain has been put on safety net providers, for example, free-care clinics, public and teaching hospitals, and other health care facilities that provide care to those with limited funds or insurance coverage. When a patient does not have access, then the patient's health status is at risk and further complications may occur. Vulnerable populations who often have limited access are: low-income, children and adolescents, minorities, homeless, mentally ill, uninsured, disabled, elderly veterans, immigrants, and prisoners. These populations are more vulnerable and often less "attractive" to providers and the community. Efforts have been made to resolve some of these concerns, and some of these efforts have been more successful than others. Case management can have a positive impact on the health care of vulnerable populations who frequently have complex needs and problems.

Examples of Vulnerable Populations and Health Care Reimbursement

The Mental Health Parity Act of 1996 was passed to address issues of parity for those with mental illness, but it was poorly designed legislation because it had loopholes that allowed insurers to continue limit care for people with mental illness. On October 3, 2008, President Bush signed the Mental Health Parity and Addiction Equity Act of 2008 (MHPAEA), which has improved how care will be reimbursed for this population (Centers for Medicare and Medicaid, 2008). Key changes made by MHPAEA, which was generally effective for health insurance plans, began in October 2009. The following are critical aspects of this legislation.

- If a group health plan includes medical/surgical benefits and mental health benefits, the financial requirements (e.g., deductibles and copayments) and treatment limitations (e.g., number of visits or days of coverage) that apply to mental health benefits must be no more restrictive than the predominant financial requirements or treatment limitations that apply to substantially all medical/surgical benefits.
- If a group health plan includes medical/surgical benefits and substance use disorder benefits, the financial requirements and treatment limitations that apply to substance use disorder benefits must be no more restrictive than the predominant financial requirements or treatment limitations that apply to substantially all medical/surgical benefits.
- Mental health benefits and substance use disorder benefits may not be subject to any separate cost sharing requirements or treatment limitations that only apply to such benefits.
- If a group health plan includes medical/surgical benefits and mental health benefits, and the plan provides for out-of-network medical/surgical benefits, it must provide for out-of-network mental health benefits.
- If a group health plan includes medical/surgical benefits and substance use disorder benefits, and the plan provides for out-of-network medical/surgical benefits, it must provide for out-of-network substance use disorder benefits.
- Standards for medical necessity determinations and reasons for any denial of benefits relating to mental health benefits and substance use disorder benefits must be made available upon request to plan participants.

- The parity requirements for the existing law (regarding annual and lifetime dollar limits) will continue and will be extended to substance use disorder benefits.

Case managers frequently work people with mental illness or with patients who have medical illnesses and mental illness. These changes in reimbursement mandated by law are very important in ensuring equitable care to a vulnerable population. The health care reform legislation of 2010 will help to increase mental health parity and make changes in this reimbursement. (See Chapter 3, Box 3-6.)

Another group that has problems with access are adolescent children with special needs. Confidentiality is an issue with adolescents, particularly those who may use mental health, substance abuse, contraceptive, or abortion services. Insurers maintain databases of services, and these data may be shared. Many teens need to receive services at clinics that often have difficulty obtaining funding to maintain their services. This affects adolescent access to needed services.

Access for special populations needs to be addressed whenever changes are made that may limit their access to care. In addition, organized efforts are needed to address current barriers to care for this population. Case management is one method for helping vulnerable populations get quality, timely care when needed.

Outcomes Management

Outcomes and analysis of outcome variances are critical components of case management because outcomes have an effect on costs and the quality of care. It is important to recognize how outcomes are used in case management to identify patient and treatment goals for evaluation. Where is the treatment going, and how will the patient and case manager know if there is improvement? Examples of expected outcomes directly related to the patient's health are to:

- Avoid adverse effects of care
- Improve the patient's physiological status
- Reduce signs and symptoms of illness
- Improve the patient's functional status and well-being

Case managers are also concerned with treatment setting, LOS outcomes, cost of care, and other outcomes related to the financial aspect of care.

As health care providers and organizations have become more experienced in assessing quality, they have turned more to performance-based quality care evaluation. Did the patient benefit from the care received? If so, how? These questions are critical and form the basis of outcomes. It is necessary to first develop indicators that identify areas of potential problems or improvement of care. This is the content or focus of assessment or evaluation. An indicator is a defined, measurable dimension of quality, specifying patient care activities, event occurrences for outcomes that can be monitored. Box 5-4 identifies some indicator components.

BOX 5-4

Components of Quality Indicators

- Accessibility
- Appropriateness
- Continuity
- Effectiveness
- Efficacy

- Efficiency
- Timeliness
- Patient perspective issues
- Safety of care environment

Indicators must also include a quantity element: the threshold. This is a pre-established level that indicates the need for more intensive assessment. Indicators can emphasize relative rate or trends that need further investigation. For example: The initial, preoperative, and postoperative pain assessments include (a) localization of pain, (b) type of pain, (c) duration of pain, (d) time of onset, (e) factors associated with pain, and (f) interventions taken and the results, with a threshold of 92%. The threshold indicates when further evaluation needs to be done—if more than 8% of the patient assessments do not meet this indicator, further investigation is required. Other indicators focus on sentinel events or events that always require investigation (e.g., suicide attempt, cardiac arrest in labor and delivery, lack of referral to specialist and patient dies).

Examples of some outcome focus areas are mortality rates, LOS, adverse incidents, complications, readmission rates, patient/family satisfaction, referral to specialists, patient adherence to the discharge plan or treatment plan, and prevention adherence (e.g., mammogram, Pap smear, immunizations), and costs. Indicators may also focus on process (actual activities done by health care providers) or structure (facilities, equipment, staff, finances), but the outcome focus (short-term and long-term results, complications, health status and functioning) has become more important.

Performance management and reimbursement are interconnected and can be demonstrated in patient outcomes. After outcomes are identified and care is implemented, data should be collected and variance analysis used to better understand the outcomes or care results. A variance occurs when something happens that is not expected, either positive or negative. Outcome variances require investigation and analysis to determine the intervention that is required and to prevent negative variances from reoccurring. Best practice can also be identified with outcome data. What worked? What didn't? When approaches were changed, what happened? Chapter 7 discusses variances in relationship to clinical pathways.

Case Management Program Evaluation

Case management programs need to be evaluated on a regular basis, preferably annually. This evaluation needs to include review vision and mission statements, the goals and objectives, the organizational chart, accessibility of needed resources to meet goals and objectives, budget, documentation, outcomes, staff records, and tools or methods used to manage care. Vann (2006) identifies some sample questions that need to be considered (p. 150).

- What specific activities and services do case managers perform? Are others required?
- How do case managers distribute their time between specific activities and interventions?
- Who is served by the case management program? Which patients? What communities and populations?
- Have the case managers received sufficient education and training to optimally case manage the clients/patients?
- What are the outstanding educational and training needs of the case managers?
- Is the case management program meeting the stated programmatic goals and objectives?
- Is the case management program cost effective? Are financial resources adequate to meet program requirements?
- Are case managed patients appropriately selected? Does the case management program target the patients in greatest need of services and those with the best potential for improved outcomes?
- Is the intensity or level of care received by patients appropriate?

- How are families and/or significant others included in the case management process?
- Are patients and families satisfied with services? What are the strengths and weaknesses?
- Are patients discharged from case management services when clinically appropriate?
- What are the program strengths and weaknesses?

The case manager position description should be reviewed to ensure that it describes the work that is done. Policies and procedures should be examined for support of EBP. Getting feedback from all stakeholders better ensure a more comprehensive review.

ACCREDITATION OF THIRD-PARTY PAYERS

Accreditation is the process that is used to evaluate HCO and insurer performance. This process is based on established minimum standards. There are two major reasons for accrediting insurers. Health care purchasers want objective data to make informed decisions about health plans to support a good return on their investment. Accreditation data from accreditation and accreditation status provide objective data. In addition, consumers have become more interested in data about health plans when they make their own decisions about health plans annually. Purchasers and consumers are interested in two critical elements: cost and quality. They want greater accountability for the quality of services. **Report cards** describing quality and outcomes data have become more common and accessible through the Internet.

The following discussion focuses on the types of accreditation that are available to insurers and issues related to their use and their effectiveness. It is important to note that accreditation is voluntary; however, many purchasers/employers do not contract with unaccredited insurers. The federal government requires accreditation to award contracts to managed care organization Medicare beneficiary health care coverage.

National Committee for Quality Assurance (NCQA)

The **National Committee for Quality Assurance (NCQA)** is an independent, nonprofit organization that began in 1990 but originated from an organization that was founded in 1979 by two managed care trade associations. Its mission is to improve the quality of health care insurance plans. It accredits the following. (National Committee for Quality Assurance, 2009a):

- Health Plans
- Wellness and Health Promotion
- Managed Care Organizations
- Preferred Provider Organizations (PPOs)
- New Health Plans
- Disease Management
- Quality Plus

The NCQA also provides certification for a variety of programs such as utilization management. The NCQA, though a nongovernment organization, does collaborate with government agencies such as the HCFA and state regulatory agencies. Insurers are regulated by both federal and state agencies, making this a very complex area. The NCQA evaluates health plans by conducting both on-site and off-site surveys. Insurers pay for the surveys, just as health care facilities pay for theirs.

Accreditation Process

The NCQA accreditation process includes two major steps. The first step is an on-site two-day survey, similar to accreditation surveys of hospitals (National Committee for Quality Assurance, 2009c). A team of trained surveyors, typically composed of physicians and an NCQA staff member, visit the insurer's central office, all its contracted hospitals, and selected provider components (excluding those accredited by other bodies), and practitioners to evaluate compliance with NCQA standards. The survey provides opportunities for the team to interact directly with staff. The survey also includes the NCQA's Interactive Survey System (ISS), which is a Web-based tool, which helps to reduce the time it takes to complete an accreditation survey. The NCQA has developed over 60 standards; details about current accreditation standards can be found on the association's website.

Health Plan Employer Data and Information Set (HEDIS)

The **Health Plan Employer Data and Information Set (HEDIS)** is used by more than 90% of U.S. health plans to measure performance (National Committee for Quality Assurance, 2009a). The NCQA continues to develop and use the HEDIS. It recognizes the need to standardize how health plans calculate and report performance information. HEDIS provides an opportunity for benchmarking to compare similar health plans. Various methods for benchmarking are described on the NCQA website. The NCQA describes quality health care as: "the extent to which patients get the care they need in a manner that most effectively protects or restores their health. This means having timely access to care, getting treatment that medical evidence has found to be effective and getting appropriate preventive care. Choosing a high-quality health plan—and a high-quality doctor—plays a significant role in determining whether you'll get high-quality care" (National Committee for Quality Assurance, 2009). Report cards are also available to assess health plans via the NCQA website. Some of the performance measures noted in 2009 are (National Committee for Quality Assurance, 2009a):

- Advising smokers to quit
- Antidepressant medication management
- Breast cancer screening
- Cervical cancer screening
- Child and adolescent access to primary care physician
- Child and adolescent immunization status
- Comprehensive diabetes care
- Controlling high blood pressure
- Prenatal and postpartum care

The types of evaluative programs provided by the NCQA are broad and are described on its website (National Committee for Quality Assurance, 2009b).

UTILIZATION REVIEW ACCREDITATION COMMISSION (URAC)

The American Health Care Commission's **Utilization Review Accreditation Commission,** commonly referred to as **URAC,** is a private, nonprofit, independent accrediting and certification organization for utilization management programs, which began in 1990. Utilization management companies assist third-party payers and health care providers in managing and evaluating the necessity, appropriateness, and efficiency of health care services. The purpose of URAC is to promote quality and preserve patient rights. URAC has 22 accreditation and certification programs (URAC, 2009).

The URAC website provides details about URAC case management accreditation standards and process (http://www.urac.org). With the increasing use of case management, it is important that case management programs adhere to standards that demonstrate their quality and cost effectiveness.

Joint Commission

Accreditation is the process by which organizations are evaluated on their quality, based on established minimum standards. The major organization that accredits HCOs is the Joint Commission, a nonprofit organization that accredits more than 17,000 HCOs, including hospitals, long-term care organizations, home care agencies, clinical laboratories, ambulatory care organizations, behavioral health organizations, critical access hospitals, disease-specific care, health care staffing services, and office-based surgery practices. The accreditation process is complex, time-consuming, and costly. Participation is voluntary, though few HCOs could survive without this accreditation. The Joint Commission emphasizes quality and safety through a continuous quality improvement (CQI) process. HCOs go through a survey every three years and may also have unscheduled surveys. Periodic Performance Review is also required with submission of specific reports. During the survey and with updated reports, the Joint Commission determines if patients are achieving expected outcomes, and, if not, why. Examples of some outcomes that the Joint Commission assesses are: mortality rates, LOS, adverse incidents, complications, readmission rates, patient/family satisfaction, referrals to specialists, patient adherence to the discharge plan or treatment plan, and prevention adherence (e.g., mammogram, Pap smear, immunizations). All of these outcomes are of interest to insurers and case managers. The Joint Commission standards cover multiple service areas (Joint Commission, 2009a). All are listed on its website.

The Joint Commission also certifies disease management programs and services by providing comprehensive evaluation of the services. "While accreditation ensures an organization's overall commitment to quality, certification demonstrates excellence in fostering better outcomes by the integration and coordination of care" (Joint Commission, 2009b). The disease-specific conditions that are covered are listed on its website.

Other information about the certification program can be found on the Joint Commission's website. The website for the Joint Commission Quality Check™ can be used to search for information about specific health care organizations through the website http://www.qualitycheck.org/consumer/searchQCR.aspx. This site lists both Joint Commission-accredited, and certified HCOs and HCOs not accredited or certified by the Joint Commission.

Quality Report Cards

Health care report cards provide specific performance data about an organization at specific intervals, focusing on quality care. The report can be used by the HCO to compare its outcomes with report cards published by other HCOs or a large state or national database. Some of these report cards are now accessible through the Internet and can then be used by the consumer (patients, families). Case managers can use the reports to assess one HCO with another similar HCOs. The goal is to examine performance based on clearly defined criteria, and the data provide this information.

Quality report cards provide specific performance data about an organization. The organization may then compare these data with data from other similar organizations. The goal is to provide information that is helpful to the purchaser of health care services, the consumer of health care services, and health plans. Employers are primarily interested in differences in quality related to the costs of plans. Patients or consumers are interested in quality comparison among plans and their providers.

Health plans also want this performance information for marketing purposes. Key questions related to report cards identified by Bindman in 1997 and still relevant today include:

1. Who should be evaluated—hospitals, physicians, health plans?
2. What should be evaluated, and is it a valid indicator of health care quality?
3. Are the performance measures reliable, available in a timely manner, and sensitive to differences in the types of patients a plan covers or a provider sees?
4. How should performance measures be disseminated and used?

In 1998, the American Nurses Association (ANA) established the National Database of Nursing Quality Indicators (NDNQI). As of 2007, over 1,000 hospitals participate in this database. This initiative "provides each nurse the opportunity to review the evidence, evaluate their practice, and determine what improvements can be made" Montalvo & Dunton, 2007, p. 3). The database includes a large number of hospitals increasing the pool of evaluation data. The ANA classifies key nursing quality indicators by (Montalvo & Dunton, 2007, p. 1):

- *Nursing Workforce:* Measures of the supply of nursing (e.g., total nursing hours per patient day); nursing skill (percentage of nursing hours provided by registered nurses [RNs])
- *Nursing Processes:* Risk assessment; protocol implementation
- *Patient Outcomes:* Fall rates that are related to nursing hours; hospital-acquired pressure ulcer rates that are related to skill mix

The indicators are (Montalvo & Dunton, 2007, p. 173):

- Nursing Hours per Patient Day (RNs, LPNs/LVNs, UAPs)
- Patient Falls
- Patient Falls with Injury (injury level)
- Pediatric Pain Assessment, Intervention, Reassessment (AIR) Cycle
- Pediatric Peripheral Intravenous Infiltration Rate
- Pressure Ulcer Prevalence (community acquired, hospital acquired, unit acquired)
- Psychiatric Physical/Sexual Assault Rate
- Restraint Prevalence
- RN Education/Certification
- RN Satisfaction Survey Options (job satisfaction scales, practice environment scale [PES])
- Skill Mix (percentage of total nursing hours supplied by RNs, LPNs/LVNs, and UAPs; percentage of total nursing hours supplied by agency staff.)

The indicators are changed based on needs and current data.

Report cards, however, are not perfect. They are costly from the perspective of data collection, data analysis, and data sharing. A report card may indicate improvement in the indicators used to determine the content, but there is no assurance that this affects other aspects of care. If a report card indicates that an insurer's plan is particularly good at providing care to a specific patient population that is sicker and expensive to care for, the insurer may not want this information shared. It may not want to increase its membership with sicker patients, who may wish coverage when they learn that a particular plan provides excellent care, which may be costly to the plan. There is, however, no guarantee that releasing this information affects quality or the employer's and the consumer's choices. Many decisions that consumers make about their health care are not always based on quantitative data. Understanding the new data and finding the data may not always be easy. Patients often seek out information and guidance from family members and friends, who have their own personal views and values that may not be based on facts. A key problem with understanding the effect of managed care on the quality of care is the need to compare managed care plans with traditional plans in before-and-after studies. This is very difficult research to conduct, and it is difficult to obtain appropriate samples. Managed care plans vary, making comparisons somewhat difficult.

Utilization Review/Management

Utilization management (UM) is the process of evaluating the necessity, appropriateness, and efficiency of health care services used by the enrollees/patients who receive care from a provider. Utilization review (UR) data are used by HCOs to assess access and usage of services; cancel services that are no long needed; identify need for a new service; review the relationship of data to patient outcomes, and monitor financial risk to the organization. Data describing the use of services, number of patients, LOS and length-of-treatment can be useful in budget decision making.

UR has been used in acute care settings for a long time; however, it is also very important to insurers. Nurses are frequently hired as UR staff. They have the clinical skills and knowledge necessary to evaluate patient needs and services to determine necessity, appropriateness, and timeliness of services. Insurers are particularly interested in UM because it is a tool used primarily to control costs. Case managers are very involved utilization of UR data.

Authorization, the major method used in UM, is the approval by the third-party payer for a health care provider to provide specific care. The payer or insurer identifies what services or benefits require authorization. This is done at the time the plan is purchased. Plans that have the greatest amount of control have a tight authorization system. To be truly effective in controlling costs, an insurer must be able to influence provider utilization behavior. For example, if an insurer cannot find a way to decrease a provider's number of hospital admissions or the number of referrals to specialists, costs will continue to be a problem. Insurers are particularly active in controlling authorization. The purchaser of the plan, the employer, does not like the idea of health care costs increasing and may decide to drop the insurer and contract with another, more cost-effective insurer.

Who can authorize services is a critical decision. This decision is made in several ways. Probably, the most recognized method is to have authorization done by the primary care provider/physician (PCP). If an enrollee wants to see the PCP, no authorization is required. Some PPOs and managed indemnity plans require that plan staff authorize services. In this case, the physician or other type of provider would call a plan representative and describe the patient's problems and the need for services. The staff representative compares this information with predetermined criteria. This representative may be a case manager. The nurse case manager discusses the patient's needs with the provider and determines whether authorization can be provided. If the provider does not agree with the decision, the provider is referred to a supervisor or the medical director. Some plans use a different system. They have the enrollee call the plan directly, using a nurse advice line or a case manager. The enrollee does not have to go to the PCP to use a specialist but rather uses the advice line to gain authorization.

Predetermined criteria are used to assess the enrollee's needs. Insurers have been trying to find new methods to expedite authorization. Providers have found this to be a time-consuming process and have been particularly insulted that "staff" in the plan are making medical decisions. As insurers have grown more sophisticated, they have moved toward using more nurses in these roles in order to decrease these criticisms. Insurers also recognize the advantages of using health care professionals who can discuss the medical issues with providers and then make clinical decisions, and providers prefer talking with other health care professionals about patients. Predetermined criteria are important; however, it is also important to have professional experience to understand medical problems, application of the criteria, and recognize when there might need to be exceptions. The three common methods that are used to collect authorization data and make the decision are paper-based, telephone-based, and electronic systems. There is a move away from paper-based systems to telephone and electronic systems, recognizing that these systems are faster and more efficient.

Several different categories of authorization are used by insurers and have been associated with hospital UR for a long time: prospective, concurrent, retrospective, pended (for review), denial (no authorization), and subauthorization (Kongstvedt, 2009).

- *Prospective authorization* or *precertification* is the most common type of authorization. This authorization is given before care is provided. For example, an insurer requires approval of all surgery is approved prior to the surgery or approval of all hospital admissions prior to admission. In ambulatory care, authorization is often required for referral to a specialist or for certain types of laboratory tests or procedures. Second opinion is also a form of prospective authorization, which requires that the patient obtain an assessment from a second physician prior to a service or procedure in order to receive reimbursement. This is typically done for surgical procedures. The purpose of prospective authorization is to intervene before care is provided to determine if that care meets the criteria for medical necessity and, consequently, avoid unnecessary costs.
- *Concurrent authorization* is given as the care is provided. An example is the requirement that hospital admissions must be reported to the third-party payer within a specific time period, such as within 24 hours. In this type of authorization, there is some opportunity to intervene with treatment decisions but not the initial decision to treat. Hospital UR nurses play a critical role in concurrent authorization. Their work involves three major areas: admission reviews, LOS, and discharge planning. Staff other than nurses may be used in UR. Questions that are asked during the hospitalization include:
  - Was the admission or the procedure appropriate based on the patient's condition?
  - Is the LOS appropriate for the patient's diagnosis and clinical status?
  - What is the expected LOS for a specific diagnosis, and is the patient within that range or an outlier?
  - Was discharge planning begun on admission?
  - Is the discharge plan appropriate and realistic?
  - Was the expected LOS taken into consideration when the discharge plan was developed?
  - Have the patient and his or her family been involved in the discharge planning?
  - If the patient has had frequent admissions, what makes this discharge plan different from other recent admissions so that readmissions can be reduced?
- *Retrospective authorization* is given after the care is completed. This type of authorization was the more common focus of treatment audits in hospitals some years ago. Medical records are reviewed after the patient is discharged. After this review, the payer can decide not to reimburse for the care that has already been provided. Reimbursement denial at this point can be a major drawback for the provider, who still must pay for any expenses incurred in providing the care. This type of authorization is unusual today, and its use usually requires a decision from high up in the payer's chain of command, such as the medical director. Clearly,

with this type of authorization, the payer has no influence on the medical decision-making process because the care is already provided.

- A *pended authorization* is not a positive situation for the provider. The case has been put into a review category with no decision made. In fact, authorization may never be given. This indicates that there are problems with the past authorization process. For example, the PCP may not have met the requirements to obtain prospective or concurrent authorizations. Once the care is provided, a pended case may then be given a retrospective authorization.
- *Denial* indicates that the care will not be authorized, and thus there will be no reimbursement for that care.
- *Subauthorization* is a specific type of authorization that allows one authorization to piggyback onto another. The best example is that when authorization is given for surgery, authorization for anesthesia and pathology is automatically included. In other words, the PCP or surgeon does not have to ask specifically to have anesthesia and pathology authorized separately from the surgical authorization.

UR and discharge planning (DP) are two functions in hospitals that are interconnected. Case managers may be involved in both functions, and in some cases the two functions may be combined. It is becoming more common for UR to be more important than DP. Why is this so? "This predominance of UR over DP evolved partly by the initiative to defend 'medical necessity' and 'appropriateness,' and partly because of the way hospitals contract with—and are paid by—third party payers" (Birmingham, 2007, p. 17). Many of the UR and DP activities are the same, such as admission review, continued stay review, and assessment of readiness for discharge. There are, however, some critical components associated with DP that should not be ignored. Some of these are routine monitoring of changes in the plan and counseling the patient and family about the discharge plan. Today, with the acuity of patients and staffing shortages, nurses have less and less time to prepare patients for discharge. Patients and their families who are not involved in the DP process are more likely to have problems in the next level of care. This is costly for all concerned.

MANAGED CARE CONTRACTS AND PROVIDER PERFORMANCE EVALUATION

With the growth of managed care over time, there has been a greater emphasis by all types of insurers on provider performance evaluation. Insurers contract with providers. Written contracts state insurer responsibilities and what the provider will do within a specific time frame. An important element of the contract process is the evaluation. Health care providers are more dependent on these contracts. Prior to offering a contractual agreement the insurer evaluates new providers. The insurer also reevaluates its providers prior to renewing contracts. This is a relatively new experience for providers. In the fee-for-service (FFS) environment, the third-party payer was not unduly concerned with evaluating the provider. The patient saw the provider, the provider billed for services, and the third-party payer paid for the services. A patient's decision to continue seeing a provider was seen as a form of evaluation. This evaluation often was not based on any organized evaluation and might simply be based on whether the patient liked the provider. Later, as HMOs developed, there was more interest in the evaluation of providers who are hired as staff physicians or selected for provider panels. As costs for care have risen, questions about utilization have become more important. Utilization is the focus of that evaluation and part of the contractual process for many types of insurers.

Summary

Quality care is a critical issue today in the U.S. health care delivery system. What is quality care and how to improve care require data, monitoring, and interventions that can have an impact on care for individual patients, populations and communities, and the nation as a whole. Costs and quality are intertwined. Case management is directly involved in QI.

Chapter Highlights

1. Quality care has always been difficult to define. There is, however, consensus that it has three components: structure, process, and outcomes.
2. The customer is the person, organization, or business that purchases care, and the consumer is the person who receives the health care services.
3. The changes brought on by managed care have increased interest in quality care.
4. Outcomes have become the focus of the evaluation of care. Indicators are used to define a measurable dimension of quality.
5. Just as accreditation of HCOs is important, so is the accreditation of insurers. Employers that contract with insurers, providers, the government, and consumers are interested in the insurer accreditation.

Several organizations provide accreditation, and this has made it more complicated.

6. The NCQA, with its use of the HEDIS, is the most recognized of the managed care accrediting organizations.
7. Quality report cards, which provide specific performance data about an HCO or an insurer, are now available to providers and the public. These reports are used when purchasers of plans consider their choices. A key concern with the reports is whether the reader is interpreting and understanding the results correctly.
8. Typical methods that are used to monitor health care and for the accreditation process are standards of care, credentialing, UM, clinical guidelines, clinical pathways, benchmarking, EBP, risk management, and assessment of access.

References

Aliotta, S., et al. (2007). The impact of CMSA's case management adherence guidelines and guidelines training on case managers—reported behavior change. *Professional Case Manager, 12*(5), 288–295.

Berwick, D., Enthoven, A., & Bunker, J. (1992). Quality management in the NHS: The doctor's role—II. *British Medical Journal, 304*(6822), 304–308.

Berwick, D., & Nolan, T. (1998). Physicians as leaders improving health care. *Annals of Internal Medicine, 128*(4), 289–292.

Bindman, A. (1997). The challenge of measuring and monitoring quality. In J. Wilkerson, K. Devers, & R. Given (Eds.). *Competitive managed care: The emerging health care system.* San Francisco: Jossey-Bass Publishers.

Birmingham, J. (2007). Case management: Two regulations with coexisting functions (utilization review + discharge planning = case management). *Professional Case Management, 12*(1), 16–24.

Bodenheimer, T. (1999). The American health care system: The movement for improved quality in health care. *New England Journal of Medicine, 340*(6), 488–492.

Bower, K. (1992). *Case management by nurses.* Washington, DC: American Nurses Publishing.

Case Management Society of America. (CMSA). (2009). Case management adherence guidelines. (CMAG).

Retrieved from http://www.cmsa.org/Individual/Education/CaseManagementAdherenceGuidelines/tabid/253/Default.aspx on August 22, 2009.

Centers for Medicare and Medicaid Services. (CMS). (2007). Never Events. Retrieved from http://www.cms.hhs.gov/apps/media/press/release.asp?Counter=1863 on August 17, 2009.

Centers for Medicare and Medicaid Services. (CMS). (2009). Retrieved from www.cms.gov on March 2, 2009.

Case Management Society of America. (CMSA). (2002). *Standards of practice for case management.* Little Rock, AK: Author.

Donabedian, A. (1980). *Explorations in quality assessment and monitoring.* Vol. I: *The definition of quality and approaches to its assessment.* Ann Arbor, MI: Health Administration Press.

Institute for Healthcare Improvement. (IHI). (2009). Institute for Healthcare Improvement. Retrieved from http://www.ihi.org/ihi on June 30, 2009.

Institute of Medicine. (IOM). (1990). *Clinical practice guidelines: Directions for a new program.* Washington, DC: National Academies Press.

Institute of Medicine. (IOM). (1993). *Access to health care in American.* Washington, DC: National Academies Press.

Institute of Medicine. (IOM). (1999). *To err is human.* Washington, DC: National Academies Press.

Institute of Medicine. (IOM). (2001a). *Crossing the quality chasm.* Washington, DC: National Academies Press.

Institute of Medicine. (IOM). (2001b). *Envisioning the national health care quality report.* Washington, DC: National Academies Press.

Institute of Medicine. (IOM). (2003a). *Health professions education: A bridge to quality.* Washington, DC: National Academies Press.

Institute of Medicine. (IOM). (2003b). *Keeping patients safe. Transforming the work environment for nurses.* Washington, DC: National Academies Press.

Institute of Medicine. (IOM). (2004). *Insuring America's health.* Washington, DC: National Academies Press.

Institute of Medicine. (IOM) (2008). *Knowing what works in health care. A roadmap for the nation.* Washington, DC: National Academies Press.

Joint Commission. (2009a). 2009 Standards. Retrieved from http://www.jointcommission.org/AccreditationPrograms/Hospitals/Standards/09_FAQs/default.htm on August 19, 2009.

Joint Commission. (2009b). Certification of Disease Management Programs. Retrieved from http://www.jcaho.org on April 4, 2009.

Kongstvedt, P. (2009). *Managed care. What it is and how it works.* Boston: Jones and Bartlett Publishers.

Montalvo, I., & Dunton, N. (2007). *Transforming nursing data into quality care: Profiles of quality improvement in U.S. health care facilities.* Silver Spring, MD: American Nurses Association.

National Committee for Quality Assurance. (NCQA). (2009a). Report Cards. Retrieved from http://www.ncqa.org/tabid/60/Default.aspx on May 2, 2009.

National Committee for Quality Assurance. (NCQA). (2009c). Health Plan Accreditation. Retrieved from http://www.ncqa.org/tabid/689/Default.aspx on August 19, 2009.

National Guideline Clearinghouse. (2009). Clinical Guidelines. Retrieved, from http://www.guidelines.gov/ on April 16, 2009.

Pike, J., Jansen, R., & Brooks, P. (2002). Role and function of a hospital risk manager. *Journal of Legal Nursing Consultants, 13*(2), (3–13). Washington, DC: National Academies Press.

Plsek, P. (2001). Redesigning healthcare with insights form the science of complex adaptive systems. In Institute of Medicine, *Crossing the Quality Chasm* (pp. 309–322).

Reason, J. (2000). Human error: Models and management. *British Medical Journal, 320*(7237), 768–770.

Six Sigma. (2008). Retrieved from http://main.isixsigma.com/ on February 27, 2008.

URAC. (2009). URAC. Retrieved from http://www.urac.org/ on August 2, 2009.

Vann, J. (2006). Measuring community-based case management performance. *Lippincott's Case Management, 11*(3), 147–157.

Questions and Activities for Thought

1. What are two examples that demonstrate the increasing interest in the quality of care?
2. What does "quality" mean to you?
3. How are outcomes related to the assessment of care and accreditation?
4. Why is accreditation of insurers important?
5. What is the value of quality report cards?
6. Compare and contrast the organizations that accredit insurers.
7. Do you think case managers can have an impact on the quality of care? If so, how would this occur? Provide examples.

CASE

You have taken your first position as a case manager working for a hospital. You are the 200-bed rural hospital's first case manager. As you begin to think about your new position and the hospital, you consider how you are going to use QI Develop an outline of a plan for your first year. Consider all the possible methods described in this chapter. Include timelines and sources of data.

Internet Links

1 http://www.ahcpr.gov
Visit this site and click on "Quality & Patient Safety." What can you learn about *Americans as Health Care Consumers: The Role of Quality Information*?

2 http://www.ncqa.org
Visit this site and click on "HEDIS and Quality Measurement." What is the current news about the HEDIS? Access any HEDIS benchmarks that are

available. Does the HEDIS supply useful information? How might it be used in the managed care environment?

3 http://www.ncqa.org

Visit this site and click on "About NCQA." What is the NCQA? What information is available about accreditation? What does *meaningful improvement* mean in accreditation? Search for "QI Effectiveness: Defining 'Meaningful Improvement.'" What is the NCQA Quality Compass?

4 http://www.ahcpr.gov

Visit this site and click on "Quality & Patient Safety." Review the Department of Health and Human Services report *The Challenge and Potential of Assuring Quality Health Care for the 21st Century*. What problems does the report identify? What recommendations are suggested for solving these problems?

5 http://www.ahcpr.gov

Visit this site and click on "Research Findings" and then "Research Activities." What is the Nationwide Inpatient Sample? How might an MCO use this information in its QI effort?

6 http://www.urac.org

What is URAC? Click on "Consumers" and then "Accreditation." What is the accreditation process that is described? Why do MCOs want to be accredited? Why is a modular approach used for accreditation? Who develops the standards?

7 http://www.hcqualitycommission.gov

What is the main focus of this site? What has happened to the consumer rights effort? Review information on the report *Quality First: Better Health Care for All Americans*.

8 http://www.jcaho.org

Who sponsors this site? What is the report procedure for a complaint about an HCO? What is ORYX? Describe the accreditation process improvement provided by Joint Commission for managed care.

OTHER LINKS RELATED TO HEALTH CARE QUALITY

- Institute of Healthcare Improvement
  http://www.ihi.org
- Centers for Medicare and Medicaid Services/ OASIS Program
  http://www.cms.hhs.gov/OASIS/
- Joint Commission
  http://www.jointcommssion.org
- Clinician-Consumer Health Advisory Information Network (CHAIN)
  http://www.chainonline.org/content.cfm?menu_id=119
- The Joint Commission, Quality Check
  http://www.jointcommission.org/QualityCheck/06_qc_facts.htm
- Case Management Adherence Guidelines
  http://www.cmsa.org/Individual/Education/CaseManagementAdherenceGuidelines/CMAGWorkbooks/tabid/255/Default.aspx
- National Quality Forum. (NQF). (2009)
  http://www.qualityforum.org

CHAPTER 6

The Consumer and The Case Manager

OBJECTIVES

After completing this chapter, the reader will be able to:

- Describe the history of health care consumerism.
- Examine recent consumer legislative efforts.
- Define *consumer*.
- Distinguish between the employer and employee as health care consumers.
- Analyze the relationship between patient education and health care consumerism.
- Describe how consumers are involved in evaluating the quality of care.
- Discuss the case manager's role as patient advocate.
- Describe the following methods for increasing consumer participation: demand management, disease management, and case management.
- Explain the effect of technology on the health care consumer.
- Apply knowledge of health care coverage and reimbursement to assist the patient's understanding of health insurance.

KEY TERMS

Advocacy, p. 138
Benefit package, p. 147
Choice, p. 139
Consumer, p. 137
Consumer rights, p. 138
Copayments, p. 138
Covered services, p. 147
Deductibles, p. 138
Demand management, p. 143

Formulary, p. 143
Gatekeeper, p. 152
Grievances, p. 143
Macroconsumer, p. 139
Member services, p. 142
Microconsumer, p. 139
Out-of-pocket expenses, p. 146
Preexisting conditions, p. 147
Provider directory, p. 146

INTRODUCTION

What has happened to the **consumer** as health care has undergone major changes and managed care has had a major impact on health care reimbursement and delivery? This chapter addresses the needs of the consumer, particularly the enrollee or patient. The role of the consumer/enrollee/patient has become more important in the health care delivery process. By its very nature this process should place the patient and the patient's family in a major role throughout the process. As was mentioned in Chapter 1, patient-centered care is a health care core competency. Patient **advocacy** has long been an important component of nursing care. Nurses who are case managers can easily understand this process and the needs of patients. Patients as consumers of health care services have been gaining strength as they speak out about their health care, and they are concerned about the cost and quality of care. Changes that might occur would have an impact on case management.

There is no doubt that the patient is paying more for care as employers pay less. Premiums, **copayments**, and **deductibles** are increasing. Recognition of consumer priorities and understanding the criteria that consumers use as they evaluate their health care services are critical to maintaining a positive relationship between the employer and the employee. This requires that the employers, who select the plans that are offered to their employees, and third-party payers listen to their employees and enrollees and increase consumer involvement in decision making. **Consumer rights** and protection are front-page news as state and federal health care legislation escalates. Legislation, however, may lead to more problems, and thus must be considered carefully. There must be a balance between meeting the needs of all consumers, patients/enrollees/employees, employers, the government, providers, and insurers. The new health care reform legislation of 2010 emphasizes patient-centered care.

Helping the consumer to understand health care reimbursement, health care organization, choices the consumer can make, and the importance of an active role in managing one's own health care is an important contribution that case managers can make in their daily practice. Patients often turn to their case managers for guidance. Case managers should be prepared to answer their questions or know how to help patients seek the answers. Patient-centered health care means the case manager must be more aware of customer/patient needs, including the struggle that patients and their families are having with the complex health care reimbursement system. There is no doubt that managed care health plans are much more complicated than other types of third-party plans. Assessing their quality as a consumer is a confusing process. The reasons consumers, whether employers or employees, select one health insurance plan over another or discontinue a plan is very complex. Helping consumers as they make health care decisions is also complex. Case managers that work with Medicare or Medicaid beneficiaries also have to provide consumer guidance. This chapter discusses consumer education about health care coverage and the information that consumers/enrollees/patients need as they find their way through the health care reimbursement maze in order to select the right health care coverage for themselves and their families/significant others. Consumers also need to know how to effectively manage the use of the health care plan to maintain health and quality of life.

THE CONSUMER

Who Is the Consumer?

The consumer's role has changed as health care has undergone major changes, and managed care has become the dominant approach to health care reimbursement and delivery. This chapter addresses the role of the consumer or the patient in the health care delivery system. By its very nature the nursing process places both the patient and the patient's family in a major role. Patients as consumers of health care services have been gaining strength as they speak out about their health care. They are concerned about the quality of care and its cost. Nurses have had a role in this as well. Patient advocacy is an important component of nursing care. Nurse care managers understand the process and patient needs.

There is no doubt that the patient is paying more for care as employers pay less. Premiums, copayments, and deductibles are higher. It is important for employers, who select the plans that are offered to their employees, and third-party payers listen to their employees and enrollees and increase consumer involvement in decision making. Health care delivery organizations also need to know more about consumer issues. What does the patient expect? Is the outcome what the patient wanted? Case managers also need to take time to understand what is important to health care consumers. This will bring the consumer into the decision-making process and should improve patient outcome. As mentioned above, consumer rights and protection are front-page news today with changes brought about by state and federal legislation. Legislation, however, may lead to more problems, and thus must be considered carefully. A balance must exist between meeting the needs of all consumers, patients/enrollees/employees, employers, the government, providers, and insurers. Patient-centered health care means the nurse case manager must be more aware of customer/patient needs and also bring the patient into the process. There needs to be greater recognition of patient values and preferences, cultural issues, medical history and status, family and significant others, economic and social concerns, and other similar factors that impact each patient's life daily.

Consumers can be described in a variety of ways. A **macroconsumer** is a consumer who is a large purchaser of health care (e.g., employers, government). The macroconsumer may also be called the customer. Clearly, this type of consumer has a major voice in health care decisions owing to its size, and it acts as a liaison between insurers and employees. Much of the content in this text has focused on the macroconsumer. A microconsumer is the employee, the employee's family, and also people who buy insurance as individuals. They all become enrollees, members or beneficiaries, and patients. They are the users of the health care services. This chapter focuses on the **microconsumer**, the patient. All consumers, whether macro or micro, make decisions about the purchase of health care coverage. **Choice** is an important aspect of health care, and some consumers feel that their choices have diminished (e.g., choice of health plan has decreased as employers offer fewer plans and more tightly control the types of plans; limits on choice of providers; when the provider can be consulted have been affected; and the choice of using specialty care has diminished). As health care reimbursement has changed, choice has become an important consumer issue and one that is integral in many consumer complaints. In many instances the consumer's voice has helped to ensure consumer control over provider choice in the past few years. Third-party payers need to be aware of consumer needs and consumer satisfaction with the product or health care services, recognizing that the consumer can have an impact. Table 6-1 compares some of the consumer and customer needs.

TABLE 6-1   Customer and Consumer Needs

Customer	Consumer
Best value	Services
Affordable care	Access
Healthy employees	Choice
No hassle	Affordability

History of Health Care Consumerism

Health care consumerism evolved over many years. With the development of managed care, consumerism became even more important. Quality and access to services have been important issues throughout the history of the health care consumer movement and are even more important in the current health care environment. As managed care became the dominant player in the health care system in the 1990s, what happened to health care consumerism? Consumers were not as active in the early 1990s as they became at the end of the decade. Managed care developed on the West Coast and then moved to the East Coast. After that, managed care moved slowly across the country with some areas not feeling its effect until the mid-1990s. As this was occurring, managed care did not affect enough consumers to cause consumers to organize and protest against it. The media were not as cognizant of the changes, and managed care was not a front-page item. As more consumers were affected by managed care and managed care became stronger and had a major impact on health care delivery, consumers became concerned when the changes affected their personal care.

The sudden surge in health care consumer marketing was not the caprice of a few thousand executives who all attended the same industry conference. It signaled the changing demographics of America, as the typical consumer grows older, more affluent, and more educated. The baby boom generation has, in effect, been subsidizing the managed care system, paying more in premiums than it has taken out in claims. Now, this is changing with baby boomers entering retirement and a period of increased need for health care services. With the increasing focus on and access to communication technology, the consumer is demanding more and more information.

There is no doubt that as consumers experience problems with third-party payers and managed care, consumers often criticize managed care and demand changes. There are, however, aspects of managed care that are positive, such as its increased emphasis on preventive care, health promotion, and continuity, but it is easy to lose sight of the positive aspects of managed care and health care insurance in general. Emotions sometimes undermine rational policy changes and criticism. If the goal is to control costs, provide quality care, and increase care delivery to those who cannot afford care, it will be critical to find a balance and identify the strengths and limitations of managed care while building on its strengths.

Currently, insurers and providers recognize the need to listen to consumer criticisms and are more willing to make changes that address these criticisms. Today, patient-centered care is the focus. The recent Institute of Medicine (IOM) reports have highlighted this and even identify that providing patient-centered care is a core health care profession competency (Institute of Medicine, 2003). More effort has been made to provide the consumer with information. The need to obtain contracts from employers is one driving force. Insurers also want consumers to have more understanding about their health care needs in order to be informed purchasers of care and informed users of health care services. They believe that an informed health care consumer will reduce health care costs. At the same time, consumers are turning to government and legislation to influence health care policy-making and get their needs met.

Consumer Rights

Consumer rights have slowly become a major issue in health care policy, particularly owing to dissatisfaction with managed care. States are active in establishing requirements related to information that the insurer must supply to the consumer and to identify grievance and appeal requirements. The Patient Self-Determination Act of 1990 (PDSA) is a law that applies to all health care organizations (HCOs) (hospitals, long-term care facilities, and home health agencies) that participate in Medicare or Medicaid by receiving reimbursement from these government sources (American Cancer Society, 2008). What does this law require? All of these facilities must provide their patients with information about patients' rights, which are typically referred to as a Bill of Patients' Rights. Some of the rights that organizations typically develop relate to: (a) confidentiality, (b) consent, (c) right to make medical decisions, (d) right to be informed about diagnosis and treatment, (e) right to refuse treatment, and (f) use of advance directives.

The consumer rights issue is highly controversial. If too many consumer rights are recognized, how will this affect the ability of insurers to meet their goals to reduce health care costs? Reducing costs is a concern for all, not just the insurers. What effect will patient rights have on health care provider organizations? For example, the changes in patient privacy protection are costly to implement and yet they represent a consumer issue. Consumers also want costs lowered; however, the critical factor is what must be given up to reach this goal. HCOs such as hospitals, clinics, long-term care facilities, and home care agencies must consider how particular patient's rights might impact care and costs. Although probably initiated by dissatisfaction with managed care, many of the consumer-driven changes had little to do directly with managed care and in reality focused more on health care in general, leading to demands for a more patient-centered health care delivery system today.

The Consumer Assessment of Healthcare Providers and Systems (CAHPS) is a public-private program that develops patient surveys to assess patient perspectives of their ambulatory and facility level care (Consumer Assessment of Healthcare Providers and Systems, 2009). CAHPS is funded and administered through the Agency for Healthcare Research and Quality (AHRQ). The goals of this program are to assess patient-centeredness, compare contract performance, and improve quality of care. The data provide benchmarking opportunities for comparison of health plans (commercial plans, Medicare, and Medicaid), clinician groups, and hospitals. The CAHPS website is a valuable resource about consumer views of their health care. The site provides an interactive benchmarking database. A quality improvement (QI) process is described on the site that includes content related to plan strategy, development and testing of strategy, monitoring strategy, and reassessment and response. The level of content and resources this site provides indicates that consumer viewpoints about their health care are much more important than they were ten years ago.

CASE MANAGEMENT AND THE CONSUMER

Advocacy has always been a major aspect of the nursing role with the consumer. There are two important components of advocacy: (1) providing information that is useful to the patient and (2) supporting the patient's decision, which may not be the decision the case manager desired but nonetheless must be supported. Case managers who are nurses are particularly effective as advocates. The advocacy role with the third-party payer system and with case management must include helping the patient use the health care system and the patient's reimbursement system to the best advantage for the patient. To be successful, collaboration must be part of this process. The nurse case manager provides services through a collaborative relationship with the patient and the patient's family and advocates for the patient. To be an advocate, the case manager needs to be persuasive with the patient and with others with whom the case manager may interact on behalf of the patient. Advocacy does not mean that the case manager takes over for the patient, but rather that the case manager helps the patient to be independent, recognizing that the patient is a stakeholder in the care process. Changes in reimbursement such as the expansion of managed care has certainly affected physician–patient relationships. The physician may be involved in making decisions based on financial issues rather than as an advocate for the patient's needs. How has this also affected the case manager's role as advocate? Nurse case managers can guide the patient, for example, to use grievance and appeal processes or to understand how the primary care physician (PCP) makes decisions about specialty referral. An advocate must also recognize limits. A nurse is not a health care insurance expert; however, a nurse case manager can combine nursing expertise with case management expertise.

Advocacy needs to be part of daily case management practice. A perspective of advocacy described by Gilkey, Earp, and French (2008) describes advocacy as a continuum.

- The individual level focuses on informing patients, and considers "interventions that target the personal beliefs, attitudes, and knowledge needed to achieve health" (p. 17). This would include self-management and patient education. Chronic illness, discussed earlier in this book, is a critical concern. E-health has become increasingly important as consumers turn to the Internet for information.
- The next level is the interpersonal level focusing on supporting and empowering patients. Interventions such as "advice giving, emotional support, and provision of resources and other help" (p. 18) are an integral part of this level, and all require interpersonal interactions. Families and significant others need to be brought into this process.
- The third level is the organizational and community level focusing on transforming culture. What are organizations and communities doing to support patient advocacy?
- The fourth level is the policy level focusing on translating consumer voice into policies and laws. "In patient advocacy, important policies are those that (1) control access to patient care; (2) regulate health care organizations, especially with regard to patient safety surveillance; and (3) protect health care consumers" (Gilkey, Earp, & French, p. 21).

THE CONSUMER AND HEALTH CARE REIMBURSEMENT

Role of the Consumer: Employer and Employee

The role of the employer in the selection of health care coverage is very important. The employer takes the first step toward health care coverage for its employees by selecting the plans that will be offered for employees to purchase. What does the employer look for as plans are reviewed? The employer is interested in information about the provider network or panel, quality of care and outcomes, customer or **member services,** medical management and utilization, information systems, financial performance, and cost to the employer. Case management services should also be of interest to employers as they review plan options. The employer wants the best value for the price. Insurers need to demonstrate that their plans can ensure quality care and control costs. The employer wants as little ongoing involvement in the reimbursement process as possible and also wants limited complaints about health care coverage from its employees. After the employer selects the plan options, employees have the opportunity to enroll in the plan of their choice from the plan options. Employers review plan options and contracts annually with insurers. Their decisions directly affect employees' choices and may mean that employees must make changes in insurers and even providers. Consumers also need to be more responsible and accountable for their own health care and make more informed health care decisions. They need to be more aware of costs and resource utilization. In some situations, employees are involved in the employer health plan selection process of health care coverage options. In unionized businesses, unions play an active role in this process. Some employers include employees on the committee that evaluates the plans. Complaints and **grievances** from employees about their coverage are also influential. Third-party payers know that member satisfaction is important and should not be ignored. Enrollee satisfaction may mean the difference between getting a contract and losing a contract.

New Efforts to Increase Consumer Participation

The growth of managed care provided the opportunity to develop new models and methods of care to increase consumer participation. Case management is certainly one of the methods. Other examples are demand management and disease management.

- *Demand management* focuses on services or support that assist the consumer (member or enrollee) and includes self-help tools, nurse advice telephone services, and preventive services with the goal of decreasing demand for services (Kongstvedt, 2009). Demand management seems to accomplish two goals. It increases patient satisfaction and decreases utilization of services, bringing the consumer into the process to make informed health care decisions. This approach supports patient-centered care.
- *Disease management* (DM) also increases patient participation and satisfaction and provides better control over utilization of services. The focus is on patients with chronic illness, whose care can be very costly. Disease management is "the process of intensively managing a particular disease" (Kongstvedt, 2009, p. 218). It is similar to case management but is much more focused on prevention and maintenance. Case management may be used in a DM program. Consumer education also plays a significant role in DM, as it does in all efforts to increase consumer participation. More information about DM is found in Chapter 7.

The Medicare Consumer

The Medicare consumer can now obtain comparison information about plans on the Internet. The Balanced Budget Act of 1997 required the HCFA provide this information to consumers. The HCFA also works with senior advocacy groups to determine the best methods for informing seniors about their new Medicare+Choice options. The lack of plan consistency, however, makes it difficult for the beneficiary to compare plans. Consumers may not understand the meaning of the terminology that is typically used in plan descriptions, such as **formulary,** *cap,* and *description of benefits*. The HCFA must approve insurer marketing material in an effort to ensure consumer understanding, but even this has not guaranteed consistency. It also takes time to ensure the quality of the materials. The Ombudsman Center, Centers for Medicare and Medicare Services (CMS) offers current information to Medicare (and Medicaid) beneficiaries (http://www.cms.hhs.gov/center/ombudsman.asp). Box 6-1 provides some facts to help consumers who receive federal benefits.

BOX 6-1

Federal Benefits

FAST FACTS Got Quality Healthcare?

Are you searching for information to help you choose a quality health plan for you and your family?

- How well does your health plan help you and your family stay healthy?

- Do you get the best care available when you're ill?
- What do your co-workers, friends and doctors say about the plans available to you?

We know that when choosing a health plan you carefully consider cost, whether your doctor is in the plan, and what is or is not covered. You should also pay attention to indicators that measure health plan quality: This information can help you avoid making an uninformed decision that could put your family's health at risk.

Current research tells us that:

- Quality varies from one plan to another
- Quality can be measured accurately and fairly
- The plan you choose can determine the quality of care you get

Here are three ways to evaluate health plan quality:

1. Consumer Surveys
2. Effectiveness of Care
3. Health Plan Accreditation

1. *Consumers Assessment of Healthcare Providers and Systems* (CAHPS) is a satisfaction survey designed by national experts in healthcare quality. CAHPS captures data on quality from the patient's point of view that is, topics for which enrollees and patients are the best sources of information. These items address consumers' experiences with health care providers and with the health plan itself (including customer services), but not the Federal Employees Dental and Vision Insurance Program. Individual FEHB plan results are found in the *Guide to Federal Benefits* at www.opm.gov/insure/health/planinfo/guides/index.asp and in the plan comparison tool at www.opm.gov/insure/health/search/.

Do enrollees in the health plan say, for example:

- They are satisfied with their health plan
- They got the care they felt they needed
- They received the information or help they needed from the plancustomer service department

CAHPS results answer these questions and more.

2. *Effectiveness of care* is measured by the Healthcare Effectiveness Data and Information Set (HEDIS), an important measure of services provided in your doctor's office and in hospitals, based on information such as members' medical records. HEDIS measures how well your plan prevents and treats conditions

HEDIS results for individual plans answer questions such as:

- Are patients receiving preventive care (e.g., immunizations for children, and eye exams for diabetics)?
- Do pregnant women get all the prenatal care they need?
- Are patients with high blood pressure regularly screened?
- Go to our website at http://www.opm.gov/insure/health/planinfo/quality/hedis.aspx to see the many measures we report and to see how your plan compares against the FEHB average and other plans.

3. *Health Plan Accreditation* is conducted by independent national organizations, not the health plans, that evaluate the systems that plans have in place to ensure and improve healthcare quality. Health plan accreditation is a "seal of approval" from the accrediting organization. Has your plan received the highest accreditation level available, something in the middle of the pack, or even something lower? Different organizations accredit health plans using different rating scales and even offer different types of accreditation; what's important is that the health plan has submitted itself to the rigors of an external, independent evaluation.

Check your health plan's brochure for its accreditation level or look for the Health Plan Accreditation link at www.opm.gov/insure/health/planinfo/quality/index.asp.

Source: U.S. Office of Personnel Management. Retrieved from http://www.opm.gov/insure/fastfacts/qualityhealthcare.pdf on August 15, 2009.

HOW DOES THE CASE MANAGER HELP THE CONSUMER WITH HEALTH CARE COVERAGE?

Most consumers need to know more about health care coverage, selection of a health plan, use of the plan, and evaluation of the plan. It is important for case managers to know this information and be ready to discuss it with patients and families. Case managers today are working in settings that demand that they know about changes in the health care environment and how these changes affect patients and practice. Patients expect the case manager to be their advocates. This content provides a framework for discussing health care plans with patients as consumers of health care. The content relates to content found in Chapters 3 and 4, but in this chapter this content is described from the consumer perspective and in a manner that makes it useful for a case manager to use with patients and families.

Selecting the Right Health Care Plan

The typical way that people select their health care coverage today is to check to see if their key provider(s) is in the "book" or on the approved provider list. What does this mean, and why is it done? Selecting the right health care plan is a complex decision; however, with information and guidance, consumers can be prepared to make a decision that meets their health care needs. Choosing coverage today is different from in the past when the common choice was a traditional indemnity insurance plan. A person would select the plan and then continue to see his or her own family physician or a specialist. Typically, either the physician would bill the insurer or the patient would pay the physician and then be reimbursed by the patient's insurer. The patient would pay any required deductibles and copayment. If the patient had to go into the hospital, the patient and the patient's physician would decide on the best choice for the patient, but a critical factor would be where the physician had admission privileges. Today, this type of traditional coverage, fee-for-service (FFS), is difficult to find and expensive.

What is the employer's role in plan selection? Employers now play a major role in the selection process by selecting the plans from which the employee may choose. Some employers offer several types of plans for their employees, and some offer only one choice, often a health maintenance organization (HMO). The latter eliminates employee choice, but this does not mean that the employee does not need to learn how the HMO can benefit the employee as a plan member. Critical information that consumers need to know concerns costs, degree of provider (e.g., physician, hospital) choice, the benefit plan, the plan's reputation, access to care, convenience, utilization review and authorization, quality, and responsiveness to plan members. The first step is to understand what types of plans the employer has selected.

Types of Plans and Managed Care Models

The various types of health plans and managed care models that health plans use can seem complicated and may overwhelm consumers. Chapter 4 described some of the types of plans in more detail. Cost and choice are the important distinctions used to compare the different managed care models. Generally, when cost is low, consumers experience less choice. For example, HMOs cost less, and the patient has less choice of providers (e.g., physician/advanced practice nurse, hospital, laboratory). Some HMOs provide all of their services in one location, which does limit some of the enrollee/patient choices, but for some this may be viewed as more convenient. The name *health maintenance organization* implies an organization interested in maintaining health, and HMOs have typically covered health promotion and disease and illness preventive care. It should be noted that now other types of managed care organization (MCO) and insurer models also provide some preventive services, so it is important to review the benefit description. Other plans may cost more but may provide more choice for the consumer. Preferred provider organizations (PPOs) have become more popular because they allow more flexibility in choosing a physician or provider; however, if the patient uses a provider outside the approved PPO list of providers, including hospitals, the patient pays more for services from these providers. Another common model is the point-of-service (POS) plan. This type of plan allows the patient to make a decision about a provider when a specific health care service is needed. For example, if the enrollee becomes ill and needs to see a specialist, the enrollee can decide at that time to use one of the specialists approved by the plan or go outside the plan providers. If the latter is chosen, it will cost the patient more. There are differences in plans such as some use carve-outs, which are medical services that are separated from the general plan. Examples of services that may be carved out are dental, mental health, and substance abuse treatment. A health plan does this to better control utilization and costs for these services. If an enrollee thinks these services might be needed in the future, the enrollee needs to learn more about the carve-out provision. These benefits and authorization for their use may be very different from those provided for general health needs.

Choice

Choice is an important aspect of health care coverage. The first issue related to consumer choice is the choice of health plan(s), which is controlled by the employer, who identifies which plans will be offered to employees. Each employer selects the health plans it will offer to its employees. If individuals are buying their own insurance, they may choose any plan for which they qualify and wish to pay. There are other important choice issues. Is there a **provider directory** or panel, and if so, does the approved provider provide enough choice? Are there providers in the directory that the consumer recognizes or has used? This is particularly important if the consumer's current physician is not listed in the directory. Does the plan give a choice of hospitals? If there is only one approved hospital, its reputation may be of critical concern when a plan is compared with another plan option that has several approved hospitals. Is the panel of specialists a large one, providing the consumer with greater choice? After a consumer joins a plan and becomes an enrollee, some plans require that the enrollee select a primary care provider. If the selected provider leaves the provider panel of plan, a new provider must be selected, so it is important to review the directory for more than one provider. Providers and plans are not required to notify patients/enrollees of these changes, and few do. A patient may call the office for an appointment only to find out that the physician or nurse practitioner is no longer reimbursed by the patient's health plan. If a consumer joins a plan that uses POS, he or she has more choices to make when services are needed, for example, to use a provider on the plan provider list or a provider who is not approved by the plan.

Cost

How does the plan pay for health care? To become enrollees of a health plan, consumers pay an insurance premium to join. Since the U.S. health care insurance system is driven mostly by employee health care insurance plans, this is paid monthly via an enrollee's employer. If an individual is purchasing insurance for himself or herself, the individual pays the premium directly to the insurer. There are other **out-of-pocket expenses.** The enrollee must pay a deductible, which is the amount of covered expense that is paid before the insurer will pay for health care services. After the designated deductible is paid for the year, the enrollee does not pay any more deductible for that year. Many plans also have a copayment. This is the amount that must be paid for every service, and it is another out-of-pocket expense. A copayment may be a specific amount regardless of the service received. For example, the insurer may cover prescriptions, but the patient must pay $4 for every prescription. If the enrollee must share some of the cost with the plan, this is called coinsurance. A typical arrangement is 80/20: The insurer pays 80%, and enrollee/patient pays 20%. The plan may not reimburse for use of providers that are not approved by the plan or may require that the patient pay a higher copayment if nonapproved providers are used. This means that the insurer continues to reimburse for the care, but the patient has a higher out-of-pocket payment and thus must cover more of the total cost. Today, insurers want their enrollees to be more aware of the costs of care and hope that this awareness will make enrollees/consumers more careful health care shoppers. Plans also protect enrollees by setting annual limits on how much enrollees pay in total. Health care reform legislation of 2010 will eliminate annual limits when the law is implemented. HMOs operate differently because they cover all of the care approved by the HMO. Some HMOs require that enrollees pay a small copayment for visits.

How does the insurer pay the provider? Some plans still pay providers for services as they did on an FFS basis. Managed care, however, has made capitation a more common form of reimbursement. Insurers that use capitation pay physicians and other providers a specific amount per month per member enrolled. The provider will be paid this amount whether the enrollee receives care or not. How does this affect the provider's decisions and how much time the physician spends with the patient? There may be an incentive for the provider to do less, and this is a growing concern about capitation. Hospitals can also be reimbursed on a capitation basis. They may be reimbursed a specific amount for each hospital day. If a patient is hospitalized longer than expected, it will cost the hospital more because the insurer will not pay more for the care. This serves as an incentive to discharge the patient. Since there is variation in plans, it is difficult to describe only one approach. Case managers need to understand an individual patient's health plan.

Benefit Package

The **benefit package** is very important because it tells enrollees what health services the plan covers, what it does not cover, and what it covers partially or with limitations. The package should be described in the plan information that is provided to enrollees prior to making a final enrollment decision. **Covered services** are health services that the plan will cover if they are considered to be medically necessary. In determining medical necessity, the insurer assesses appropriateness of the treatment for an individual patient/enrollee based on diagnosis and needs. The insurer's decisions are based on standards that the insurer develops as well as on professional standards. The plan may also limit who may provide the service (e.g., type of professional), where service is provided, and number of visits, treatments, days of care, and so forth. The physician, nurse practitioner, or nurse midwife has a role in this decision making. This takes considerable provider time, particularly if there is a question about medical necessity. The basic services that most plans cover are:

- Physician's/provider's office visits
- Hospital room and board
- Inpatient and outpatient surgery
- Services provided by nurses, such as home care nurses, nurse practitioners, or nurse midwives
- Diagnostic and radiology testing
- Ambulance services
- Medical equipment rental for the home

There are some services that vary a great deal from plan to plan. Dental and vision are usually not covered, but some employers offer carve-out plans for these services. Other types of plans sometimes cover health promotion and disease and illness preventive care, which are more common with HMOs but are increasing with other types of insurer models. Expensive procedures may require special permission from the insurer.

There are other terms that are important in the benefit package, for example, exclusions, limitations, and **preexisting conditions.** The plan identifies diagnoses, conditions, and services that it will not cover or reimburse; however, as health care reform of 2010 is implemented, insurers will not be able to use preexisting conditions to limit insurance coverage. These are the exclusions and limitations. In the past, enrollees or family members who had a mental or physical condition prior to purchasing a plan often experienced problems with preexisting condition clauses. Issues around preexisting conditions are very problematic.

Special Care Issues

Special care issues are important as an enrollee selects a plan. Examples of several special care issues follow.

MENTAL HEALTH AND SUBSTANCE ABUSE TREATMENT. Historically, insurers have been more restrictive with mental health and substance abuse services and may also use carve-outs to cover them. Carve-outs are plans that are different from the general medical plan. Frequently, insurers require that these services have different and more stringent authorization, higher out-of-pocket expenses for the enrollee, and different provider panels. An increasing number of insurers are covering less treatment for these problems. The Mental Health Parity Act of 1996, a federal law, went into effect in 1998. Its purpose was to ensure equal treatment for physical and mental illness by banning annual and lifetime caps on mental health benefits; however, insurers were still able to limit the number of outpatient visits or hospital days. This manipulation of treatment continued to make mental health reimbursement different from general medical care reimbursement. As a result of the concerns about treatment manipulation to limit outpatient and inpatient treatment, another bill was passed in 2008 (the Mental Health Parity and Addiction Equity Act). This law went into effect January 2010 and applies to all types of health plans. "The Mental Health Parity and Addiction Equity Act does not require health insurance plans to provide mental health or substance use disorder benefits. However, for group health plans with 50 or more employees that choose to provide mental health and substance use disorder benefits, the Act does require parity with medical and surgical benefits" (Human Resources News, 2009).

What are some of the issues related to mental health treatments that are important to consider as a health plan is selected? If an enrollee or a family member has been receiving services from a particular provider, it is important to check if that provider is on the provider panel as well as the number of provider choices that are available. If visits are limited, this may be very important. How are appointments to see a mental health provider to be made? Is a referral from a PCP required? How long does it take to get an appointment? What hospitals are included in the provider list? If a patient experiences problems receiving this care, an advocacy organization may be a helpful resource, such as the National Alliance for Mental Illness, http://www.nami.org/. Case management is used in mental health care.

MATERNITY CARE. If maternity care may be required, a review of these benefits is important. Maternity care has become highly personal, involving, for example, choosing to use birthing centers and nurse midwives, and consideration of the philosophy of family in the birthing room. Consequently, enrollees need to investigate if the plan supports their special needs and viewpoints of childbirth. If the enrollee or family member has been seeing a provider prior to joining the plan, is it possible for this relationship to continue during pregnancy? Is the physician or nurse midwife on the provider panel? What hospitals are on the panel, and do they meet the patient's needs? What neonatal services are provided for the newborn? If the newborn experiences critical problems, do the hospitals in the panel provide neonatal intensive care services, or would the baby need to be transported to another hospital? If a provider is chosen from outside the panel, how much will this cost the enrollee? Consumers who require fertility specialists may find that this coverage is limited or does not exist. This care can be very expensive. If the enrollee or family member has a chronic illness such as diabetes or knows that the pregnancy will be high risk, it is important to know what benefits are covered and who is on the provider panel with expertise that will meet the special needs. The issue of the length of hospitalization after delivery has become very important. Insurers are now required to cover at least 48 hours of hospitalization for vaginal delivery and 96 hours for a cesarean section. There may be circumstances in which the baby or the new mother stays in the hospital longer. How does the plan cover this situation? Some plans are now providing a home visit soon after discharge to check on the new mother and baby. Finding out the answers to these questions will alleviate stress later. Case management may be used for complex, high-risk pregnancies.

CHRONIC ILLNESS.   If an enrollee or a family member has a chronic illness, selecting a health care plan that meets these specific needs is important, particularly choice of PCP, specialty care required, medications, and medical equipment. Is the enrollee's present physician(s) or provider on the provider panel? The plan's formulary and its rules are also important. If the plan uses generic or therapeutic substitution drugs, this might be a problem if the patient uses a particular medication that has been effective and is not in the plan formulary. The plan may not reimburse for the medication or may require higher copayment from the patient. If special medical equipment is required for care at home, does the plan reimburse for its use? What are the limitations? Some plans now use case management and disease management plans that focus on specific chronic illnesses such as diabetes, asthma, or arthritis. These programs may help monitor the illness and provide up-to-date consumer education about the illness and its treatment, and to increase self-management.

ALTERNATIVE/COMPLEMENTARY THERAPIES.   Interest in alternative therapies has been increasing, and some insurers are reimbursing for some of these therapies. If research on their effectiveness is positive, this coverage will probably increase. Examples of these therapies are acupuncture, Oriental medicine, naturopathy, massage, herbal therapies, relaxation, and healing touch. If an enrollee has used these therapies or is interested in trying them, it is necessary to find out if these services are covered. For example, if an enrollee has been using a chiropractor, some plans will not cover this service.

EXPERIMENTAL TREATMENT/CLINICAL TRIALS.   Experimental treatment or clinical trials may not be something that comes up regularly; however, there may come a time when it is considered, for example, cancer treatment or clinical trials for new cardiac medications. Plans vary in their coverage of this treatment. Before approving the use of experimental treatment insurers consider cost, possible outcomes, complications, and length of treatment. There have been changes in this area, and some insurers are now more flexible about experimental treatment. The National Institutes of Health (NIH) has a website that focuses on clinical trials (http://clinicalresearch.nih.gov/). This site answers questions such as:

- How does clinical research work?
- Who participates in clinical research?
- What do I need to know if I am thinking of participating?
- Where can I find clinical trials?
- What happens after a clinical trial is completed?

Ethical issues are also discussed on the site. This is a useful site for case managers, patients, and families.

Member Services

Insurer member services is synonymous with customer services or consumer affairs. It is a very important department. The focus of member services is typically not on membership enrollment but rather on helping the enrollee or member with problems and grievances, tracking consumer issues and resolutions, and improving member satisfaction.

Basically, member services help enrollees use the plan to reach the best outcomes, cost, and quality. This department has frequent contact with enrollees, and thus its performance needs to be evaluated regularly. This evaluation may include telephone responsiveness, timeliness of response, and productivity of department and individual service representatives. Staff from this department are often involved in outreach or making contact with new enrollees to explain how the plan works. The goal is to reduce enrollee complaints and need for assistance. Patients may need additional guidance as issues arise, and the case manager may be involved in meeting these needs.

Complaints and Grievances

Complaints and grievances occur with any insurer. Complaints usually relate to concerns about staff attitudes and administrative service problems. These are usually settled by member services. Examples of complaints might be poor response to telephone calls to the insurer or provider, delayed receipt of printed material, and so on.

Grievances are more serious and focus on issues such as denial of claims for payment and requests for exceptions to the benefit contract. If an enrollee is dissatisfied with a decision, the enrollee may appeal the decision. The plan's printed information should explain the grievance and appeal processes, but frequently this information is confusing. Following the designated time limits is critical because the appeal opportunity can be lost if the time limits are not met. A grievance filing requires detailed information such as providers, description of the event or situation in detail, follow-up, and other relevant information. It is important to know to whom to address grievances, how long the enrollee has to file a grievance, how long the plan has to respond, whom to call if the enrollee does not get a response, and the appeal process. The patient's physician may be directly involved in the grievance even the grievance is not against the physician. Medical information may need to be provided by the physician. Grievances are stressful, but there are times when they are necessary.

TECHNOLOGY AND THE CONSUMER

With the increased interest in quality and cost of health care, there is an increasing amount of information available to consumers about health care. The Internet is particularly helpful if more current information is required; however, the quality and reliability of the information varies. It is important to know who has developed the Internet site and its content. National organizations and the government often provide the best information. Health literacy is also a topic the IOM addressed in its report (2004). The report highlights that health outcomes and the provision of high-quality care requires clear and effective communication. Even well-educated patients do not always understand medical information. The report states that 99 million people have problems understanding the information. The definition of health literacy from the IOM is: "The degree to which individuals have the capacity to obtain, process, and understand basic health information and services needed to make appropriate health decisions" (Ratzan & Partker, 2000 as cited in Institute of Medicine, 2004, p. 4).

Technology has revolutionized consumer access to information. Interactive technology has certainly changed the availability of information, particularly electronic mail, websites, intranets, and interactive voice response systems. These new technologies offer additional ways to communicate with current customers and to collect, manage, and utilize health care information that will help insurers keep current with customers and also recruit new ones. This technology is now used by third-party payers all types of health care providers, the government, and consumer organizations.

Technology opens up new roles for the case manager in the health care system and reimbursement. Nurse case managers may play an active role in the development and maintenance of these sites for providers and insurers who want to make them available to members. Content needs to be accurate and useful, and nurse case managers have the clinical expertise and ability to develop this content for consumers. To focus on customer service, large companies may hire nurse case managers in full-time positions, or they may be contracted to assist in developing this content on an as-needed basis. Case managers who participate in these projects need to understand reimbursement, clinical needs, educational principles, the use of technology to provide information and teach, and they need to be creative. Computer expertise is a plus, but in most cases, it is not required. Most providers and insurers who develop sites have computer experts to assist in this aspect of the project.

National organizations and the government often provide the best information. *Healthy People 2010* addresses the issue of communication and emphasizes the need for appropriate communication at individual and community levels (U.S. Department of Health and Human Services, 1998). Information and education play vital roles in promoting health; preventing, managing, and coping with disease; and supporting appropriate decisions across the spectrum of health care. For individuals, effective health communication can help raise awareness of health risks, provide motivation and skills to reduce them, bring helpful connections to others in similar situations, and offer information about difficult choices, such as health plans and providers, treatments, and long-term care.

USING THE HEALTH CARE PLAN

Self-Managing Care

Consumers should be able manage their own care. Even if they choose not to receive provider care, they have made a decision about the importance of their health. The best way to prevent problems and reduce health care costs is to practice self-management, health promotion, and disease and illness prevention. Collaborating with health care providers to understand treatment choices, understand patient and health care provider responsibilities, and follow the treatment selected is critical to positive health care outcomes. If patients are involved in their health care decisions, they will be more satisfied with their health care. Seeking information to increase understanding is very important. In addition, enrollees need to collaborate with their insurers who play a major role in their health care decisions.

Authorization is part of the insurer-enrollee process (Kongstvedt, 2009). As patients manage their own care, it is important to understand why authorization is done and how it is done. When patients cannot get the care that they believe is needed, it can be very frustrating and stressful. There are ten reasons why an insurer uses authorization (Kongstvedt, 2009):

1. Verify eligibility for the service coverage
2. Certify that the enrollee receives the benefits in the contract
3. Pay claims to contracted providers
4. Validate the medical necessity and appropriateness of care
5. Screen for procedures that require a second opinion
6. Screen for medications that are not in the plan formulary
7. Screen for the appropriate treatment setting
8. Provide information for case management
9. Track utilization patterns
10. Control costs and financial management

Who authorizes care? There can be wide variation among plans as to who must authorize care, and it can be very complicated. The PCP, as **gatekeeper,** may authorize treatment. An interdisciplinary team within the health plan or an outside organization referred to as a utilization management/review (UM/UR) organization may authorize treatment. Some insurers use their own staff to authorize care. Another approach is to identify treatments and services that have automatic authorization, for example, Pap smears, hernia repair, vaccinations, and mammograms. The common services requiring authorization are hospital admission, emergency room care, continued stay in the hospital, transfer to another facility, access to alternative care settings, experimental procedures, expensive diagnostic procedures, nuclear diagnostic procedures, treadmill stress tests, invasive diagnostic and therapeutic procedures, inpatient surgery, same-day surgery, and any high-cost service (Kongstvedt, 2009). The health plan should identify which services require authorization. What happens if the patient misses an appointment for an authorized service? Some plans may require that the service be reauthorized.

Primary Care Physicians and Specialists

Managed care has made the term *provider* important and uses this term for a variety of providers of care. For example, physicians, nurse practitioners, nurse midwives, hospitals, home health agencies, and long-term care facilities are all providers. One of the most critical providers is the PCP, which is used by many plans but not all. Usually, this is a physician, who is often referred to as the gatekeeper and is responsible for overseeing and coordinating the patient's care. Some plans require that the PCP approve the use of specialists before specialty care will be reimbursed. Can any physician be a PCP? Certain types of physicians are recognized as PCPs by the insurer. Typically, these are general practitioners, family practice physicians, internal medicine physicians, and pediatricians; and recently, more plans are including obstetricians and gynecologists. Some plans now accept nurse practitioners and nurse midwives as PCPs. Because most medical decisions are made with the PCP (e.g., medications, laboratory testing, frequency of exams, hospitalization, home care), the PCP is very important. The PCP manages the patient's needs throughout the continuum of care with the patient to ensure that needs are met. Typical services that are provided are:

- Health promotion and education
- Disease and illness prevention
- Urgent/immediate care
- Routine ambulatory care
- Diagnosis or treatment by ancillary services (e.g., physical therapy, respiratory therapy, occupational therapy)
- Acute inpatient care
- Intensive care
- Subacute skilled nursing care
- Home care nursing
- Assisted living
- Long-term care
- Hospice care

The physician does not work alone. Other professionals who often work with physicians are nurses, advanced practice nurses, nurse midwives, physician assistants, certified registered nurse anesthetists, and many other health care professionals. Physicians who are selected for the plan's approved provider panel must meet criteria established by the plan. These criteria usually include board certification, which indicates that the physician has met specific standards and passed an exam. This is in addition to the physician's medical board exams. The insurer is also interested in whether the physician has been involved in a malpractice suit and the results of the suit. Professional references are also required. Many plans also assess the physician's practice and services. HMO physicians are usually employees of the HMO; however, other types of plans contract with their physician providers. These contracts are for specific time periods, and thus this allows the plan to review the physicians periodically during contract renewal. At these times, plans evaluate specific practice or performance issues, such as hospitalization rates, prescription history, laboratory testing, complications, medical record review results, compliance with standards, and patient satisfaction. In order to renew a contract, physicians and other providers are now evaluated carefully, and sometimes contracts are not renewed. In fact, some experts believe that physicians' performance is evaluated better than performance was evaluated in the FFS system. It is important to recognize that some physicians choose not to renew a contract with a managed care or insurer plan. Why would they make this decision? Typical reasons include:

- The number or types of patients that the physician expected to be referred by the plan did not materialize.
- The payment rates were not satisfactory.
- The plan's administrative services were not what the physician expected.
- The physician did not feel comfortable with the plan's authorization and medical decision-making process.

Referral to specialty care has been changed by many health plans. In the past, patients often consulted their physician about the need for a specialist or might even have decided for themselves that the problem required a specialist. The insurer did not usually tell enrollees if they could see specialists. Now, the insurer may tell enrollees when and what type of provider to see or even determine if enrollees really need specialty care. Some plans require approval for every visit to a specialist and may require approval of all of the specialist's medical decisions, such as medication, laboratory testing, and hospitalization. As discussed in Chapter 3, special physicians called intensivists or hospitalists, who may provide all hospital care instead of the patient's PCP or specialist. This means that the physician who cares for the patient in the hospital may be a stranger who will have contact with patient's ambulatory care physician or PCP, but will make all decisions about the patient's hospital care. The patient may speak to the case manager about this different approach to medical coverage in the hospital. The case manager would have contact with both the patient's physician and the physician covering the patient's care in the hospital and can provide critical information and help to coordinate services, particularly at the time of discharge.

Medications and the Plan Formulary

If a patient takes medications regularly, he or she will want to inquire about the plan's formulary and policies about generic substitution and therapeutic substitution. The plan formulary identifies the prescription drugs that the plan reimburses for its enrollees (Kongstvedt, 2009). The plan considers medication safety, effectiveness, cost, and cost effectiveness of the drugs it selects for its formulary. The plan may also consider how medications affect quality of life or the ability to carry on normal activities. Providers are informed about the formulary and encouraged to follow it. Some plans track the prescription of formulary drugs versus nonformulary drugs. An important question is whether the formulary is open, closed, or incentive. The types of formularies were discussed in Chapter 4.

Medications are a very important treatment intervention today, and an increasing number of new medications are coming in the market. Many will be very effective but expensive. This will undoubtedly increase the importance of plan formularies. If the plan allows generic substitution, the provider may prescribe medications that are a replacement for another medication containing the same active ingredient in the same amount and dosage form. These are sold by different pharmaceutical companies and are usually cheaper. Therapeutic substitution may also occur. Some plans and hospitals allow pharmacists to substitute medications that are different from those prescribed by an enrollee's physician. The substituted medications must be in the same pharmacological or therapeutic class. The substitutions are usually in the hospital or plan formulary. How is this different from generic substitution? These drugs may have different side effects, biological effects, and interactions. In addition, the physician may not even know the substitution has been made. The plan may not only manage the enrollee's prescriptions, but it may also designate which pharmacy may fill the prescriptions. How convenient is the pharmacy? This affects accessibility of treatment and can be very important.

Hospitalization

The plan also selects the hospitals enrollees may use. Some plans have several hospitals that they have approved for reimbursement, whereas others have only one. This clearly affects patient's choices. As was true in the past, providers need to be credentialed to practice in the selected hospitals. Prior to a plan's contracting with a hospital, the plan evaluates the hospital, accreditation status, its services, and performance data. Competition among hospitals for these contracts is intense. The end-of-chapter Internet Links list provides a link to compare hospitals through an interactive database provided by the U.S. Department of Health and Human Services.

What happens when an enrollee is out of town and needs to go to an emergency room or be hospitalized? Will the insurer cover this care? If it is a minor problem, the enrollee might try using an urgent care center that treats less serious emergencies. Whenever care is received out of town, the enrollee needs to take his or her health plan identification card and notify the plan about the care received within 24 hours of treatment or the time period required by the insurer. Copayments and deductibles are still required when enrollees receive out-of-town care that is approved for reimbursement by the insurer. The enrollee should also take his or her physician's telephone number and address because this information may be required. The enrollee will need to have documentation of any treatment received sent to his or her PCP for the enrollee's medical record. International care is typically not covered, but it may be purchased as needed for travel.

Consumer Evaluation of the Health Care Plan

Evaluation of health care plans occurs when consumers are selecting coverage to purchase, as they receive care covered by the plan, and when they reenroll in a health care plan. The consumer now has many resources for obtaining information about a health care plan, and the availability of this information is increasing. Some of the issues and data that consumers need to consider in evaluating health care plans are its accreditation status, report cards, and consumer satisfaction data, discussed in Chapter 5.

Patient Satisfaction and Quality

Patient satisfaction and quality have become more important in today's highly competitive health care delivery environment (Stumpf, 2001). Health care providers and insurers compete for patients and enrollees. Patients do report greater satisfaction with their care in shared governance organizations, which tend to have greater staff retention and work satisfaction (Stumpf, 2001). So the context in which staff work and patients receive care are interrelated and affect patients' views of their care. However, some problems do exist with patient satisfaction. Besides these issues with the process of determining satisfaction, other issues should be considered.

Can the patient, as a health care consumer, judge "good" care effectively? How does the patient's illness affect the patient's impression of the treatment, and how does the patient express the evaluation? Along with this issue, Zimmermann (2001) also notes that the patients who complete surveys are patients who are able to do this—alert, typically English-speaking, and often younger. This eliminates many other patients. As is true for many problems that may be identified in the evaluation process, staff tend to trivialize complaints by saying the patient was annoying or a constant complainer. This is a way of avoiding complaints and not working on improvement. Patient satisfaction data are also an important component of report cards. As more is learned about the type of data that are really helpful, report cards should become more useful and reliable for the patient, employer, all types of providers, and third-party payers. It is important to recognize that the variables of satisfaction need to be identified by the patient, not the health care professional, and this is a problem. Box 6-2 identifies some consumer tips for safe health care.

Examples of Current Consumer Issues

The health care delivery system is complex, and consumers must cope with its complexity and barriers. Some consumer concerns are: (a) self-managing care, (b) use of PCPs and specialists, (c) medications, and (d) hospitalization. Patient education and patient advocacy, two key case management functions, require many leadership competencies such as effective communication, coordination, collaboration, decision making, and so on are important strategies to help patients gain strength as consumers.

Consumers manage a lot of their own care—even if they choose not to receive health care, they have made a decision about the importance of their health and what they want to do about it. The best way to prevent problems and reduce health care costs is to practice self-management, health promotion, and disease and illness prevention. Collaborating with health care providers to understand treatment choices, understanding patient and health care provider responsibilities, and following the treatment selected are critical to positive health care outcomes. If patients are involved in their health care decisions, they will be more satisfied with their health care. Seeking information to increase understanding is very important. In addition, enrollees need to collaborate with not only their health care providers but also with their insurers, who also play a major role in their health care decisions. Case management can play a critical role in helping patients to self-manage their own care.

BOX 6-2

Consumer Tips for Safe Health Care

- Speak up if you have questions or concerns.
- Keep a list of all medications you take.
- Make sure you get the results of any test or procedure.
- Talk with your doctor and health care team about your options if you need hospital care.
- Make sure you understand what will happen if you need surgery.

Source: Reprinted from Agency for Health Resources and Quality (AHRQ). *Five Steps to Safer Health Care* (Publication No. OM 00-0004, available on the Web at http://www.ahrq.gov/consumer/5steps.htm).

Summary

With the growth of managed care and its impact on changing health care reimbursement, the consumer is much more involved in health care. This is due mostly to problems that the consumer has experienced with the changes caused by managed care. There are, however, other reasons for this increased involvement. Consumers are now more involved in all aspects of daily living—not just health care. Consumer organizations have grown. Consumer written material is more available. The Internet plays a major role in providing current information for the consumer. Health care professionals must now recognize that they have an important role in patient advocacy. Nurses have always recognized this and can serve as effective case managers supporting patient advocacy. This means that nurse case managers must be more knowledgeable about managed care and reimbursement to help the patient or consumer.

Chapter Highlights

1. *Consumer of health care* can be a confusing term. It can mean the patient who receives the care; however, it can also be the employer or government who purchases the care.
2. The history of consumerism has evolved, and health care consumerism is growing rapidly. Managed care has affected its growth.
3. Nurses have long been patient advocates, and nurse case managers can serve as effective patient advocates.
4. Consumers are learning that they must voice their needs and concerns in the public policy process.
5. Consumer rights is a critical topic today in health care policy and in the health care delivery system.
6. Health care insurance is complex and difficult for the patient and family to understand.
7. New efforts have been developed to increase consumer participation in health care. Examples of these are demand management and disease management (DM).
8. Technology has made it easier for consumers to participate in health care. For example, e-mail and the Internet provide new methods for communication with providers and increased the amount of current information that is easily accessible.
9. The nurse case manager can help the consumer/patient understand health plan selection, use the health care plan, and evaluate the health care plan.

References

American Cancer Society. (2008). The Patient Self-Determination Act. Retrieved from http://www.cancer.org/docroot/MIT/content/MIT_3_2X_The_Patient_Self-Determination_Act.asp?sitearea=MIT on June 20, 2009.

Consumer Assessment of Healthcare Providers and Systems. (CAHPS). Consumer Assessment. (2009). Retrieved from https://www.cahps.ahrq.gov/default.asp on August 20, 2009.

Gilkey, M., Earp, J., & French, E. (2008). What is patient advocacy? In: J. Earp, E. French, & M. Gilkey, *Patient advocacy for health care quality* (pp. 3–28). Boston: Jones and Bartlett Publishers.

Human Resources News. (2009). Mental health parity act effective date delayed. Retrieved from http://employmentlawpost.com/hrnews/2009/02/18/mental-health-parity-act-effective-date-delayed/ on June 30, 2009.

Institute of Medicine. (2003). *Health professions education*. Washington, DC: National Academies Press.

Institute of Medicine. (2004). *Health literacy: A prescription to end confusion*. Washington, DC: National Academies Press.

Kongstvedt, P. (2009). *Managed care. What it is and how it works*. Boston: Jones and Bartlett Publishers.

Ratzan, S. & Parker, R. (2000). Introduction. In: *National Library of Medicine Current Bibliographies in Medicine: Health literacy*. NLM Pub. No. CBM 200-1. Selden, C., Zorn, M., Ratzan, S., Parker, R. (Eds.). Bethesda, MD: National Institutes of Health, U.S. Department of Health and Human Services.

Stumpf, L. (2001). A comparison of governance types and patient satisfaction outcomes. *Journal of Nursing Administration, 31*(4), 196–202.

U.S. Department of Health and Human Services. (1998). *Healthy People 2010*. Washington, DC: Author.

Zimmermann, P. (2001). The problems with health care customer satisfaction surveys. In: J. Dochterman & H. Grace (Eds.), *Current issues in nursing* (6th ed., pp. 255–260). St. Louis: Mosby, Inc.

Questions and Activities for Thought

1. How has health care consumerism changed?
2. What are the differences between the employer as consumer and the employee as consumer?
3. What is the effect of consumer rights on health care policy, delivery, reimbursement, and health care professionals?
4. Why is a nurse case manager particularly effective in working with consumers (patients, enrollees, members)? How have patient rights changed?

5. What is the nurse case manager's role as patient advocate?
6. If you worked for an insurer as a case manager, what methods would you use to increase consumer participation in health care?
7. How are patient education and health care consumerism related?
8. What health care consumer efforts have occurred in your local community?

Case

You are employed by a health insurance company. Data for consumer satisfaction surveys indicate that consumer dissatisfaction with the insurer is increasing. Consumers or members are particularly confused about their insurance plans and how to use them effectively. You are working with a team of case managers to develop information that all of you will use to increase your patients' and their families' understanding of their insurance plans. What would the team include in the information? This information will not be handed to the patients but will rather used by all of you as you introduce new patients to case management services.

Internet Links

1 Consumer information is found on many Internet sites. The following are examples of sites: URL: http//www.healthfinder.gov URL: //familydoctor.org
Who sponsors the site? What information does each site provide? Is it helpful for the consumer? Is the information easy to access? Can you search for specific information? Is the information accurate? As a health care professional, how might you use the site? Can you find any information related to managed care, reimbursement, health care delivery, quality care, or patient rights? Why is the site's content related to this chapter's content?

2 URL: //www.ahcpr.gov
Visit this site and click on "For Your Health." What information is available for consumers as they choose their health plans? What information is available for consumers as they use their health plans?

3 URL: //www.ncqa.org
Visit this site and click on "HEDIS & Quality Measurement." What is CAHPS? Does it provide helpful information? How might an MCO use this information? How might a health care professional or organization use this information?

4 URL: http://www.hospitalcompare.hhs.gov/Hospital/Search/Welcome.asp?version=default&browser=IE%7C7%7CWinXP&language=English&defaultstatus=0&pagelist=Home
Search the site for U.S. Department of Health and Human Services "Hospital Compare" and use the interactive database to compare and contrast health plans, hospitals, and so on. How might you use this site with patients as a case manager?

CHAPTER 7

Case Management
Documentation and Tools

OBJECTIVES

After completing this chapter, the reader will be able to:

- Define *clinical pathway*.
- Describe the historical development of clinical pathways.
- Explain the purpose of clinical pathways and advantages and disadvantages of their use.
- Describe the pathway development process.
- Analyze liability and ethical issues related to the use of clinical pathways.
- Explain why variance analysis is an important component of clinical pathways.
- Illustrate how clinical pathways might be implemented in a clinical setting, and both the positive and negative consequences of doing so.
- Describe practice guidelines.
- Discuss the importance of practice guidelines.
- Compare and contrast the use of practice guidelines and disease management (DM) in managed care.
- Explain why standards of care, utilization review, benchmarking, and evidence-based practice (EBP) are considered tools to increase collaborative care.
- Discuss the reasons for including health promotion and disease and illness prevention in this content.

KEY TERMS

INTRODUCTION

Using methods or tools to manage care, such as **clinical pathways, practice guidelines,** and **disease management (DM) programs,** requires **collaboration** with providers, third-party payers, patients, families, and case managers. Collaboration is important within clinical settings and between organizations. Because health care is complex, working together to reach goals is more successful and usually more efficient. Collaboration is needed to develop the tools to manage care, and it is also critical to continue collaboration when the tools or methods are implemented. This chapter describes these tools or methods and how their implementation benefits the patient, provider, and third-party payer. Clinical pathways are discussed in more detail to provide an example of how this type of tool is developed and implemented.

CLINICAL PATHWAYS

Collaborative care and interdisciplinary care are intertwined. As noted by the Institute of Medicine (IOM), core competencies both are critically import to improving the quality of care (Institute of Medicine, 2003). The development of clinical pathways and their implementation requires interdisciplinary collaboration. This section describes clinical pathway development, definitions and purposes, the clinical pathway development process, implementation, the effect of pathways on outcomes, and providers' responses to clinical pathways.

Definition of Clinical Pathway

A clinical pathway is a written guide that provides specific direction for the care required to meet the needs of specific medical problems. A pathway includes sequencing and timing of interventions. Reviewing a variety of definitions is helpful in appreciating the differences and similarities so that care can be received in a timely and appropriate manner. The pathway lays out the care process with expected outcomes and interventions so that the interdisciplinary team can use it to coordinate care. It is helpful to the case manager to ensure outcomes and efficient use of resources. The critical descriptors for a clinical pathway are:

- Provide guidelines for practice
- Define outcomes
- Focus on timelines
- Use of resources efficiently
- Emphasize the need for coordination, communication, and collaboration
- Enhance interdisciplinary work

Over time, pathways have changed so that they no longer focus only on nursing interventions but rather focus much more on interdisciplinary treatment and the effect of interventions on cost and quality. Electronic versions are also used now. Another major change is the move to ensure that clinical pathways are based on the best evidence available, **evidence-based practice (EBP).** What do research results say about the best care? Pathways must also consider the other four EBP elements: (1) clinical expertise, (2) patient history and (3) assessment data, and (4) patient values and preferences.

An issue that has not been resolved with the evolution of pathways is the best term to use. Initially, they were called critical pathways. Now, pathways may be called care paths, CareMaps®, case management plans, anticipatory recovery plans, care guides, collaborative plans, coordinated plans, integrated plans, plans of action, and probably the most common name, clinical pathways. This does cause confusion because some health care professionals may think that each of these terms represents a unique tool, yet they are all basically the same. As is discussed in later sections in this chapter, there are other tools that add to this confusion, for example, **algorithms,** practice guidelines, and DM programs. How are pathways different from these other tools? In some cases, clinical pathways are used with other methods, for example, with DM programs. The major characteristics of pathways are their comprehensiveness, timeliness, and emphasis on coordination and collaboration. They are used by case managers.

Practice guidelines focus on general treatment for a specific illness or condition whereas pathways are more specific and are unique to the health care agency or insurer. Pathways are also individualized for patients and meet the practice concerns of providers. These characteristics also make it more difficult to use pathways developed by other institutions and organizations (e.g., health care organizations [HCOs], insurers). Pathways need to be adapted to meet the individual needs of the institution, its providers, and its patient population.

A common misperception is that clinical pathways and case management are the same. How did this come about? The case management plan that is used by case managers confuses the issue. This plan focuses on case manager responsibilities, and the clinical pathway focuses on shared accountability of the interdisciplinary team. More case managers are using pathways as they coordinate care with the interdisciplinary team.

Purpose of Pathways

Pathways provide direction in the coordination of care and ensure that outcomes are met within a designated time frame, emphasizing efficient use of resources to reach outcomes and control costs. **Variances** occur when patients do not follow the expected trajectory. Variance data are used to analyze what went wrong and consider what needs to be improved. In some cases this analysis may lead to interventions to prevent further variances and to better ensure the patient outcomes are met and costs are controlled. An interdisciplinary focus better ensures that all aspects of the patient's care are addressed to meet identified outcomes. Pathways can also be used to demonstrate compliance with **standards of care,** accreditation, and regulatory requirements. These tools are often used to assist staff during orientation. Some institutions have developed patient versions of pathways that are given to the patient/family on admission or when treatment begins to help the patient and family understand the patient's care and what to expect. Case managers could use them for this purpose, too. What are the advantages and disadvantages of using clinical pathways?

Critics of pathways question whether pathways are not rigid requirements that allow for limited individuation. This could be a major disadvantage; however, insurers and health care organizations have considered this potential problem. They usually require assessment of pathway content each time the pathway is used with a patient to ensure that individual patient needs are met. The physician, nurses, case managers, and other providers need to document changes or adaptations. Another disadvantage is the cost and time required to develop and implement pathways. Insurers often find that the use of clinical pathways can reduce costs due to the impact they can have on effective planning and implementation of plans, meeting outcomes more effectively. For any HCO, the development of its first pathways is the most expensive part of the project. It takes time to develop the process, policies and procedures, forms, conduct research to get the information, and time to educate the project committee, interdisciplinary teams, and other relevant staff. This process is described later in the chapter.

Selection of the illnesses or conditions that require pathways should be done carefully. Case managers need to target the patients whom they frequently have in

BOX 7-1

Pathway Development Process Project Committee Selected

- Assessment of environment for change
- Identify target populations
- Design pathway format
- Medical record and documentation issues
- Develop variance tracking and analysis requirements
- Develop policies and procedures
- Select interdisciplinary teams for specific pathways
- Provide education about pathways to the teams
- Develop and implement general staff education

Interdisciplinary Teams

- Research to prepare content for specific pathway
  - Retrospective chart review
  - Current practice patterns
  - Benchmarking
  - Standards of practice
  - Literature review

- Review pathway samples from other institutions and literature
- Review financial data
- Review utilization data
- Review outcome studies
- Request expert opinions
- Identify outcomes, length of stay, and timeline
- Define required content
- Pilot test
- Make changes based on pilot test data
- Repeat pilot as necessary

Final Approval of Pathway by Project Committee and Administration

Implementation of Pathway

Variance Tracking and Analysis

Continue Overall Project Evaluation

their caseload and to consider the same red flags mentioned in Chapter 2. If there are few patients in a category (illness or condition), it may not be cost effective to spend time developing pathways that may make little difference in care, outcomes, and effective cost control.

Pathway Development and Implementation Process

Pathway development requires an interdisciplinary committee/team that is willing to discuss issues openly, use research information, be receptive to change, and is committed to the project. The committee should follow the development phases highlighted in Box 7-1 to guide their work. The case manager may be the team leader or committee chair.

Before beginning the project, the committee or interdisciplinary team needs education about project development, clinical pathways, and change. Content should include:

- Project development and organizational change
- Definition and purposes of a pathway
- Advantages and disadvantages of pathways
- Implementation of pathways
- EBP and research resources
- Variances and variance analysis
- Project evaluation

The committee or team uses resources such as current articles on pathways, books, and even sample formats from similar organizations. They need access to data such as length-of-stay (LOS), common admission diagnoses, laboratory tests, and incident data. Some staff may not know what data are available, so including management information system staff that can assist the committee. Data from pathway utilization should be a source of quality improvement (QI) data. As pathways are developed, they need to be considered as sources of data about QI.

BOX 7-2

Scope of Clinical Pathways

- *Inpatient Care.* Focus is on admission to the inpatient setting to discharge. This is the most common.
- *Complete Episode of Care.* Focus is on the time that care is requested at the physician's office to termination of posthospitalization treatment.
- *Specialized Applications.* Focus is on the patient's special needs (e.g., renal dialysis, ambulatory surgery, management of outpatient treatment of a problem).
- *Life and Health Management.* Focus is on management of chronic conditions (e.g., asthma, hypertension, diabetes). These are very similar to disease management programs.

Sources: Author; content summarized from Coffey, R. (1992). An introduction to critical paths. *Quality Management Health Care, 1*(1), 45–54; and Coffey, R., et al. (2001). Critical paths: Linking outcomes for patients, clinicians, and payers. In: P. Kongstvedt (Ed.), *The managed health care handbook*. Gaithersburg, MD: Aspen Publishers, Inc.

Development of the Pathway Format

It is best if there is a standard pathway format that is used throughout the organization. Reviewing formats used by other organizations is a good way to understand what can be done, and many examples are found in the literature. The committee may also want to contact similar organizations and ask about their pathway formats and their experiences with using clinical pathways. The format that is chosen needs to be easy to use and clear.

What is included in the clinical pathway format? The scope of clinical pathways can vary; for example, a pathway might focus on inpatient care, a complete episode of care, specialized applications, or health management. Box 7-2 describes these scopes in more detail. Figure 7-1 describes the connection among the types of information found in clinical pathways. Specific pathway content may also vary among organizations; the most common categories of information that are included in pathways are identified in Box 7-3.

A pathway does not have to include all of these categories. The committee selects the categories that are important for its purpose, patient population, and organization. A pathway that a case manager might use in assisting a patient through ambulatory care would have different emphasis from a pathway used by a case manager in a hospital.

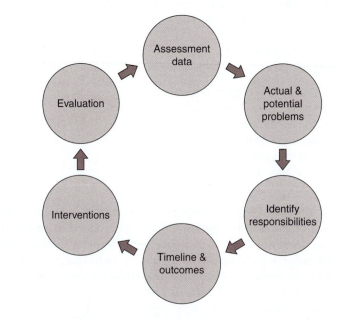

FIGURE 7-1 Types of Clinical Pathway Information

BOX 7-3

Pathway Content Categories

- Assessment and monitoring
- Psychosocial assessment
- Actual and potential problems
- Treatment interventions: prevention and therapeutic
- Tests and procedures
- Expected outcomes
- Consults
- Required observations
- Predetermined length of stay

- Timeline with trigger points
- Key indicators
- Medications
- Patient activity
- Nutrition
- Intravenous therapy
- Patient/family education
- Variance tracking
- Delineate responsibilities of interdisciplinary team

Key indicators are a very important part of the pathway. These indicators are the interventions that must be implemented in order to attain outcomes. During the development phase, it is important to understand the key indicators; however, overemphasis on indicators can be a problem. This usually happens when there is concern that there is missing information. The goal is to focus on the most important care needs. The development phase should be documented so that there are records to show how the pathway was developed. Box 7-4 identifies some of the advantages of using clinical pathways. These advantages relate to all of the major aspects of patient care delivery and help to explain why clinical pathways have become so common.

- Organize data logically.
- Prepare staff for computerization of clinical data.
- Ensure coordination when patient is transferred or moves from acute care to the community (transition and handoffs).
- Reduce readmissions.
- Reduce home care visits.

BOX 7-4

Advantages of Clinical Pathways

- Improve outcomes
- Reduce resource utilization
- Provide teaching tools for staff
- Improve collaboration
- Provide a consistent, interdisciplinary approach to patient care
- Identify trends
- Identify early indication of clinical variances and unique patient needs
- Provide a simple system for documentation that meets Joint Commission on Accreditation of Healthcare Organizations' interdisciplinary standards
- Provide earlier, more effective patient education
- Increase patient satisfaction

- Improve quality of care
- Eliminate redundancy, fragmentation, and duplication of services
- Delineation of responsibilities
- Improve communication
- Improve inventory management and reduce inventory control
- Organize data logically
- Prepare staff for computerization of clinical data
- Ensure coordination when patient transferred or moves from acute care to the community
- Reduction of readmission
- Reduction of home care visits

Sources: Author; content summarized from Griffin, M., & Griffin, R. (1994). Critical pathways produce tangible results. *Health Care Strategic Management, 12*(7), 1, 17–23; Critical paths concept evolves into more comprehensive system. (1992). *Hospital Peer Review, 17*(2), 27–30; Hague, D. (1996, May). Clinical pathways: The care plans of the 90s. *Ohio Nurses Review,* 15–19; and Cesta, T., Tahan, H., & Fink, L. (1998). *The case manager's survival guide: Winning strategies for clinical practice.* St. Louis: Mosby-Yearbook, Inc.

- Improve outcomes.
- Reduce resource utilization.
- Provide teaching tools for staff.
- Improve collaboration.
- Provide a consistent, interdisciplinary plan.
- Improve quality of care.
- Eliminate redundancy, fragmentation, and duplication of services.
- Delineate responsibilities.
- Identify trends.
- Identify early indication of clinical variances and unique patient needs.
- Provide a simple system for documentation that meets the Joint Commission's and other accreditation organizations' interdisciplinary standards.
- Provide earlier, more effective patient education.

Pathway data obtained about patient outcomes can be used in a variety of activities and have an impact on patient care, such as:

- Impact of pathways on the quality of care: coordination, collaboration, and patient-centered care
- Utilization of family education, outcomes, and data assessment
- Decrease in costs, meeting expected LOS, increasing consistency, and improving care
- Decrease in risk management issues
- Increase in compliance with accreditation and regulatory requirements
- Providing data for research
- Serving as staff education tools.

Patient satisfaction is an important factor in the evaluation of the use of pathways. This evaluation should consider three key questions.

- Does the patient/family feel involved in the care?
- Were the patient's goals met?
- Did staff discuss the patient's progress with the patient?

Patients need to first understand what a clinical pathway is and how it is used. Case managers who use clinical pathways need to explain their use to their patients. Factors that might impact the effectiveness of clinical pathways are patient satisfaction, patient education, continuity of information, continuity of care, quality of care, LOS, and reduction of costs.

Staff satisfaction should also not be overlooked in pathway evaluation. Important questions to consider include:

- Do you understand the reasons for using pathways?
- Did you feel prepared to use the pathways?
- If you participated in the development of the pathways, do you feel that your input was respected?
- How has the use of pathways affected your daily practice/work?
- How has the use of pathways affected your relationship with your patients/families?
- Do you think that pathways support interdisciplinary collaboration? If so, how?
- How has the use of pathways affected your documentation?
- What would you like to see changed with pathways and their implementation?
- Are staff using the pathways and using them correctly?

These questions are particularly important for HCOs that use temporary nurses, part-time staff, and travel nurses, which may make it difficult to ensure that all staff are knowledgeable about the pathways and are committed to using them. Full-time staff may carry the burden of ensuring that pathways are used correctly. This can lead to increased staff stress and affect patient care delivery.

There are many questions that can be asked in the evaluation process. Case managers should also regularly ask themselves these same questions. HCOs and insurers need to develop questions relevant to their environment, patients, and staff. Gathering data can be overdone, so question selection and related data should be carefully considered. When evaluation is complete, a summary of the results and any pathway revisions must be shared with the staff. In many organizations, staff find out about changes when they are affected by them, but this is too late. Staff should not pick up a copy of a pathway when they need to use it and find out it has been changed. This does not allow time for staff to understand the changes and how they affect patient care delivery.

Identification of the Target Population

Identification of the target population is a critical decision for the project committee. Time should not be wasted on the wrong population. Selecting the focus for pathways should consider the following as the typical illnesses or conditions in patient population are reviewed:

- High volume
- High risk
- Complex care requirements
- High cost
- Variations in LOS compared with the "norm" or benchmarks
- Variations in practice patterns
- Payer request or interest in the illness or condition
- Opportunity for improved care

Development of the Content

The team selected to develop specific pathway content needs to be qualified in the particular clinical area or some aspects of the delivery of care. This could be a team of case managers, or case managers may lead the team or committee. For example, within an HCO a pathway for a surgical condition should include surgeons; registered nurses from surgical units, operating room, and recovery room; and representatives from anesthesia, transportation, pharmacy, laboratory, medical records, admission, finance, utilization review, quality improvement, risk management, and informatics. The team begins by brainstorming but must focus on the routine, not the exceptions. Developing a flowchart often provides a helpful picture of the steps in routine care for the identified illness or condition. The team considers all aspects of care, a timeline that corresponds to the LOS goal, outcomes, and the key indicators for reaching the outcomes. It is also important to review current research to ensure an EBP approach. As the team prepares to develop content, its members review medical records of cases with the same diagnosis or condition, literature, outcome data, current practice, local practice patterns (both internal and external), and seek expert opinions. Identification of outcomes is a critical aspect of the process. Outcomes need to be specific, objective, and quantitative. After a pathway is implemented, outcomes should be reviewed periodically to ensure that they are current with new research, technology, medications, and clinical practice.

Another approach to the development of pathways is to use pathways that have been developed by other health care or professional organizations or are found in the literature. It is critical that all selected pathways are then adapted to the specific organization or third-party payer needs and services. Using this type of source requires consideration of a number of factors. Who developed the pathway? Is the pathway EBP-based? Does the pathway's population match the desired population? Is the pathway complete, including all relevant categories of information? How easy is it to adapt the pathway to meet the user's needs?

Many drafts of the pathways are required as the team works through the content, discusses it with other staff, and reviews the literature. The project committee identifies the final review process that should be followed for all pathways that are developed. This process includes key persons in the organization as well as the project committee. Consensus is critical for successful implementation, but it is not always easy to reach. It may require negotiation and collaboration.

Initiation of the Pilot Testing

Clinical pathways need to be pilot tested prior to their final approval. The project committee determines the pilot testing process, including its length, the number of times the pathway is implemented with patients, and the data collection procedure. Undoubtedly, changes need to be made, and some of these may be major. If so, another pilot may be required. The pilot should consider ease of use of the pathway, appropriateness of timeline and interventions, pathway quality, accuracy of outcomes, and appropriateness for the target population. Obtaining staff feedback as staff use the pathway in the pilot is critical for success. If this feedback is ignored, staff feel left out and are less inclined to support the pathways when they are implemented. Once pathways are approved, implementation begins; however, there are two issues that are important throughout the development and implementation phases. These are collaboration with insurers, HCOs, or both, and consideration of the liability and ethical issues related to pathway use.

Collaboration with Third-Party Payer

Clinical pathways have been helpful in meeting insurer demands that HCOs provide quality care that is cost effective and meets outcomes. Third-party payers require quality and want the product (care provided to their enrollees) to meet required outcomes in a cost-efficient manner. Some insurers and health care organizations have collaborated in the development of pathways. Insurers are requesting more and more data about their providers' care. Pathways can be used to collect data. Variances that occur can then be addressed quickly, thereby reducing costs and, it is hoped, improving care. In addition, insurers review variances and ask questions about them. When insurer contracts are renewed with providers, insurers evaluate the providers' variances and improvement. Providers who can show that they are identifying variances and actively pursuing changes to resolve variances will have an easier time with insurer contract renewal. Even though demonstration of improvement is important, there is no doubt that variance review is often seen as accusation and finding fault. Providers worry that data will be used against them and limit their access to patients, decrease their revenue, or cause them to lose insurer contracts. Consequently, variance analysis is not always viewed as a method for improving care but rather limiting care or providers. Collaboration, however, can occur only if the insurer–provider relationship focuses on sharing and helping one another rather than focusing on fear, competition, and conflicts.

Liability and Ethical Issues

Clinical pathways can be introduced as evidence in court to demonstrate a standard of care or what the outcomes or timelines should be for a patient. There are two areas of concern. The first is liability of staff who developed the pathway, and the second is provider liability. Pathway developers have been named in liability cases. The critical issues are whether or not the pathway is evidence based and expert advice was used during the development of the pathway. What can be done to prevent a liability issue? The committee should be an interdisciplinary team, with representatives who have expertise in the pathway focus area. Their résumés should be kept on file in case questions arise later. Written policies and procedures about the pathway development process and implementation should be kept on file, including a clear description of how pathways are individualized and how this is to be documented. It is important that all of this material is dated. A file should be kept for each pathway that includes the pathway tool, all of its major drafts, reference material, pilot testing data, and evaluations. All relevant organizational policies and procedures need to be evaluated to ensure that there is no conflict with new pathways. It is best that risk management staff and legal counsel review final pathways, policies, procedures, and the like. Staff who prepare and use the pathways need to have appropriate education about pathway development, and attendance needs to be documented. The evaluation process needs to be clearly defined and compliance with the process documented.

What is the liability for the provider? The provider needs to ensure that the pathway is appropriate for the patient and adapted as needed. When the provider deviates from the pathway, the provider documents reasons for this deviation. If the pathway is inadequate, the provider needs to recognize this and not blindly follow the clinical pathway. An important point to make is that the provider is at risk if a pathway is blindly followed. Case managers also need to follow these same guidelines to ensure the best care for an individual patient. If a pathway contains errors or represents substandard care, the provider is still responsible for the care provided. Nothing relieves the health care professional of the responsibility of using professional judgment. If pathways are used, every health care professional who uses them must be responsible for learning how to use them correctly or take the risk of making an error. Variances are tracked and used to assess achievement of outcomes. Comments about general variance data should never be documented in individual medical records. Disclaimers may be used with pathways.

Pathway Implementation

Implementation of clinical pathways requires time and patience. Staff may be uncomfortable and have concerns about how their use will affect their practice. Pathways should not be seen as a method for improving all of an organization's problems. For example, using clinical pathways probably will not improve a long-standing problem of poor communication. During the implementation of pathways, problems are often encountered that need to be resolved to prevent project failure. Patients with **comorbidities** may not quite fit with a pathway. This requires consideration of individual assessment data and needs. No pathway should be seen as an automatic approach or a cookbook to care. There also needs to be consideration of how pathways are integrated into required documentation. Over time, pathways most likely will need to be changed based on data; for example the expected LOS, length of treatment, or timing of interventions may not be realistic. New evidence may indicate a need for change so that the pathways can be evidence based.

Physicians are usually concerned about pathways. They need to be reassured that pathways do not replace physician orders. They are also concerned about losing their autonomy. To decrease this fear, physician input is necessary during pathway development, implementation, and evaluation. Some institutions have even gone so far as to require a physician's order for the use of a pathway or when the physician may choose not to use a pathway or make major alterations. Of course, these approaches could defeat the purpose of the pathways, and the health care organization needs to monitor the use of these alternatives to ensure that pathway implementation is not sidetracked. Outcome data obtained from the pathways may also be affected by these physician options. Insurers need to consider what are the critical approvals required before new clinical pathways are used.

Pathway Evaluation

Pathway evaluation should not be a complicated process. The areas of most concern are whether costs are changing per patient diagnosis and for itemized costs, such as laboratory tests, pharmacy, physical therapy, and radiology, and whether the quality of care is compromised. Are outcomes met? Evaluation also focuses on the LOS or the length of treatment. Critical evaluation issues are patient satisfaction, staff satisfaction, and variance analysis.

Patient satisfaction is a very important factor in the evaluation of the use of pathways. Important questions to consider are: (1) Does the patient/family feel involved in the care? (2) Were the patient's goals met? (3) Did staff discuss the patient's progress with the patient? Patients need to first understand what a clinical pathway is and how it is used.

Variances and Analysis

Variances are deviations from the expected or that which is defined in the clinical pathway. They may be positive or negative. Negative variances indicate that the patient has not achieved expected outcomes or that treatment activities have not been completed. A positive variance indicates that the patient achieved an outcome or treatment activity by the expected deadline. If the trend is toward more positive variances, it may mean that the deadlines need to be reviewed and could be shortened. *System or operational variances* focus on hindrances within the system or organization that prevent the achievement of patient outcomes. Examples are delay in laboratory results, lack of bed space, hours of service, delayed transfers to a long-term care facility, lack of supplies, and so on. *Provider variances* focus on the variances that may be caused by the provider. Examples include:

- The physician does not respond to a telephone call from a nurse about a patient's condition.
- A case manager does not take required steps in a timely manner.
- A mislabeled medication is given to a patient.
- A staff member is unable to follow a procedure due to lack of experience or knowledge.
- Orders are misread, and a patient is sent for the wrong procedure.
- A lab report is not communicated in a timely manner.
- Inadequate nursing staff decreases the time a nurse requires to review a patient's history.
- A case manager does not collaborate with the patient's home care agency.

Documenting these variances can be problematic due to liability risk. Staff need to avoid blaming a staff member in the medical record, for example, to state in the medical record that because a physician did not respond to a call from the nurse about the patient's condition, as a result the patient developed a complication. A patient variance identifies factors related to the patient that prevent the achievement of patient outcomes; for example, a patient refuses medication; a patient experiences complications (e.g., elevated temperature that interferes with proceeding with treatment); a patient experiences inadequate pain relief; or a patient does not follow the case manager's directions or arrives late for his or her admission for ambulatory care surgery. It is important to avoid blame when assessing variances but rather to look at causes and resolution. Why is the patient refusing medication? Is the patient afraid of the medication and its side effects? Does the patient lack understanding of the purpose of taking the medication? Does the patient have the money to pay for the medication? Does the patient lack transportation to pick up the medication? Does the patient think the medication will help? Why did the patient not follow the case manager's directions? Jumping to conclusions is not helpful and limits true understanding as to the reason for the variance. Variance data are most critical in understanding outcome achievement or lack of achievement and also provide direction for change. Data should be shared with the pathway development team and relevant staff. Involving them in developing resolutions is also important.

Documenting variances must be done with care. Reasons for the variance, if known, need to be identified and should be based on factual data. When treatment is provided that is not in the pathway or is added or deleted, this must be documented. In HCOs, nurses document most of the variances because they have the most contact with patients, particularly in acute care, home health care, and long-term care. Case managers may also document variances. Variance documentation requires accurate and complete documentation. The HCO develops documentation policies and procedures and prepares staff on their use.

Variance analysis assists in identifying patterns of concern or problems that are seen in a number of patients. These problems may require more intensive action for every patient who experiences these problems. The variance might, however, be due to a repetitive problem in the system. Algorithms are created to resolve these variances and prevent future variances. Generally, algorithms are not developed until variance data indicate a need. Algorithms are developed in the same way as pathways. Typically, they are formatted as decision-making trees. For example, if a patient experiences an elevated temperature, then specific treatment is begun.

DISEASE MANAGEMENT PROGRAMS

Disease Management (DM)

Disease management (DM) is another service strategy or method used by third-party payers to control costs and improve care. DM focuses on the whole patient who has a specific disease or illness, typically a chronic, long-term illness. Examples of illnesses that are often targeted for DM are asthma, arthritis, cancer, diabetes, hypertension, osteoporosis, high-risk pregnancy, congestive heart failure, depression, high cholesterol, and human immunodeficiency virus/acquired immune deficiency syndrome (HIV/AIDS). Box 7-5 highlights some of these common diseases.

BOX 7-5

Disease Management Programs: Common Diseases

- Asthma
- Cardiovascular diseases (e.g., coronary artery disease, congestive heart failure, angina, lipid irregularity)
- Depressive disorders
- Diabetes
- Ambulatory infectious diseases (e.g., otitis media, urinary tract infection, community-acquired pneumonia)
- Pain
- Upper gastrointestinal disease (e.g., peptic ulcer disease, reflux esophagitis)
- Women's and children's health

Sources: Author; content summarized from Gurnee, M., & Da Silva, R. (1997). Constructing disease management programs. *Managed Care*, 6(6), 8–16.

Disease management is "a system of coordinated health care interventions and communications for populations with conditions in which patient self-care efforts are significant" (DMAA, 2009). Why would an insurer develop a DM program, which takes time to develop and is expensive to develop and offer? The following are some DM program goals that help to understand the advantage of using this strategy to (Kongstvedt, 2009):

- Improve patient outcomes.
- Encourage self-management and patient-centered care.
- Reduce costs.
- Support preventive care.
- Increase patient adherence to recommended medical care.

DM programs are similar to continuous quality improvement (CQI) programs that have been used by organizations to improve their functioning. CQI programs focus on identification, intervention, and measurement, just as do DM programs. DM programs can vary from one insurer to another, but they usually include all or some of these elements:

- Prevention
- Early detection/diagnosis
- Treatment
- Management

Some programs just monitor medication treatment. Other programs offer only patient education or behavior modification. The more complex DM programs use case management for their patients in order to provide coordinated care over a long period of time and to ensure that there is collaboration within interdisciplinary teams. Health management organizations (HMOs) offer more control over the physician and can more easily encourage physicians to use DM programs. Usually, the role of the physician is to continue to provide appropriate interventions for the patient; however, other healthcare professionals, often nurses or case managers, provide education that focuses on prevention and health maintenance based on the disease and individual needs of the patient. The major goal is to prepare the patient to understand the disease and increase the patient's self-management of the disease.

Even though it seems that DM programs could be highly effective programs for patients, there are reasons for not developing a DM program. As an insurer makes decisions, it must always consider the costs and long-term benefits of its decisions. Employers usually give their employees the option to change their enrollment in health plans annually, and many employees do change their health plans. This flux in enrollment means that an insurer may go to considerable lengths to identify the needs for DM. These programs are based on enrollment data collected at a specific time. The insurer may then find out that there are changes in the data because enrollees are moving in and out of various benefit options or changing plans. The other problem is that an insurer could develop a reputation for providing excellent management of a particular disease, and this might attract more enrollees with this disease. As discussed in earlier chapters, chronic illness is on the rise. DM often focuses on chronic diseases. Does the insurer want to attract more enrollees who are sick? No, it does not, so this presents a dilemma for insurers as they develop DM programs. Figure 7-2 describes the Chronic Care Model that can be used as a framework to develop programs and services for chronic illness.

Health Promotion and Disease and Illness Prevention

Health promotion and disease and illness prevention are strategies that focus on encouraging the enrollee to become a partner in maintaining his or her health. Education is a key method for accomplishing this partnership. Each time an insurer develops

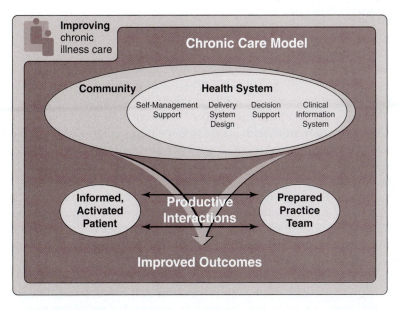

FIGURE 7-2   Chronic Care Model
There are six fundamental areas identified by the Chronic Care Model describing a system that emphasizes high-quality chronic disease management.

Source: Reprinted with permission from the Institute of Healthcare Improvement. Retrieved from http://www.ihi.org/IHI/Topics/ChronicConditions/AllConditions/Changes/ on May 26, 2008.

health promotion and disease and illness prevention services, it reassesses the costs and benefits of these services. The HMO is the managed care model that is more likely to cover preventive services, such as immunizations, well-baby care, and physical examinations; however, more insurers are covering some preventive services. **Primary prevention** focuses on health promotion by "maintaining or improving the general health of individuals, families, and communities" (Greiner & Edelman, 2006, p. 15). Examples of interventions are health education and immunizations.

The goals of health promotion are to help people modify their lifestyles and make choices to improve their health and quality of life. Health education is very important in helping enrollees/patients to accomplish this goal. There are three types of disease and illness prevention: primary, secondary, and tertiary. Primary prevention focuses on wellness behaviors and prevention of illness or prevention of the natural course of an illness. Examples of interventions are prenatal clinics, stress management courses, AIDS education, nutrition education, and seatbelt safety. **Secondary prevention** focuses on early diagnosis of symptoms and treatment after the onset of disease or illness and recognizes that early treatment may decrease complications. Examples of interventions are mammograms, parent education, and screening for diabetes or glaucoma. **Tertiary prevention** focuses on rehabilitative strategies to decrease disability from a disease or illness. Examples of interventions are chemotherapy education for a cancer patient and bladder training for a stroke patient.

How do insurers determine which services or interventions to offer? The Agency for Healthcare Research and Quality (AHRQ) publishes up-to-date prevention guidelines on a variety of topics through its website (http://www.ahrq.gov/clinic/prevnew.htm). This resource provides information about preventive services categorized by age and sex. Examples of some of the topics covered are:

- Skin cancer
- Colorectal diseases

- Prostate cancer
- Promoting breastfeeding
- Sexually transmitted diseases
- Behavioral health

The U.S. Preventive Services Task Force publishes a preventive guide that can be accessed through its website at http://www.ahrq.gov/CLINIC/uspstfix.htm. Preventive services are frequently inadequately provided. Some of the reasons for this have been inadequate reimbursement, fragmentation of health care delivery, and insufficient time with patients. Even when these factors have been removed, the services are often not provided. This is partially due to lack of knowledge about what to provide and questions about their effectiveness. Patients may also be unaware of their needs for preventive services and thus do not request them. Some preventive services are best provided on a community basis rather than with an individual focus in a clinical setting. This may become more common in the future. In addition, insurers may develop their own clinical guidelines for preventive services, which increases the variability of these services.

After insurers identify the health promotion and disease and illness preventive services to offer, they must develop the services, ensure that providers provide the services, and then communicate preventive services availability to enrollees. Insurers use newsletters, personal letters, information provided at the worksite, and the Internet to share information with their enrollees. The National Committee for Quality Assurance (NCQA) includes some preventive services in its quality indicators, for example, vaccination rates, cervical cancer screening, mammography, and retinal exams for diabetics. The inclusion of preventive services by the major quality assessment organization for insurers is an indication of the importance of these services to managed care. Models of managed care other than HMOs, such as preferred provider organizations (PPOs), may cover the services or may set a dollar amount for preventive services. In the latter case, the enrollee has more choice as to how to use the money that is set aside for health promotion and prevention. Some plans may require copayments and deductibles for these services. Health Care Reform of 2010 places a greater emphasis on health promotion and prevention.

As insurers determine which preventive services to offer, cost effectiveness is an important consideration. "Cost-effectiveness analysis is a method for assessing and summarizing the value of a medical technology, practice, or policy. Underlying the methodology is the assumption that the resources available to spend on health care are constrained, whether from the societal, organizational, practitioner, or patient point of view. Cost-effectiveness information is intended to inform decisions about health care investments within this finite budget. The cost-effectiveness ratio summarizes information on cost and effect, allowing interventions to be compared on the basis of their worth and priority to the patient, society in general, or some other constituency. Although the cost-effectiveness ratio takes the form of a price—that is, a dollar cost per unit of effect—it is generally interpreted in the inverse manner, as a measure of the benefit achievable for a given level of resources" (U.S. Preventive Services Task Force, 2001).

The central purpose of cost-effectiveness analysis (CEA) is to compare the costs and the values of different health care interventions in creating better health and longer life (Agency for Healthcare Research and Quality, 2009). Many new medical devices, procedures, diagnostic tests, and prescription drugs are expensive. CEA can help to evaluate whether the improvement in health care outcomes justifies the expenditures relative to other choices. This understanding of the costs and outcomes of comparative interventions is essential for public and private sector decision makers to make informed decisions about using health care resources efficiently.

There is a need to allocate resources efficiently or to get the most out of the resources. Insurers need to factor into the CEA the value of providing services that will keep enrollees healthy when the long-term benefit will be gained by another insurer. Why is this a concern? It is common for enrollees to change health plans, and thus an insurer's membership is rarely constant over a long period of time. As is true for all of the tools or methods used to manage care in case management and in the reimbursement area, much more needs to be learned about their cost effectiveness and impact on outcomes.

PRACTICE GUIDELINES

Third-party payers are interested in practice guidelines. Health care provider organizations, the federal government, and health care professional organizations are also involved. This interest in tools to manage care stems from the need to decrease costs and yet provide quality care. Guidelines have been used in conjunction with clinical pathways. The goal is to narrow the gap between an organization's current care and optimal care. Practice guidelines are used to assist with treatment decision making and to evaluate care. The Joint Commission does not require the use of practice guidelines but does require that hospitals consider their use and application to the hospital's services and processes.

Practice guidelines are systematically developed statements used to assist practitioners in making decisions about appropriate health care for specific clinical conditions that should be evidence based (National Guideline Clearinghouse, 2009). As with clinical pathways, practice guidelines are called by many names. Some of the more common ones are appropriateness indicators, practice parameters, medical review criteria, and standards. The purpose of using guidelines is to pull together research information from the literature, evaluate these results, and access expert opinion about the clinical condition. This better ensures that care is evidence based. This information is then prepared in a usable form. Practice guidelines are different from standards of care in that guidelines do not define treatment but rather provide information and options.

Development of Practice Guidelines

Public and private sector organizations develop practice guidelines, including professional organizations, HCOs, and researchers. Condition-specific organizations (e.g., American Heart Association, Arthritis Foundation) have also developed guidelines. Nurses have been active in the development of guidelines. Governmental agencies that have been involved in the development are the AHRQ through the National Guideline Clearinghouse, the National Institutes of Health (NIH), the Centers for Disease Control and Prevention (CDC), the U.S. Preventive Services Task Force, Centers of Medicare and Medicaid Services (CMS), and the Department of Health and Human Services (DHHS). Active participation from many types of organizations indicates the level of interest in practice guidelines. AHRQ guidelines are well-known sets of statements that may be used to assist practitioners and/or patients in making health care decisions for specific clinical problems. Interdisciplinary panels of experts develop these guidelines. The AHRQ guidelines are evidence based and accessible through the Internet at http://www.guideline.gov.

Physicians are using practice guidelines, but the level of use is variable. How might physicians and other providers such as advanced practice nurses use these guidelines? Examples of their purposes that are important for practitioners are to guide screening, immunizations, use of diagnostic tests, and management of specific types of chronic illnesses. What are the problems or factors that are keeping providers, such as physicians and nurse practitioners, from using practice guidelines? One major problem is the accessibility of the information while the provider, such as a physician, nurse, or nurse practitioner, is with the patient. If the provider has access to a computer in the examining room, then this information could be discussed with the patient in the examining room. This would save time and be more relevant to the patient. With so many guidelines in existence, making decisions about which ones to use is problematic. Information overload is a major complication today, and it can actually increase stress rather than decrease or control it. A common approach made by providers is to amalgamate the guidelines by considering providers' personal experiences and approaches with the specific condition. Nonadherence to guidelines can often be traced to limited provider input in guideline development, and then the provider does not accept the guidelines. Change that is instituted from outside is rarely successful. In addition, change that brings limited rewards often fails. Some insurers encourage guideline use by paying incentives to providers who use them and by tracking their use when they evaluate provider performance. A final concern with practice guidelines is coverage of comorbidities, which is also true with clinical pathways. For example, what does the provider do when a patient has a cardiac condition and diabetes and there are separate guidelines for the cardiac condition and for diabetes? The guidelines may not consider the impact of one illness on the other and may actually offer conflicting treatment options. Often, the provider chooses not to use any practice guideline rather than deal with conflicting and confusing recommendations.

Insurer Interest in Practice Guidelines

Why would insurers be interested in using practice guidelines? The common reasons for their use are to:

- Reduce health care costs.
- Improve the quality of care.
- Ensure consistency of care.
- Provide performance data for comparison with other insurers, as well as comparison of individual provider performance levels.
- Comply with accreditation and regulatory requirements.

Typically, insurers select practice guideline content based on services or conditions that have high cost, high liability risk, and a high incidence in their particular enrollee population, which are the same key criteria used to select pathway focus and also for case management. If an insurer has few enrollees with renal problems, it does not make sense for it to expend efforts to institute the use of practice guidelines for renal problems. The insurer must reduce its costs but must also consider the expenses that are incurred to make changes that might reduce costs. In addition to cost reduction and quality issues, another force that is pushing insurers to use practice guidelines is accreditation.

Most insurers, however, do not develop their own practice guidelines. They review guidelines that have been developed by professional organizations, the AHRQ, or other resources. Guidelines are then selected and adapted to meet the needs of the insurer. This is less costly, expedites the development process, and, more important, helps to ensure that the final product meets the individual needs of the insurer, its providers, and its enrollees. For example, lengthy guidelines—and there are many that are quite long—have not been found to be as helpful to the provider. Many providers do not even take the time to read them. Some guidelines may make recommendations that the insurer considers too costly. The insurer must recognize that once it adapts a practice guideline, it is no longer the same guideline and thus loses the integrity of a published guideline as agreed upon by the publishing organization or authors. The insurer must then take the responsibility of periodic evaluations to ensure that the content is current and accurate.

STANDARDS OF CARE

Standards of care provide minimal descriptions of accepted actions expected from a health care organization or professional with specific skill and knowledge levels. Standards were discussed in Chapter 5 as important in quality improvement, but they are also an important in establishing expectations for care. Standards are developed by professional organizations, legal sources such as nurse practice acts and federal and state laws, regulatory agencies such as accreditation bodies and federal and state agencies, and health care facilities, and are supported by scientific literature and clinical pathways. Standards act as guides for care.

UTILIZATION REVIEW/MANAGEMENT

Utilization management (UM) is the process of evaluating the necessity, appropriateness, and efficiency of health care services for specific patients or patient populations, as discussed in Chapter 4. UM has been used in acute care settings for a long time; however, it is also very important in other types of delivery settings and to insurers. Third-party payers and MCOs are particularly interested in UM because it is used primarily to control costs. UM data are used when tools are developed to access outcomes.

EVIDENCE-BASED PRACTICE

Today, EBP is incorporated into an increasing number of health care delivery systems. The recent IOM reports on quality and safety emphasize the need to apply EBP in practice. EBP has been defined as "developing changes and improvements with a firm foundation of the best data that exist at that time from the science, the individual performing the services, and the consumer of the service" (DePalma, 2002, p. 55). EBP helps to identify and assess high-quality, clinically relevant research that can be applied to clinical practice as well as the development of health policy. As one travels from one area of the country to the other, or even within one community, there can be great variation in practice and delivery. Problems are approached differently and often with no rationale that is based on sound evidence. EBP synthesizes results found in professional research so that they can be used to improve care or the delivery of health care services, but it also focuses on other key elements: clinical expertise, patient values and preferences, and the patient's health history and assessment.

The two key goals of EBP and also evidence-based policy development that organizations consider are to: (a) challenge others to provide evidence for their practice or their policy decisions and (b) critically assess to find and use evidence (Mooney, 2001, 9, 17). Today, patients are more knowledgeable about their illnesses and treatment.

Technology has made much more information accessible to consumers. Information increases control, and now more and more patients want the best. In order to meet these goals, it is important to (Mooney, 2001, p. 17):

- Frame a clinical question (delivery, or policy question).
- Search for the evidence.
- Evaluate the evidence.
- Implement the evidence.

EBP requires that information is available for specific questions. The research literature is reviewed using explicit scientific methods and includes all relevant research. This valuable information is then available to practitioners and should be helpful in directing their care decisions. An obvious question is, how does the case manager get this information and then, how does the case manager know what information is valid and reliable? Evidence-based reviews act as gatekeepers of the knowledge (Evans & Pearson, 2001). Criteria need to be used to determine what type of evidence will be useful. The hierarchy of evidence is described in three levels (DePalma, 2002; Rutledge & Grant, 2002).

1. The highest level is published research differentiated by methodology such as randomized, controlled studies, and then qualitative studies.
2. The middle level is theoretical evidence, which is based on propositions that may not have been tested.
3. The lowest level is nonresearch evidence. Examples of this type of evidence are: benchmarking data, cost analyses, regulatory and legal opinions, ethical principles, case reports, quality and risk data if systematically obtained, principles of pathophysiology, standards of care, and infection control data, if systematically collected.

Mooney (2001) recommends that not only should staff or the reviewers evaluate the information based on its scientific merit, as indicated in the previous hierarchy, but the following questions must also be considered: Have the results been replicated? This helps to establish credibility. Are the results relevant to the practice, policy, or delivery? What are the risks and benefits of incorporating the results into practice, policy, or delivery? Just adopting ideas without considering these factors can be costly. What is the feasibility of incorporating the new evidence? This is tied to the previous question because it can increase costs or limit benefits. Now, what happens after evidence is collected? It could be overwhelming, because the result is often a large amount of information and there may be contradicting information. Typically, a panel of stakeholders is selected to review the information and come to a consensus about it (DePalma, 2002).

The U.S. Preventive Services Task Force, which is an interdisciplinary group that works under the AHRQ, evaluates research and publishes guidelines based on their reviews. This can be a source of information to support EBP. "The AHRQ Evidence-Based Practice Center (EPC) Program sponsors and disseminates state of the art systematic reviews on important topics that provide the evidence bases for guidelines, quality improvement projects, quality measures, and insurance coverage decisions. They sponsor both methodological investigations and publications of systematic reviews" (Cronewett, 2002, p. 4). Cronewett (2002) notes that EBP reports from the AHRQ are typically developed by scientists from single disciplines and thus provide one point of view rather than an interdisciplinary view, which is a disadvantage. Clinicians, patients, and advocacy groups are not usually involved. The EBP reports include analyses, evidence tables, references, and search strategies. Cronewett (2002) has some criticisms of AHRQ EBP reports due to incomplete literature, possible database publication biases, and the emphasis on using evidence from randomized controlled trials, which can skew the information, and making the conclusions relevant only to the patient populations included in the studies.

INFORMATION TECHNOLOGY, TELEHEALTH, AND OTHER MEDICAL TECHNOLOGY

With the rapid growth of information technology, the management and provision of health care have been radically changed. Health care informatics has become very important today in the health care delivery system. Information is available via many different types of technology, giving health care providers the opportunity to track patient information across health care settings and virtually anywhere in the world. Information technology has provided opportunities to expand health care into new areas such as the use of the Internet to communicate with providers, HCOs, and consumers. **Telehealth** is also used in some areas, particularly rural areas that have limited access to health care experts. The use of interactive video and telephone conferencing has opened new doors for health care providers. Medical testing, such as electrocardiograms, continuous cardiac monitoring, and pulmonary function tests, may even be done in the patient's home with the results sent to the provider.

Telephone patient advice is also growing. Insurers are finding that this is an excellent triage method, allowing patients to speak directly with a health care professional, who is often a nurse or case manager. Questions can be answered, and this may prevent the need for a physician office visit or even hospitalization. Patients can also be assessed and referred to the best resource for service. Patient education and guidance can also be provided. The telephone is used for patient follow-up. For example, the insurer can call patients who have failed to keep appointments or call to obtain satisfaction data. Staff from a day surgery unit call patients before surgery to discuss preoperative requirements and after discharge to determine their status and whether they are following discharge advice. Most health care providers are using the telephone, e-mail, and even text messaging to contact patients and remind them of appointments to decrease the number of patients who do not show up for appointments. When patients miss appointments, it is expensive for providers because this time could have been used to see other patients. Health care providers, particularly hospitals, are using the telephone to obtain initial intake information and thus reduce admission time and at the same time provide the patient with pertinent information. The telephone is certainly not new; however, health care providers are now using this technology more to their advantage. Information is a critical need in the health care insurance industry on a day-to-day basis.

Telemedicine uses computers, telephone lines, video cameras, and special monitoring equipment to enable health care providers to "visit" patients in their homes while the provider remains at the clinic, hospital, or home health agency. Thus far, telemedicine has been used more for physician–physician consultation, but this is expected to change. Advanced practice nurses are active in using telemedicine. Home health agencies and other providers who monitor patients with chronic illnesses may use telehealth. Prevention and early intervention are powerful outcomes of telemedicine and reduce medical costs. Case managers may also find greater use of this technology in their practice.

Information management is the process of collecting, manipulating, analyzing, and storing information. An important component of the management information system (MIS) is the exchange of information, both internally and externally, for example, from an independent provider to the insurer, from a hospital to the insurer, from the insurer to its providers, and of course, information exchange within the insurer. Computers have solved many problems related to the exchange of information, accuracy, timeliness, and the need to store large quantities of information. This information is an important part of financial management and clinical management. Cost and utilization data are a requirement for an insurer. Monitoring specific provider performance provides important data for provider panel selection and panel contract renegotiation.

MISs are not only important internally for the insurer, but have also become much more important for providers. Hospitals have long had some type of computer system, but these systems are now even more critical for each hospital's success. These systems must provide the information that is required by all insurers who have contracted with the hospital. In most cases, each hospital has many insurer contracts, and data requirements may vary. This can be a burden for the hospitals, and it is expensive. In addition, physicians have a greater need to use efficient computer systems to manage their data;

however, many medical practices have a long way to go before they have reliable, comprehensive systems in place. Though costly it is required for their success with insurers. The government payment systems, such as Medicare and Medicaid, collect large amounts of data that need to be managed via the information management system to make this information useful.

As these information systems are developed, it is important to consider all of the linkages that are required—provider, payer, and medical supplier, and others. In many cases, the patient should also be considered. Planning for MISs should consider the following questions.

- Who needs the data?
- What data are needed?
- How will these data be used?
- What format should be used to collect the data?
- Is the data easy to access?

Data validity is always important. Data can be manipulated to prove or support a decision, and this can lead to problems, both ethical and legal. To affect decision making and reduce costs, the MIS needs to produce accurate data in a timely manner. Typical employer, enrollee, and provider data that are required include (Kongstvedt, 2009):

- Enrollment information
- Eligibility lists
- Claims and claims payments
- Referrals
- Hospital authorizations
- Premium and capitation statements and payments
- Medical records
- Provider information
- Member education materials
- LOS
- Length of treatment
- Prescription practice
- Medical procedures

The increasing use of e-mail has affected the management of information. E-mail is now used to inquire about prescriptions, confirm physician instructions or ask questions, and receive health promotion information from HCOs and individual providers such as physicians. E-mail is faster than other types of sending written information, and it is more permanent than oral communication. E-mail provides a written record that can be inserted into a patient's record. Telephone tag can be eliminated, and thus the patient feels that his or her needs are met. E-mail provides a written record of patient education information that has been provided to the patient and a record of questions that have been asked and answered. Security and confidentiality are still concerns with systems that include confidential information. To decrease this concern, before using e-mail with a provider, the patient may be asked to sign guidelines describing the use of e-mail. This serves as a form of informed consent. The use of e-mail for prescriptions requires a sophisticated record-keeping system, but it can be successful. Prescriptions via e-mail are now also available through various groups with prescriptions mailed to the home. Fax is also used for prescriptions. The use of all of these methods will undoubtedly increase as this technology becomes more accessible for more people.

In addition to e-mail, computers have opened up other communication opportunities for insurers, providers, and patients. With the increased usage of computers by consumers, software has been developed to assist patients in monitoring their own health care. This software provides a format for maintaining a health diary. This information can then be easily accessible to the patient and can be shared with the health care provider. In addition, the Internet has created opportunities for insurers to provide information about their organization and its services. Some insurers are also providing Internet health care information. The Internet already has a tremendous amount of health care information, and it increases daily. Enrollees can access information about health prevention practices, such as Pap smears, mammograms, colorectal examinations, prostate examinations, and other screenings. Some software systems provide patient follow-up communication to encourage regular screening. These efforts will undoubtedly increase. One might wonder that if computers had not developed into user-friendly resources, would MCOs be where they are today, particularly with their need for data management? Many MCOs are becoming much more concerned with outcomes. Data are required to assess outcomes, and systems that help do this reduce the time and cost of this effort. "The information system constitutes the backbone of the MCO's (insurer's) operations" (Kongstvedt, 2009, p. 152). To ensure patient's privacy, when an MIS is developed and other electronic communication methods are used, HIPAA regulations must be followed.

Summary

Tools to manage care, such as clinical pathways, practice guidelines, and DM programs, have increased as the health care insurance industry has put more pressure on health care providers to improve care and provide more cost-effective care. These tools offer health care providers the opportunity to determine the best approaches to clinical problems based on current research and expertise. As long as individual patient needs are not ignored, clinical pathways, practice guidelines, DM programs, and other similar tools provide many benefits for patients and providers. They increase the ability of health care providers to monitor the quality of care as outcomes are identified and evaluated.

Using these methods or tools and informatics and technology to manage care requires collaboration from providers, case managers, third-party payers, patients, and families. Collaboration is important within clinical settings and between organizations. Because health care is complex, working together to reach goals is more successful and usually more efficient. Collaboration is needed to develop the tools to manage care, and it is also critical in implementing the tools.

Chapter Highlights

1. Collaborative care is a critical component of case management and requires the use of a variety of tools that help manage care, for example, clinical pathways, practice guidelines, and DM programs.
2. Clinical pathways provide guidelines for practice by defining outcomes, timelines, and interventions that support efficient use of resources, and assist in the coordination and communication of needs during the care process.
3. Pathways focus on the interdisciplinary team and total patient care needs. For example, a pathway describes the expected medical care, nursing care, physical therapy, social service, and so on.
4. There is concern that tools such as clinical pathways may become "cookbooks" and individualized care and needs will be ignored. These tools need to be adapted to individual patient needs.
5. Insurers recognize that clinical pathways and other similar tools assist in reducing costs and improving care.
6. Providers who follow pathways or other types of guidelines are still required to use professional judgments and are not immune to liability when they are using pathways, guidelines, and the like.
7. Variance analysis is an important part of using clinical pathways. This analysis provides data about

problems, changes that need to be made in care and in pathways, and improvement in care.

8. Practice guidelines assist health care professionals in making clinical decisions. They provide current information and research on a specific problem or diagnosis. HCOs, professional organizations, and the federal government develop guidelines.

9. Disease management programs are growing. These programs focus on specific populations who have specific needs, such as patients with diabetes or rheumatoid arthritis. The focus is on providing information, education, and preventive care.

10. The use of health promotion and disease and illness prevention has gradually increased in all areas of heath care delivery and in health care benefits.

11. Use of standards of care, UR, and EBP all provide important guidance to care decisions with consumer involvement.

12. Information technology has increased, and it is now an essential part of the health care delivery system.

References

Agency for Healthcare Research and Quality. (AHRQ). (2009). Focus on cost-effectiveness analysis at AHRQ. Retrieved from http://www.ahrq.gov/research/costeff.htm on June 15, 2009.

Cronewett, L. (2002, February 19). Research, practice and policy: Issues in evidence-based care. *Online Journal of Issues in Nursing*, http://www.nursingworld.org/ojin/keynotes/speeh_2.htm

DMAA. (2009). Disease Management. Retrieved from http://dmaa.org/ on July 6, 2009.

DePalma, J. (2002). Proposing evidence-based policy process. *Nursing Administration Quarterly, 26*(4), 55–61.

Evans, D. & Pearson, A. (2001). Systematic reviews: Gatekeepers of nursing knowledge. *Journal of Clinical Nursing,* 10, 503–599.

Griener, P. & Edelman, C. (2009). Health defined: Objectives for promotion and prevention. In: C. Edelman & C. Mandle, (Eds.), *Health promotion throughout the life span* (pp. 1–22). St. Louis: Elsevier Mosby.

Institute of Medicine. (2003). *Health professions education.* Washington, DC: National Academies Press.

Kongstvedt, P. (2009). *Managed care. What it is and how it works.* Boston: Jones and Bartlett Publishers.

Mooney, K. (2001). Advocating for quality cancer care: Making evidence-based practice a reality. *ONF28* (2 supplements), 17–21.

National Guideline Clearinghouse. (2009). Patient Guidelines. Retrieved from http://www.nationalguideline.gov on June 19, 2009.

Rutledge, D. & Grant, M. (2002). Introduction to evidence-based practice in cancer nursing. *Seminars in Oncology Nursing, 18*(2), 1–2.

U.S. Preventive Services Task Force. (2009). Cost effectiveness. Retrieved from http://www.ahrq.gov/CLINIC/uspstfix.htm on August 19, 2009.

Questions and Activities for Thought

1. Compare and contrast the different definitions of *clinical pathway*.
2. Why is collaboration so important when using tools such as clinical pathways, practice guidelines, and DM programs?
3. If you were told that clinical pathways are rigid and do not allow for individuality, how would you dispute this statement?
4. What types of patients benefit from the use of clinical pathways?
5. What questions would you need to consider if you were evaluating clinical pathways developed by another organization?
6. What are the typical staff and physician concerns that arise during the implementation of clinical pathways in an organization?
7. How can variance analysis be used to improve care or reduce costs?
8. Compare and contrast practice guidelines and disease management programs.
9. As a case manager, discuss how and why you would use clinical pathways, practice guidelines, and DM.
10. How would you integrate evidence-based practice into your daily practice as a case manager?

Case

You are a case manager working for a health insurer. The insurer has decided it needs to improve care for members with chronic illnesses, particularly those with diabetes. You supervise a team of case managers. You recommend that the team use the Chronic Care Model to develop a DM program for this population and then track outcomes. How would you apply this model to a DM program for patients with diabetes? Describe the application and the DM program the team develops. How would the team track outcomes?

Internet Links

1 http://www.guideline.gov
   This site is the National Guideline Clearinghouse that provides up-to-date, evidence-based clinical practice guidelines. What information does it have? Does it provide general information about guidelines? What specific types of guidelines are available? Review two of them.

2 http://www.ahcpr.gov
   Visit the site and click on "Clinical Information." What are EBP centers? How do they select their focus topics? Select a center and a topic. What information is provided? How might this information be used?

Case Management Reader

INTRODUCTION

The Case Management Reader provides the reader with a selection of published articles about case management. The articles focus on case manager professional issues, patient-centered care, quality improvement, case management (costs, reimbursement, and utilization review), chronic illness, and disease management. After reading each article, respond to the critical thinking questions pertaining to the article. Refer to content found in Section I.

Issue 1: Case Manager Professional Issues

Schmitt, N. (2005). Role transition from caregiver to case manager, part 1. *Lippincott's Case Management, 10*(6), 294–302.

1. Identify the antecedent conditions or motivating factors that might cause (or are causing) you to move from your current nursing role to the role of case manager.
2. What might you do to ease this role transition? What resources will you need? Who might serve as a guide or mentor for you?
3. Explore the differences in caregiver and case manager behaviors as applied to Benner's Domains of Nursing Practice (article p. 298, Table 1). What challenges might you face as you transition from caregiver on your unit to case manager?
4. A patient is being discharged from the hospital after exacerbation of chronic heart failure. Think about the care provided and actions taken by the staff nurse leading up to discharge. Now consider the role and responsibilities of the nurse case manager. What additional issues, steps, or considerations might the nurse case manager address that the staff nurse would not? What other members of the interdisciplinary health care team would the case manager need to interface with?

Schmitt, N. (2006). Role transition from caregiver to case manager, part 2. *Lippincott's Case Management, 11*(1), 37–46.

1. Identify your expectations of the role of case manager. Are they realistic? Make a list of these expectations to use when considering a position in case management. Compare and contrast with your classmates.
2. Work associated with caregiving is very different from that of case management; caregiving tasks are very focused and require completion by the end of the shift, whereas case management work is often a process that unfolds over a period of days, weeks, or even months. Examine your time and workload management skills and strategies. What are your strengths? What are your weaknesses? How do you manage work that is focused on long-term goals?

3. Working with financial issues (such as cost containment and allocation of re-sources) can often be difficult for new case managers as they can, at times, seem to be in opposition to the needs of the patient. How can the nurse case manager effectively work to address these financial issues while also maintaining the role of patient advocate?

Issue 2: Patient-Centered Care

Rosenthal, T. (2008). The medical home: Growing evidence to support a new approach to primary care. *Journal of American Board of Family Medicine, 21*(5), 427–440.

1. What are the five Medical Home principles described in this article? Discuss the potential role and functions of the case manager within each principle.
2. What strengths and unique points of view might a case manager add to the health care team (which includes physicians, social workers, nurses, physical and occupational therapists, etc.)?
3. How might you build a business case for adding case management services? We know changes in reimbursement are coming, but explore how a program might justify the salary and fringe expenses of a case manager now (consider quality, patient satisfaction, enhanced utilization of the health care team and other resources).

Carr, D. (2007). Case managers optimize patient safety by facilitating effective care transitions. *Professional Case Management, 12*(2), 70–80.

1. The author describes "five main areas of patient safety" on which case managers can have an impact. Consider just one of these areas and brainstorm ideas you might suggest to improve current practice in your work area.
2. Evaluate the process of discharge planning at your current institution. Does it begin at admission? Do you observe effective communication as "handoffs" of care occur? Discuss specific examples.
3. Review the "Essential Skills for Practitioners" outlined in Table 5. Consider a multidisciplinary team that you currently work with (or previously worked with). Are all of these skills present in the team? If you were the case manager, what might you do to assist the team to improve in at least one area?

Issue 3: Quality Improvement

Huber, D., & Craig, K. (2007). Acuity and case management: A healthy dose of outcomes, Part I. *Professional Case Management, 12*(3), 132–144.

1. Consider the four elements of intervention dose described as essential by the authors. Choose a patient in your practice and begin to analyze your case management activities using this dosage model. How can this process help your practice?
2. How is acuity measured in your current setting? Compare and contrast current system of measurement with the Case Management Acuity Tool (Table 2).
3. Identify two (or more) patients you are caring for and apply the Case Management Acuity Tool (Table 2). Then use Table 3 to score the tools. How does this information help you? Do the scores reflect your views of the patients? How might you use this information to help you and your department manage case load?
4. Explore the business metrics that are currently tracked in your department. How might the Case Management Acuity Tool assist you to "build the business case" for your services?

Craig, K., & Huber, D. (2007). Acuity and case management: A healthy dose of outcomes, Part II. *Professional Case Management, 12*(4), 199–210.
Huber, D., & Craig, K. (2007). Acuity and case management: A healthy dose of outcomes, Part III. *Professional Case Management, 12*(5), 254–269.

1. Does your facility use any tool to measure changes in acuity over time? If so, how does it compare to the AccuDiff? What are the differences? What are the strengths and weaknesses of the two tools?
2. Examine current case management case load and consider possible RDC groupings to use for your practice. What information do you need to gather about your patients to start this process? Do you discover unexpected findings during this analysis?
3. Review the concept of "reverse acuity differential." Are there cases in your practice to which this might apply? Are the cases similar? How? What does this tell you about your practice? How might you use this information?

Issue 4: Case Management: Costs, Reimbursement, and Utilization Review

Daniels, S., & Ramey, M. (2008). Faster than a speeding bullet: Changes in Medicare rules for the hospital case manager. *Professional Case Management, 13*(5), 253–261.

1. Examine your hospital's strategies and policies to address Medicare's "Present on Admission" rules. What role does case management play?
2. How do case managers interact and communicate in your health care setting? How can this be improved? What can the case manager do to facilitate enhanced communication and address some of the requirements of Medicare?
3. Visit the "Medicare" section of the Centers for Medicaid and Medicare Services (CMS) website (http://www.cms.hhs.gov/home/medicare.asp). Become familiar with the vast amount of information and resources available. Further explore rules and guidance related to topics presented in this article such as beneficiary notices and hospital-acquired conditions (present on admission indicators), as well as other areas that apply to your practice.

Issue 5: Chronic Illness

Stanton, M., Dunkin, J., & Thomas, K. (2007). Designing a system of case management for a rural nursing clinic for elderly patients with depression. *Professional Case Management, 12*(2), 83–90.

1. Monitoring outcomes for the patient population being served is a critically important function of individual case managers and the case management program as a whole. Review outcomes established by Capstone Rural Healthcare for elderly patients with depression. Now consider the patient population you currently work with. If you are the case manager, what outcomes should be established and monitored for your patients?
2. Again consider your current patient population and assume you are working as a case manager or developing a case management program. Is your population primarily urban or rural? Do most patients have access to phones and transportation, or are these significant needs? How would you propose to use on-site and telephonic case management? What additional resources might your patients need that will enhance success of case management? How can you creatively address those needs? What would be your red flags?

3. If possible, review the case management job description(s) for your facility. Are the roles and responsibilities clearly defined?

Miller, L., & Cox, K. (2005). Case management for patients with heart failure: A quality improvement intervention. *Journal of Gerontological Nursing, 31*(5), 20–28.

1. What process guides clinical outcomes improvement projects at your facility? How does that process compare to the 10-step model presented in this article?
2. Choose a clinical issue of interest to you and work through the first three steps of the improvement model. Who would you select for your project champion and team? Why?
3. As a case manager, what can you learn from the program described and ultimately discontinued? How can this help you in current and future program planning and development?

Issue 6: Disease Management

Krumholz, H., Currie, P., Riegel, B., Phillips, E., Smith, R., Yancy, C., & Faxon, D. (2006). A taxonomy for disease management: A scientific statement from the American Hospital Association disease management taxonomy writing group. *Circulation, 114*(13), 1432–1445.

1. Compare and contrast the following concepts as defined by this article: disease management (DMAA Definition, Table 4), case management, coordinated care, and multidisciplinary care.
2. If your facility offers disease management, select one program (such as diabetes, heart failure, etc.) and analyze it according to the eight domains of the disease management taxonomy presented in this article. Are all domains addressed in your facility's program? If not, identify the gaps. (See Chapter 6 for more information about disease management [DM].)

Norman, G. (2008). Commentary. Disease management outcomes: Are we asking the right questions yet? *Population Health Management, 11*(4), 183–187.

1. How does this article and the questions raised by the author impact your thoughts on the value of disease management? How can expenses associated with these programs be justified in this economic climate if hard evidence doesn't support return on investment? What other factors should be considered?
2. Why is this discussion relevant to you? What are the implications for the future of disease management?
3. The author states that "a strong case can be made that measurement for learning and measurement for judgment, at least for DM, require different perspectives" (article p. 185). After reading this article, what are your thoughts about this statement? Do you agree? Why or why not?

Lippincott's Case Management
Vol. 10, No. 6, 294–302
© 2005, Lippincott Williams & Wilkins, Inc.

Role Transition From Caregiver to Case Manager, Part 1

Nancy Schmitt, PhD, RN, CCM

This two-part article explores the process of role transition as it pertains to nurses moving from roles of caregivers to roles of case managers. Part 1 of the article presents a theoretical model that demonstrates the interplay of significant factors in the process of role transition and discusses how this model can be used to examine nurses' experience of this transition. Part 2 presents findings from a qualitative study involving interview and focus group data contributed by nurses who have made the transition from caregiver to case manager. Data point to specific tensions experienced by these nurses, which are associated with time-task orientation, interactions and relationships, business culture and objectives, and self-image and professional identity. Recommendations for preparing and supporting nurses through this role are also offered.

Case management (CM) is an area of practice engaged in by nurses and other healthcare professionals to control healthcare costs through facilitating timely and appropriate use of healthcare resources by patients, providers, and payers. Over the past 20 years, employment opportunities for nurses in this area have expanded and continue to grow (CMSA, 2004; Falter, Cesta, Concert, & Mason, 1999; Howe, 1999). Subsequently, nurses are sought after for CM positions and often make the role transition from caregiver to case manager.

As the demand for nurses as case managers expands, so too does the need to develop the means to educate and train competent practitioners. A qualitative study examining the experiences of nurse case managers (NCMs) who entered the field within the previous 3 years revealed a common theme of limited insight upon role entry regarding the role of case manager and available resources outside of their employment setting to assist them with role mastery (Schmitt, 2003). In a review of nursing and CM literature from the previous 10 years, Falter et al. (1999) found that CM education is diverse and includes not only continuing education courses and on-the-job training but also some formal undergraduate and graduate course content. Barfield (2003) reports, however, that formal training programs offered by professional organizations are directed more toward practicing NCMs, and that academic programs for preparing nurses for the practice of CM are relatively new. The extent to which each of these venues are available, utilized, or effective in preparing nurses for CM responsibilities have not been addressed.

Another study of educational approaches and issues in preparing nurses for CM indicated that although most faculty members in academic nursing programs studied had educational preparation in CM, many lacked experience in the role (Haw, 1996). This suggests that information about nurses' experiences of this role transition would provide useful information for faculty charged with constructing and delivering academic courses for nurses interested in pursuing this career option, as well as useful insight for employers of NCMs who seek to conduct effective orientation programs.

This two-part article will address significant issues in case manager role entry and learning and provide suggestions for the design of training and education programs for new case managers. Part 1 will provide and explain a model of the process of role transition that is useful in exploring the experience of professionals moving from one role to another.

Specifically, the roles of caregiver and case manager will be compared, and implications for anticipating characteristics of the transition from caregiver to case manager will be discussed. Part 2 will provide information obtained from new case managers about their experiences of this role transition, articulating their motivations and expectations in role entry, their experiences of transition and role strain, and sources of job satisfaction. Inferences are drawn from these data that form a foundation for the design and implementation of comprehensive development programs for nurses making the transition from caregiver to case manager.

THEORETICAL CONSIDERATIONS

Role theory provides a useful conceptual framework for exploration of transitions in work practices, relationships, and identities. In the role transition from caregiver to case manager, changes can include work settings, organization structures, performance expectations, and professional relationships. Murray (1998) used role theory to examine nurses' transitions from hospital-based nursing practice to home care nursing. She relates that although a significant amount of nursing literature exists that addresses the transitional experience and needs of nurses new to the practice setting, literature that addresses the transitional experience and needs of nurses who move from one area of practice to another in the course of their professional career is scarce. She further contends that educators can impact the degree of role strain experienced, and ultimately the success of role transition of nurses making practice-based career changes by incorporating role theory concepts into orientation and continuing education programs.

Biddel (1979) defines *role theory* as "a science concerned with the study of behaviors that are characteristic of persons within contexts and with various processes that presumably produce, explain or are affected by those behaviors." He points out that role theory provides us with a means of studying both the individual and the collective within one conceptual framework, because it is the "theoretical point of articulation between psychology and sociology." He offers five basic propositions that underlie this science. They are as follows:

a. Roles consist of patterned behaviors that are characteristic of persons within contexts;
b. Roles are associated with sets of persons who share a common identity;

c. To some extent, persons performing a role are governed by expectations that exist and are shared about normative performance;
d. Roles persist because of their function and perceived necessity in larger social systems; and
e. Roles are learned through socialization and people may find either joy or sorrow in performing them.

Two basic approaches to role theory have been discussed in literature, those being *structuralist* and *social interactionist* perspectives (Ashforth, 2001; Ebaugh, 1988). A debate between these two perspectives is essentially whether a person "takes" or "makes" a role. The *structuralist* approach views the role, or expected behaviors to be an objective identity or utility that a person takes on by fulfilling certain responsibilities or objectives. The *social interactionist* approach views the role as an identity or utility that is ultimately negotiated between the person engaging in expected behaviors and the context within which the role resides. The *social interactionist* view allows that the person transitioning from one role to another brings personal values, goals, meanings, and attitudes from previous roles that impact the way the new role is understood and enacted. Nurses' foundational education and experience as caregivers no doubt influences their experience of transition to the role of case manager. Exploring personal values, goals, meanings, and attitudes developed in a caregiving role may provide insight regarding tensions experienced in the transition to CM.

The concepts and propositions of role theory are useful in studying role transition because they offer a lens with which to view issues affecting persons exiting and entering different contexts, trying on new identities, and performing new behaviors. Through this lens, we can identify social, environmental, and individual aspects and processes that produce patterns of behavior, and how and why expectations about these patterns are sustained or are changed.

Allen and van de Vliert (1982) developed a Model of the Role Transition Process that incorporates the social interactionist perspective of concepts and propositions of role theory. This model accommodates a dynamic interplay of social positions, expectations, and behaviors that move individuals toward personal growth and adaptation in a role or toward role exit. Figure 1 demonstrates the sequential component parts of the role transition process, which include antecedent conditions, role transition (behavior shift), moderators, role strain, reactions, and consequences.

Antecedent conditions are motivating factors that influence individuals to move from one role to another. These motivating factors can operate on various levels. On the level of the individual engaged in transition, for example, antecedent conditions might be a change in capabilities, values, or financial needs. For nurses making a change from caregiver to case manager, a personal motivation might be more desirable compensation or schedule flexibility. On an organizational level, antecedent conditions might include a change in market share, resource availability, or mission that either attracts an individual to a new role or renders the existing role occupied obsolete or no longer acceptable to the individual. Nurses working in clinical settings as caregivers may deal with sustained staff shortages, or threatening hospital closings, or mergers by looking for alternative career options.

The *role transition process* as a component part of the model (as opposed to the model in its entirety) refers to the actual shift in behavior that occurs when individuals exit one role and enter another. According to Allen and van de Vliert (1984), there are three factors that influence this shift in terms of the permeability of old behaviors into the new role. These factors are (a) the degree of discontinuity between old and new behaviors, or how different the expected behaviors in the new role are from behaviors undertaken in the old role, (b) the accuracy of the transitioning person's anticipation of problems that will be encountered in shifting behaviors, and (c) the extent to which role entry and the assumption of new behaviors and responsibilities is formally structured and governed, as in a formal orientation, apprenticeship, or internship program.

Allen and van de Vliert (1982) and others (Ashforth 2001; Nicholson, 1984) point out that the degree of discontinuity in expected behaviors between old and new roles can influence the degree to which old behaviors are carried into the new role, and the degree to which new behaviors are accepted as more desirable. There is obviously a significant degree of discontinuity between expected behaviors of caregivers and those of case managers in terms of the provision of direct care versus the facilitation of appropriate cost-effective care.

Hordijk, Muis, and Van de Viler (in Allen & van de Vliert, 1982) found that both overly optimistic and overly pessimistic anticipation of problems associated with a new role caused more role strain than an appropriate anticipation of problems. Nurses entering the role of case manager may be aware of overt differences in expected behaviors, such as the shift from providing direct care to facilitating appropriate, cost-effective care. They may not, however, be aware of the nature of the politics involved or ethical dilemmas that case manager's face.

The remaining factor significant to the transitional shift in behavior is the extent to which the change is normatively governed; that is, the extent to which the challenges of role learning and socialization in the transitional phase are identified and planned for (Eraut, 1994). Exploring the experiences of NCMs with regard to the nature and effectiveness of their initial orientation to CM and early training agendas add to our understanding about the impact of contextual factors on this role transition.

The component of *role strain* in Allen and van de Vliert's model refers to the subjective experience of the person in the process of transition. Feelings of discomfort, disequilibrium, anxiety, and perplexity are often part of the transition process (Ashforth, 2001; Biddel, 1979; Ebaugh, 1988). Factors affecting the degree of role strain experienced by individuals may include the clarity of expectations and boundaries associated with the new role and the meaning ascribed to accomplishing the transition—as a loss or gain of function, status, or esteem. CM expectations and boundaries are not so clearly defined as clinical procedures.

Moderators are individual and environmental variables that can influence the intensity of role strain and ultimately impact other components of the process. On the level of the individual, for example, personality, locus of control, self-confidence, and social identity can moderate the transition experience to produce more or less strain. Contextual or environmental factors such as social networks, support for learning, and the availability of resources can also work to exacerbate or diminish the experience of role strain (Carkhuff, 1996; Daley, 2001). Moderators in CM may include such things as the amount and kind of clinical and life experience the transitioning nurse has to draw from, the availability of a cohort within and outside of the employing organization, and support from the organization in terms of time and reimbursement for participation in professional organizations and continuing education programs.

Reactions refer to attempts by the individual to reduce role strain. Reactions can be the activation of accommodations in self or the environment to accomplish this. Seeking out more information and working to enhance or gain specific skills are reactions to role strain. Seeking to change behavioral expectations of the new role to comply more with existing skill levels and interests is also a reaction. Exploring how nurses react to strain experienced as beginning and novice NCMs and how effective or ineffective particular reactions prove to be provide helpful insight for those interested in facilitating effective transitions into this role for nurses.

Consequences are those intended or unintended outcomes resulting from the focal person's attempts to deal with role strain. These outcomes can be an alteration in any of the other components of the process and be short or long term. For example, a nurse making the transition from caregiver to case manager may react to role strain by networking with other case managers to learn more effective practice strategies. The introduction of successful new practice strategies shifts behavior even more (role transition). Performance of new behaviors can either serve to increase or decrease role strain and produce new reactions. If role strain is increased, a subsequent rejection of aspects of the role that are intolerable may become new conditions antecedent to another shift in roles (from case manager back to caregiver, for example). If strain is decreased, the new skills acquired and success experienced may consequently become a moderator, such as a change in professional identity that serves to moderate role strain associated with any subsequent behavior changes.

To speculate about significant issues that may be associated with each of these factors in a role transition from caregiver to case manager, it is essential to examine each role for similarities and differences. Such an examination involves clearly identifying and describing behaviors, however obvious, that are characteristic of each role. Benner (1984) identified seven domains of nursing practice that serve well as an organizer for comparing characteristic role behaviors of caregivers and case managers. These domains are as follows: (a) the helping role, (b) the teaching—coaching function, (c) the diagnostic and patient monitoring function, (d) effective management of rapidly changing situations, (e) administering and monitoring therapeutic interventions and regimes, (f) monitoring and ensuring quality of healthcare practices, and (g) organizational and work role competencies. These domains encompass aspects of work for which nurses are prepared through their professional education programs essentially for caregiving. However, each domain can be viewed as a category of either a hands-on or a facilitative approach. For the purpose of this role examination, caregiving is viewed as a hands-on approach and CM is viewed as a facilitative approach. Table 1 provides a comparative survey of each approach.

NURSES AS CAREGIVERS

A basic premise of nursing care is the prevention of noxious influences and the provision of life-sustaining resources (Newell, 1996). As caregivers in the *helping role*, nurses provide comfort measures and support in coping for patients. Comfort measures include assistance with activities of daily living such as hygiene, grooming, exercise, and positioning. Coping support encompasses creating a climate for healing through control of environmental variables. Caregivers intervene in patients' environments by identifying and removing hazards, taking precautions, and introducing resources that are not only conducive to healing but stimulate or enhance patients' growth and development. Nursing interventions in this regard encompass the physical as well as psychosocial environment.

Caregivers enact a *teaching—coaching function* that includes such activities as probing to find out patients' interpretation of their illness and their readiness to learn self-care activities. "Hands-on" teaching and coaching includes providing patient education and counseling on health conditions, giving rationale for procedures and explaining the implications of illness and recovery for patients' lifestyles.

The *diagnostic and monitoring function* engaged in by caregivers includes detection and documentation of significant changes in patents' conditions through direct observations, physical examinations, and attention to patients' concerns about and experience of symptoms. Caregivers record and report patients' responses to various treatment strategies in terms of vital signs such as body temperature, blood pressure, heart rate, and respiration. Monitoring activities include measuring fluid intake and output, assessing changes in skin conditions, such as color, texture, and integrity, and noting changes in strength and joint mobility, as well as discrepancies in alertness or emotional reactions.

In providing *effective management of rapidly changing situations*, nurses as caregivers recognize emergent physical conditions and respond immediately in an effort to halt or reduce life-threatening processes and restore life-sustaining processes until physician assistance is available. This requires an immediate grasp of arising problems and the ability

TABLE 1   Comparison of Caregiver and Case Manager Responsibilities

Domains of Nursing Practice (Benner, 1984)	Examples of Caregiver Behaviors	Examples of Case Manager Behaviors
Helping role	Assistance with hygiene, grooming, positioning, and ambulation	Facilitating access to healthcare resources and available benefits
	Creating and maintaining an environment free from harm and conducive to healing and well-being	Creating an environment of open communication and understanding between patient, provider, payer, and other stakeholders in the community
Teaching—coaching function	Patient and family education and counseling about health conditions and coaching in self- and supportive care practices	Patient education about health conditions, care options, and benefit coverage
		Provider education about benefit system and available financial support
		Payer education about patients needs and the cost of necessary care
		Community education about patients' reentry needs
Diagnostic and monitoring function	Detection and reporting of significant changes in patients' physical, emotional, cognitive state through physical examination and monitoring laboratory reports	Detection of changes in patients health-care needs on the basis of patient, family, and provider feedback
		Detection of problems with insurance coverage on the basis of payer, provider, and patient feedback
Effective management of rapidly changing situations	Life-saving responses to physical and psychological emergencies	Responses to situations that threaten continuity of needed care, benefit coverage, or patient adherence to prescribed treatment
Administering and monitoring therapeutic interventions	Directly dispensing medication, fluids, and nutrition	Facilitation, coordination, and monitoring needed therapeutic interventions
	Performing procedures related to respiration, elimination, mobility, etc	
Monitoring and ensuring quality of healthcare practices	Assessment of safety and quality of prescribed treatment in light of patients' condition and responses	Assessment of safety and quality of prescribed treatment in light of established treatment protocols and patients' ability and willingness to Participate
Organizational and work competencies	Setting priorities to meet demands on time and attention from multiple patients	Recognition and understanding the needs and interests of multiple stakeholders
	Working with interdisciplinary teams and contingency planning for scarce resources needed for the delivery of care	Negotiating for the most cost-effective healthcare outcomes
		Acting as a liaison for effective communication between patients, providers, and payers

to match medical demands with available resources. Skills in cardiopulmonary resuscitation, and defibrillation, as well as knowledge of the administration of appropriate agents and procedures are essential in this role.

Nurses as caregivers directly *administer and monitor therapeutic interventions and regimes.* This includes dispensing medication, fluids, and nutrition through various means, performing procedures such as wound dressing, bladder catheterization, and tracheal suctioning, facilitating appropriate amounts of rest and exercise, and documenting patients' conditions and responses. Caregivers must therefore be current in knowledge and skill pertaining to advances in pharmacology, medical technology, and various treatment protocols.

Caregivers to varying degrees *monitor and ensure the quality of healthcare practices.* In this domain of nursing practice, caregivers assess the safety or merit of prescribed treatment in light of the patient's condition or response. This entails determining what can be safely omitted or added to the prescribed regime, and getting appropriate and timely responses from physicians.

The practice domain of *organizational and work-role competencies* encompasses the management and administrative responsibilities associated with providing direct care. Behaviors of caregivers in this domain include setting priorities among multiple demands on time and attention as they pertain to meeting the immediate healthcare needs of assigned patients. Characteristic behaviors may include building and maintaining working relationships with an interdisciplinary team of health professionals that all contribute to the well-being of those patients, and whose services require coordination. This domain could also include contingency planning when resources, such as staff, equipment, or supplies, are limited.

NURSES AS CASE MANAGERS

Case Management is a multidisciplinary area of practice with representation from the fields of nursing, social work, rehabilitation counseling, and occupational and physical therapy (Mullahy, 1998). A recent survey of working case managers, however, revealed that roughly 63% of respondents had a nursing background (American Healthcare Consultants, 2001). Nurses with strong clinical backgrounds are sought after to practice in this area because of their presumed knowledge of the healthcare system and understanding of care requirements associated disease and disability.

Nursing and CM literatures demonstrate numerous practice models and settings for CM (Chan, Leahy, McMahon, Mirch, & DeVinney, 1999; Conti, 1996; Falter et al., 1999; Howe, 1999; Lamb & Stemple, 1994; Mullahy, 1998; Newell, 1996; Nolan, Harris, Kuffa, Opfer, & Turner, 1998). NCMs are employed by hospitals and rehabilitation and extended care facilities to provide coordination and oversight of the needed in-patient services and to monitor patient responses to treatment protocols from admission through discharge. NCMs are employed in ambulatory clinics and health maintenance organizations to coordinate ongoing primary care of patient populations with at-risk and chronic conditions such as high-risk pregnancies, cardiac disease, diabetes, and asthma.

Third-party payers (i.e., organizations that provide healthcare insurance, disability and workers' compensation insurance, and automobile personal injury protection insurance) employ NCMs to identify healthcare needs associated with illness or injury claims, to coordinate access to appropriate, cost-effective resources, and to monitor the recovery process through full recovery or maximum medical improvement. Proprietary CM companies, or CM vendors, who enter into service agreements with insurance companies, attorneys, or private individuals to perform CM services, also employ NCMs.

The Case Management Society of America (CMSA) defines *case management* as "a collaborative process of assessment, planning, facilitation and advocacy for options and services to meet an individual's specific healthcare needs through communication and available resources to promote quality cost-effective outcomes" (CMSA, 2002). Based on this definition, essential CM activities can be explored using Benner's domains of nursing (1984) in the following way.

In the *helping role*, NCMs facilitate access to needed healthcare resources, focus on decreasing fragmentation of care, and provide advocacy for patient empowerment and favorable health outcomes. NCMs help establish an environment of open communication and understanding among multiple stakeholders, including patients, payers, providers, families, and other community members impacted by an individual's healthcare needs (Flarey & Blancett, 1996; Mullahy 1998; Newell, 1996; Powell, 1996).

In contrast with caregivers, NCMs operate in the domain of *teaching and coaching* not only by providing patients with education about health conditions but also by coaching patients regarding care options and benefit coverage. In addition, NCMs inform providers about payer systems and patients' willingness and capacity for adherence to prescribed treatment plans. They alert payers about patient health-care needs and assist with calculating the cost of necessary care. They may also provide communities with guidance in accommodating a patient's reentry into home, school, or work environments.

In the role of case manager, nurses enact diagnostic and monitoring functions on changes in patients healthcare needs by way of soliciting, interpreting, and synthesizing patient, family, and provider feedback.

They identify problems with insurance coverage, healthcare system utilization, and patients' health literacy by way of ongoing communications with payers, providers, and patients. Nurses as case managers are charged with *effective management of rapidly changing situations* that threaten continuity of needed care, covered benefits, or patient adherence to treatment plans. They must be prepared to act as liaisons among and between stakeholders with various interests and as problem solvers able to identify and address issues before and even as they escalate.

As opposed to hands-on care, NCMs *administer and monitor therapeutic interventions* through communication, advocacy, and evaluation. They support patients in the construction of healthcare goals, choosing between available treatment options, and adherence to prescribed treatment plans. They assist with coordination of therapeutic interventions through each level and specialty of service, and track recovery progress.

NCMs participate in *monitoring and ensuring quality of healthcare practices* through keeping abreast of evidence-based treatment protocols, assessing available care options in light of patients' ability and willingness to participate, and alerting patients and providers to their concerns regarding safety and quality. CM activities aligned with the domain of *organizational and work competencies* include recognition and understanding of the needs and interests of multiple stakeholders and planning and negotiating for the most cost-effective goods and services needed to effect the best possible health outcome.

DISCUSSION

Clearly, there are identifiable differences between the roles of caregiver and case manager. Conti (1996), by way of a survey study, identified 16 behaviors characteristically engaged in by nurses performing in the role of case manager. These behaviors in order of frequency include monitoring, problem solving, expediting, public relating, communicating, educating, contacting, planning, explaining, recommending, coordinating, documenting, assessing, negotiating, educating, brokering, and researching. She also found that the majority of nurses in her study indicated that the source of learning for this role, with all identified attendant behaviors, was employment and life experience.

Prepared to be caregivers, nurses entering the field of CM encounter new role expectations, healthcare perspectives, and competing interests. Some new ethical issues that they face include patient versus payer rights, patient noncompliance, efficacy of treatment, employer involvement, cultural diversity, and underutilization of services. Litigation, insurance fraud, guardianship, conservatorship, informed consent, confidentiality, and other medical—legal issues also pose dilemmas for case managers in the course of practice (Banja, 1999, Mullahy, 1999).

Nurses practicing as caregivers may encounter a number of these issues in providing direct care to patients; however, the number of stakeholders to be considered in healthcare scenarios expands for case managers. As a collaborative process, CM necessarily acknowledges and attends to interests of both the individual in need of healthcare and the systems within which healthcare is accessed, provided, and supported (Meany, 1999).

Though it appears that Benner's domains of nursing practice (1984) incorporate some of the behaviors identified by Conti (1996) as integral to the case manager role, some significant qualitative differences are apparent. Specifically noteworthy are (a) time perspectives (more immediate for the role of caregiver; more extended timeframe for CM activities), (b) the mode of provision of healthcare goods and services (provided directly by a caregiver; coordinated and facilitated by the case manager), and (c) setting (healthcare provider organization for the caregiver; healthcare provider or payer organization for the case manager). Also, although initial formal preparation in nursing, as well as clinical experience n the caregiver role, may provide useful foundational knowledge and skill on which to build expertise in CM, there are gains to be made in terms of preparing the case manager candidate pool with clearly anticipated perspectives, approaches, and relationships that differ between the caregiver and case manager roles.

As the need for competent case managers expands, academic nursing programs need to respond by standardizing CM perspectives and role information into foundational nursing curricula, by providing supervised practicum opportunities in advanced nursing programs, and by identifying competencies necessary for graduates to function as case managers. Employers seeking to reap the value benefits of nurses as case managers need to design and deliver comprehensive orientation and training programs that are sensitive to experience of role strain that may accompany nurses making the transition from a caregiving context. They also need to be aware of how previous employment experiences may serve to enhance or diminish the learning curve for the novice case manager. Nurses contemplating career opportunities in the field of CM need also to examine role differences to appropriately prepare for role strain as they acclimate to new work expectations and plan for role mastery.

CONCLUSION

Case Manager is a growing field of practice in systems of healthcare delivery and insurance claim payment. Nurses are often sought after to fill CM positions because of valued clinical knowledge acquired through nursing education and experience as care-givers. Although foundational nursing education and experience as caregivers provide nurses with valuable insight into issues related to illness, recovery,

and healthcare systems, this background does not necessarily prepare them to anticipate and assume a role that requires the development of new skills and perspectives and application of their knowledge base in a different context. A Model of the Role Transition Process (Allen & van de Vliert, 1982) contributes a structured approach to exploring a dynamic process of change and adaptation that can inform the design and delivery education and training programs for nurses entering the field of CM.

Part 2 of this article will present interview and focus group data from a qualitative study of nurses who have made the transition from caregiver to case manager, and will further discuss implications for education and training programs for nurses entering this field.

References

Allen, V. L., & van de Vliert, E. (1982). A role theoretical perspective on transitional processes. In V. L. Allen & E. Van de Vliert (Eds.), *Role transitions: Explorations and explanations* (pp. 3–18). New York: Plenum.

American Healthcare Consultants. (2001). Case management caseload data: Results of a national survey. *Executive Summary Case Management Advisor, 12*(3), 2.

Ashforth, B. (2001). *Role transitions in organizational life*. Hillsdale, NJ: Lawrence Erlbaum Associates.

Banja, J. (1999). Ethical decision-making: Origins, process, and applications. *The Case Manager, 10*(5), 41–47.

Barfield, F. (2003). Working case managers view of the profession. *The Case Manager, 14*(6), 69–71.

Benner, P. (1984). From novice to expert: Excellence and power in clinical nursing practice. Menlo Park, CA: Addison-Wesley.

Biddel, B. (1979). Role theory: Expectations, identities and behaviors. New York: Academic Press.

CMSA. (2002). *Standards of practice for case management, revised 2002*. Little Rock, AR: Case Management Society of America.

CMSA. (2004). Contemporary trends in case management. *The Case Manager, 15*(2), 45–47.

Carkhuff, M. (1996). Reflective learning: Work groups as learning groups. *The Journal of Continuing Education in Nursing, 27*, 209–214.

Chan, F., Leahy, M., McMahon, B., Mirch, M., & DeVinney, D. (1999). Foundational knowledge and major practice domains of case management. *The Journal of Care Management, 5*(1), 10–30.

Conti, R. (1996). Nurse case manager roles: Implications for practice and education. *Nursing Administration Quarterly, 21*(1), 67–80.

Daley, B. (2001). Learning and professional practice: A study of four professions. *Adult Education Quarterly, 52*, 39–54.

Ebaugh, H. R. (1988). *Becoming an ex: The process of role exit*. Chicago: University of Chicago Press.

Eraut, M. (1994). Developing professional knowledge and competence. London: The Falmer Press.

Falter, E., Cesta, T., Concert, C., & Mason, D. (1999). Development of a graduate nursing program in case management. *The Journal of Care Management, 5*(3), 50–78.

Flarey, D. L., & Blancett, S. (1996). *Handbook of nursing case management*. Gaithersburg, MA: Aspen.

Haw, M. A. (1996). Case management education in universities: A national survey. *Journal of Care Management, 2*(6), 10–21.

Howe, R. (1999). Case management in managed care: Past, present and future. *The Case Manager, 10*(5), 37–40.

Lamb, G., & Stempel, J. (1994). Nurse case management from the client's view: Growing as insider-expert. *Nursing Outlook, 42*(1), 7–13.

Meany, M. (1999). Building a professional ethical culture in case management. *The Case Manager, 10*(5), 63–67. Mullahy, C. (1999). Case management: An ethically responsible solution. *The Case Manager, 10*(5), 59–62.

Mullahy, C. (1998). *The case manager's handbook* (2nd ed.). Gaithsburg, MD: Aspen.

Murray, T. A. (1998). Using role theory concepts to understand transitions from hospital-based nursing practice to home care nursing. *The Journal of Continuing Education in Nursing, 29*(3), 105–111.

Newell, M. (1996). Using nursing case management to improve health outcomes. Gaithersburg, MA: Aspen.

Nicholson, N. (1984). A theory of work role transitions. *Administrative Science Quarterly, 29,* 172–191. Nolam, M., Harris, A., Kuffa, A., Opfer, N., Turner, N. (1998). Preparing nurses for acute care case manager role: Educational needs identified by existing case managers. *The Journal of Continuing Education, 29*(3), 130–134.

Powell, S. (1996). *Nursing case management.* Philadelphia: Lippincott- Raven.

Schmitt, N. L. (2003). *Role transitions for nurses: From care giver to case manager.* Unpublished doctoral dissertation, Michigan State University, East Lansing.

Nancy Schmitt, PhD, RN, CCM, is currently the coordinator of the URAC-accredited case management program at Citizens and Hanover Insurance Companies. In addition to case management, her work experience includes rehabilitation nursing, curriculum development for patient education and professional continuing education programs, and medical education administration.

Address correspondence to Nancy Schmitt, PhD, RN, CCM, 4142 Highcrest Drive, Brighton, MI 48116 (nancys@ ismi.net).

Lippincott's Case Management
Vol. 11, No. 1, 37–46
© 2006, Lippincott Williams & Wilkins, Inc.

Role Transition From Caregiver to Case Manager—Part 2

Nancy Schmitt, PhD, RN, CCM

This two-part article explores the process of role transition as it pertains to nurses moving from roles of caregivers to roles of case managers. Part 1 of the article presented a theoretical model that demonstrated the interplay of significant factors in the process of role transition and discussed how this model could be used to examine nurses' experience of this transition. Part 2 presents findings from a qualitative study involving interview and focus group data contributed by nurses who have made the transition from caregiver to case manager. Data point to specific tensions experienced by these nurses, which are associated with time—task orientation, interactions and relationships, business culture and objectives, and self-image and professional identity. Recommendations for preparing and supporting nurses through this role are also offered.

INTRODUCTION

Nurses are filling a growing demand by healthcare provider systems and insurance companies for case managers who oversee, recommend, and coordinate utilization of services (Chan, Leahy, McMahon, Mirch, & DeVinney, 1999; "What's in the Future?" 2003). The healthcare and insurance industries are looking to case managers for assistance in containing healthcare costs and improving healthcare outcomes. Fulfilling responsibilities of this role not only requires a familiarity with the clinical aspects of healthcare, but also a knowledge base and skill set for dealing with broader healthcare issues such as service access and utilization, insurance regulations and policy provisions, and cost-containment and quality outcomes (Chan et al., 1999; Conti, 1996; Falter, Cesta, Concert, & Mason, 1999).

Case management (CM) has emerged over the past 20 years as an area of practice that appears well suited to the nursing profession. The growing number of such positions being filled by nurses provides evidence for this. A survey of practicing case managers demonstrated that 60% are registered nurses (American Healthcare Consultants, 2001). Education and training agendas, however, are only beginning to address requisite knowledge and skills for case management in undergraduate and advanced practice nursing curricula and nursing literature (Barefield, 2003; Case Management Society of America, 2004; Conti, 1996), and information about the experience of transition for professional nurses entering this field is sparse.

Part 1 of this article explained how role theory and a model of role transition (Allen & van de Vliert, 1982) can assist in the exploration of nurses' experience of the transition from caregiver to case manager. The roles of caregiver and case manager were compared and contrasted, and the premise was offered that identification of disparities in role perspectives and behaviors have implications for effective learning agendas for nurses contemplating or engaging in this transition. This information provided a conceptual framework for the design of a qualitative study involving new NCMs and their experiences associated with transitioning from caregiver to case manager. Part 2 of this article presents findings from this study and draws inferences that provide specific suggestions for the design and development of CM education, and education and training programs.

STUDY DESIGN

Eleven nurses, who were educationally prepared and principally experienced as caregivers and who had recently assumed roles as case managers, were interviewed about their motivations, sources of role strain and job satisfaction, and experiences associated with assuming case manager roles. Table 1 highlights demographic data pertaining to each participant.

A qualitative study was determined to be appropriate for seeking out characteristic motivations, tensions, satisfactions, etc. from participants because it allows for exploration and description of personal experience and meaning in specific contexts (Creswell, 1994). The methods of inquiry and analysis used are based on the conceptual framework of *symbolic interaction*, which holds that people create

TABLE 1   Participant Demographics

	Age	Education	Years as caregiver	Clinical Experience	Years as NCM	CM Contexts	CM Model
Ann	53	BSN, MA	30	Critical care units Emergency department General practice clinic	1.5	WC carrier	Telephonic
Belinda	49	ADN	3	Skilled nursing facility General practice clinic Pediatric clinic	3	WC carrier	Telephonic
Ginger	53	BSN	30	Critical care units Emergency department	1.5	WC carrier	Telephonic
Irene	56	BSN	21	Medical/surgical units Pediatric clinic	3	WC carrier	Telephonic
Donna	46	ADN+	21	Emergency room General practice clinic Occupational health clinic	1	WC carrier	On-site
Hannah	41	BSN+	14	Orthopedic unit Oncology unit Home care	1.5	CM vendor	On-site
Cathy	29	BSN+	5	Medical/surgical units Oncology unit Public health clinic Home care	1	CM vendor	On-site
Judy	43	ADN+	9	Medical/surgical units Home care	1.5	CM vendor	On-site
Karen	44	BSN	20	Medical/surgical unit Orthopedic unit Home care Utilization review	1.5	HMO	Telephonic
Fran	44	ADN	10	Medical/surgical units Pediatric unit Critical care units Obstetrics and gynecology unit Emergency department Utilization review	2	HMO	Telephonic
Evelyn	47	BSN+	29	Pediatric unit Pediatric clinic Public health clinic	3	HMO	Telephonic

Note: NCM = nurse case manager; CM 3 case management; WC 3 Workers' Compensation; HMO 3 health maintenance organization. Participant names are changed or are pseudonyms.

meaning from experiences through interactional responses to situations (Bogdin & Biklin, 1998).

A *purposeful sample* with consideration to maximum variation in cases was determined to be appropriate for participant recruitment and selection in this study. Purposeful sampling is based on the assumption that a criterion-based sample selection serves the need for in-depth study of information-rich cases. Maximum variation in cases selected contributes to the identification of the relative strength of shared patterns that emerge from data, even in small samples (Merriam, 2001).

Selected participants were practicing NCMs who each had at least 3 years of hospital- or clinic-based experience beyond foundational nursing education and training prior to taking on the role of case manager. They also were required to have practiced in the role of case manager from 1 to 3 years. Case management practice settings represented were limited to payer environments. Age, gender, or ethnicity was not part of the selection criteria.

FINDINGS: EXPERIENCES OF TRANSITION

Data were collected through loosely structured individual and focus group interviews with participants. Through dialogue on contextual variables, and reflections on transition and learning experiences, insight was gained as to how these professionals experienced role transition and learned how to function as case managers. Primary areas explored include (1) motivations, (2) expectations, (3) sources of role strain, and (4) job satisfaction.

Motivations

For most participants the motivation for making this career change stemmed from dissatisfaction with their current work situations. Rather than aspiring to become a case manager with a true appreciation of what the role entailed, a majority of participants explained that a position in case management offered them an alternative to work conditions they could no longer tolerate. These conditions included (a) long hours and inflexible work schedules, (b) low staff/high patient ratios, (c) policy and regulation changes that influenced caregiving practices, (d) job insecurity, (e) inadequate compensation, (f) physically taxing duties, and (g) inadequate intellectual challenge.

The hospital setting was described as undesirable because of the long hours and inflexible work schedules that routinely included weekends and holidays. Although many nurses enjoyed providing care, the low staff/high patient ratios prevented them from delivering the kind of care they felt the patients needed. Some participants felt uncomfortable with the excessive volume and scope of their responsibilities while on duty, which increased the risk of malpractice and ultimately placed their nursing license in jeopardy.

For example, two participants, Ginger and Ann, felt overburdened with professional responsibilities in the hospital setting on the one hand, and yet uncomfortable with the type of tasks being assigned to underqualified personnel to make up for staff and funding shortages on the other hand. Although Karen left her role as a caregiver initially because of a back injury, she left her role in utilization review in a hospital setting because she too felt overutilized.

Judy and Hannah cited changes in Medicare regulations as fueling their motivation to leave their positions in home care. They described what they saw as sudden changes that significantly affected their practice and ultimately their job satisfaction.

Two participants who left clinic settings for CM positions identified their motivations for making the transition as a need to enhance income and a fear of impending position reductions. Irene and Belinda both had several years of experience in pediatric clinics and enjoyed working with children and providing support and advice for parents. After her divorce, Irene required more income and benefits than a position at a pediatric clinic offered. Although she was very satisfied with her role as a pediatric nurse, she found CM to be a more lucrative alternative.

Fran and Cathy were the only participants in search of a more stimulating occupation when they made the transition to CM. Fran explained that her reason for moving from the role of caregiver was a desire for more flexibility in her employment options. She felt that her moves first into UR, then to CM, expanded her capabilities. Cathy found a CM position in pursuit of a more intellectually stimulating career.

Although participants' motivations to make the transition from caregiver to case manager varied, most shared the characteristic of being fueled more by a desire to find a port in the storm, so to speak, than a desire to advance in their nursing career. Looking to improve the conditions of employment, most participants were willing to take a leap of faith that even the unknown aspects of the case manager role would be more tolerable than the undesirable aspects of previous roles.

Expectations

Participants' expectations about the role of case manager were closely tied to the promise it held for providing relief from the undesirable conditions of the roles they were exiting. These expectations included (a) more flexible work schedule, (b) less physically taxing job responsibilities, (c) manageable workloads, (d) opportunities to utilize nursing knowledge, (e) better compensation, and (f) job security. These expectations were fed by second-hand reports most participants received from personal friends or professional acquaintances that alerted them of open case manager positions while they were contemplating making a career move.

Ann and Belinda were approached by friends who alerted them to open positions and encouraged them to apply. Irene, Donna, Ginger, Judy, and Hannah stumbled on open positions through conversations with professional acquaintances. Evelyn and Cathy saw ads in local newspapers, applied for the positions out of curiosity, and were informed about the role in their job interviews. Fran and Karen, knowing that case management was an employment option that they wanted, submitted resumes to a health maintenance organization (HMO) asking to be considered for an interview when a position opened up.

At 56 years of age, Irene was desperate for employment that offered a suitable compensation package that would help her prepare for retirement. Although she was confident that her current position with a Workers' Compensation (WC) insurance carrier would provide her with that, she admitted that she did not have a comprehensive knowledge of what would be expected of her in the case manager role.

Judy was looking to escape the burdensome Medicare regulations she encountered in home care. At the same time, she was enrolled in an accelerated graduate nursing program and hoping to eventually advance her position within the field of nursing. She acted on an opportunity to move into case management with a CM vendor without much prior knowledge of what the job responsibilities were, or how adequately she was prepared to fulfill the expectations of her employer. She also shared that her graduate nursing program had nothing to offer in the way of scheduled courses or independent study in the field of CM.

Donna had some interaction with NCMs in her role as an occupational health nurse. In this role, she gained exposure to work-related injuries and often communicated with WC insurance claim staff, some of who were adjusters and others who were NCMs. This provided a basic awareness of the WC claim process and, to a limited extent, the case manager's tasks. Even so, she was not aware of the expectation that as a case manager she would need to log her activities and be held accountable for a certain number of billable hours.

Karen and Fran, both having had experience in UR and discharge planning in a hospital, had the most familiarity with the case manager role. They submitted resumes without seeing an ad or having knowledge of a job opening. To them, CM seemed like the next logical step. Karen admits though that her expectations were not entirely consistent with what she was encountering on the job.

Entering the role of case manager with expectations that it would provide relief from undesirable work situations and opportunities to utilize their nursing background, participants were generally not aware of aspects of the case manager role that might prove to be problematic for them or aspects that would provide them with opportunities to grow and develop professionally.

Sources of Role Strain

Hopeful that the role of case manager would fulfill their respective desires for better work situations, participants explained that there were a number of work situations that they did not anticipate, and that their knowledge and experience as caregivers did not necessarily prepare them for. Feelings of inadequacy or incompetence associated with these situations contributed to role strain. These situations appeared to center around four major themes: (a) time-task orientation, (b) interactions and relationships, (c) business culture and objectives, and (d) professional identity and self-image.

TIME—TASK ORIENTATION.   Nurses entering the field of case management directly from hospital settings did not anticipate the need to accommodate their *time–task orientation* to fit the role of case manager. Managing cases over an extended period of time as opposed to completing care required by assigned patients on an 8- or 12-hr shift contributed to role strain for new NCMs. In caregiving contexts, the scope of task accomplishment was on administering prescribed care within the timeframe of a daily shift. Patients were assigned or scheduled on a daily basis. This assignment could vary from day to day.

Alternate staff was scheduled to work on subsequent shifts or days so that work did not routinely accumulate in their absence.

In contrast, participants described the scope of task accomplishment in the case management context as scheduling and implementing a series of tasks over time to effect longer-term objectives. Although routine accomplishment of some tasks is expected within certain timeframes, such as initial contacts with patients, providers, or employers, the ongoing tasks of case management are seen as more strategic and timeframes more discretionary.

Ann, who had worked for many years as a caregiver in emergency departments, found the need for a major shift in her inclination to respond and complete task assignments immediately to a planned approach of managing a series of tasks strategically over time. Ginger, who had an extensive background in emergency and critical care nursing, struggled with the need for a sense of closure and accomplishment as a new NCM. In the hospital, she worked long, intense hours, often without breaks. Even so, at the end of her shift, she knew her work was complete and would not carry over to her next scheduled day on duty. As a case manager, she has to deal with a progression of tasks associated with each case assignment that extends over days, weeks, and even months. This has forced her to learn new strategies for prioritizing and managing time.

The autonomy afforded NCMs with designing their own system of managing tasks and time can also contribute to role strain. Donna, an on-site NCM employed by a WC insurance carrier, has an office based in her home. She has to organize her work day to accomplish not only the appointments she has made with claimants at their homes, in hospitals, at physician offices, or with their employers, but also to complete time-sensitive file documentation and manage a number of other clerical tasks without any administrative support. Her background in emergency nursing, occupational health, and outpatient clinic administration did not prepare her for this.

The caregiving experience, particularly for those participants who worked in hospital settings and to a lesser extent clinic settings, created an orientation to time and tasks associated with structure and a sense of urgency. This time–task orientation, which served to focus nurses' attention on immediate healthcare needs of the patients, was a necessary part of nursing judgment and clinical skill that they had developed over many years. The need to change this orientation in their new environment was an aspect of the case manager role that they did not expect and that contributed to a feeling of incompetence.

INTERACTIONS AND RELATIONSHIPS. The second theme associated with sources of role strain in the transition from caregiver to case manager is *interactions and relationships*. Interview and focus group discussion data suggest that new NCMs were confronted with unanticipated dynamics in their interactions and relationships with patients and physicians, and uncharted territory in interactions and relationships with non-medical colleagues, specifically claim adjusters.

In the role of case manager, nurses learn that ill or injured parties are not only patients in the sense that they require healthcare services, they are also "claimants," or in the context of an HMO, "members" of the plan who are also seeking financial support for those services. Available financial benefits associated with illness or injury creates added dimensions to nurse–patient relationships for case managers. The issue of trust in their relationships with patients is one of the first hurdles most participants had to clear.

Dealing with patients who lie to secure financial benefits, or malinger to avoid work responsibilities, created discomfort for NCMs who manage WC, disability, or automobile injury cases. They reported emotions from surprise to disgust in encounters with patients who would fabricate or embellish an injury. Belinda commented on how naïve she felt after her first few encounters with WC claimants who were less than truthful about circumstances surrounding their injury or progress in recovery, and how that affected her approach in subsequent contacts with claimants.

Establishing rapport with patients who are mistrustful was also unexpected and a source of strain for new NCMs. Participants felt that their association with insurance companies often affected patients' perception of them. Judy, whose caregiving background was in home care, noted a difference in the ease with which she could initially establish rapport with patients. "[In home care] there wasn't that self-protective mode . . . in your contact with them. [In CM] they're protecting themselves from you, almost."

Building rapport despite this initial distrust required learning strategies to "get a foot in the door." Evelyn explained how she changed her approach on introductory telephone calls after several encounters with wary parents of the pediatric population she served. "You can hear it in their voice when I call and

I say my name is [Evelyn] and I'm a case manager at [this HMO] and . . . .[they answer] 'Yes?'. . . You know what they're thinking, 'Why is someone from the insurance company calling me?'"

New NCMs also experienced discomfort about their role in legal issues associated with insurance claims. Not being versed in regulations governing WC, automobile injury protection, disability, and health insurance, they were often fearful of making a mistake in handling a case that would contribute to an unintended advantage or disadvantage to either party (the claimant or the insurer) if legal action ensued. This also created another dilemma in their relationships with patients, which is balancing advocacy with prudence. Cathy, who works for a CM vendor, found a surprising need to consider diplomacy in her communications.

In their role as case manager, nurses encountered added dimensions with their relationships to patients that caregiving had not necessarily prepared them for. In this context, patients had the added interest of securing financial benefits, and new NCMs had the added interest of protecting their employers from undue financial exposure. These factors—plus the notion that their relationships and interactions with patients could affect any ensuing legal actions associated with a claim for benefits—were considerable sources of role strain for new NCMs.

Working in a different context with physicians also contributed to role strain for some NCMs in their transition from caregiving. They were not accustomed to discussing treatment options with physicians or questioning their rationale for continuing treatment. Cathy and Belinda, for example, were uneasy about approaching physicians on a more collegial level, having been socialized to view them as the ultimate authority on all health-related issues or "the boss" in prior jobs. Ann's difficulties in relating to physicians in this new context stemmed not from the need to question or confront them in her role a case manager, but rather how to build rapport and establish credibility over the telephone.

Approaching physicians with a posture of confidence and credibility and gaining their trust is a tall order for new NCMs whether they practice on-site or telephonic CM. Successful strategies developed and used in relating to physicians as caregivers do not necessarily provide new NCMs with the knowledge and skill required to interact effectively with physicians as case managers. However, Donna, who had opportunities to relate with physicians in her previous role as manager of an industrial plant health clinic did not find interacting with physicians on a collegial level difficult.

Donna, along with a number of other participants, shared her frustration with interactions and relationships with adjusters. She experiences difficulty at times convincing adjusters of the merit of her medical perspectives on claims and also has trouble understanding the adjusters' objectives and priorities in claim-handling strategies.

Another source of strain for new NCMs in relationships with adjusters was an authority issue. The NCMs employed by WC insurance carriers believed that the adjuster had the final say in authorizing benefit payments, and when and how long the NCM was involved with the case. In essence, the NCMs felt that they were expected to submit to the adjuster. Irene and Ann both shared their frustration with what they perceived as a hierarchy in their office that gave adjusters the authority to accept or reject their recommendations on medical claim decisions.

For Judy, an NCM working for a CM vendor, the issue of adjuster relationships took on a different focus. She perceived a need to please the adjuster to secure business. She seemed less conflicted over reluctance or noncooperation from adjusters than her fear of appearing incompetent and therefore losing repeat business.

Interacting and developing working relationships with claim adjusters proved to be a source of role strain for new NCMs who were accustomed to being surrounded by medical personnel who shared similar experiences and perspectives. Participants felt tentative in arguing their cases with adjusters because of their lack of knowledge of the claim process and the regulations and strategies that drove adjusters' decisions. Some struggled with having their judgment circumvented by adjusters and others were intimidated by the "new world" of business that they had entered.

Nurses working for HMOs did not interact regularly with adjusters. In fact, the interactions were quite infrequent and dealt mostly with getting or correcting information for the file records. These NCMs interacted more with medical plan directors, who are physicians employed by the HMO responsible for reviewing claim requests for coverage that are outside of benefit package. Nurse case managers in this situation plead a case for approval for extra services, goods, or interventions that they feel are the best thing for the member. Working with adjusters was not a source of role strain for these NCMs.

BUSINESS CULTURE AND FINANCIAL OBJECTIVES. New NCMs found that acclimating to a *business culture and financial objectives* contributed to role strain. Some participants did not anticipate the discomfort they would feel in a payer setting. Nurses who were experienced in the tasks of physical care and who had been entrenched in the norms and perspectives of a healthcare provider setting found this new business culture somewhat confusing and intimidating. Among a number of environmental differences, participants perceived significant differences between support structures, work objectives, and tools used in their previous roles as caregivers and their current roles as case managers.

Participants who work in claim offices with adjusters responded that support for their role in terms of resources specific to their jobs and comradeship is just not the same as in the hospitals or clinics where they had come from. Ginger, for example, detected some resentment from adjusters who were used to handling claims without NCMs. It was difficult for her, as a new NCM, to address this issue with adjusters who did not seem to understand her role or appreciate her involvement.

Coming from clinical settings with a focus on providing patients with the intensity and duration of care prescribed by their physicians, most participants shared that cost containment remains an issue about which they feel some conflict. Although they understood that the main objective of their role is to contain healthcare costs, patients' welfare is still foremost in guiding their oversight and authorization of payment for healthcare goods and services. This at times put them at odds with claim adjusters or medical plan directors, whose main concern is holding down healthcare expenditures.

Karen remarks that it has been challenging to focus on cost containment in her role as a case manager with an HMO. As is the case presented by most participants, her previous work environments in healthcare provider settings did not require that she attend to that. "Financial concerns still kind of make me uncomfortable. I'm dealing better with them, and well you work for [an HMO] and that is an issue. And if finances aren't contained then people don't have jobs."

Many participants recognize that the bottom line is paramount in the business world. This influences philosophies about handling insurance claims, which in turn has an impact on the expectations of the case manager's role in the process. Some participants perceive this expectation as potentially confounding to their role as patient advocate. Belinda explained that she feels a tension between her role as patient advocate and the expectation that her influence on a case will result in monetary savings for the WC insurance carrier she works for and ultimately employers who pay premiums.

Another source of role strain for nurses entering a business environment is learning to use the tools available and necessary to complete tasks associated with their new role. Fran describes her adjustment to business-appropriate communications and the need to collect and compile data and demonstrate trends and outcomes.

The use of personal computers and all the electronic means of communication such as e-mail, voicemail, faxes, and cell phones as necessary tools to complete tasks at work stations were also perceived as a convention of the business culture that took some getting used to. Although Donna had experience with the business side of healthcare in roles as nursing director of general practice and occupational health clinics, she struggled with the technical aspects of setting up and managing business from an office in her home.

Coming from clinical settings where staff were medically oriented and committed to providing patients with the intensity and duration of care prescribed by their physicians, new NCMs found a certain amount of role strain associated with entering a business environment. Interacting with a majority of non-medical coworkers, attending to a business objective of cost containment, and the incorporation of clerical tasks and new tools specific to the business environment all contributed to the experience of role strain for new NCMs.

PROFESSIONAL IDENTITY AND SELF-IMAGE. The fourth theme that emerged from interview data and focus group discussions with regard to sources of role strain are experiences and perceptions associated with *professional identity and self-image*. Although most participants view CM as a legitimate area of practice within the nursing profession, some consider the case manager role to be less important or less significant than their previous role as a caregiver. Ginger, for example, refers to case management as "another phase of nursing," but does not believe a nursing background is necessary to do the work she is doing.

Belinda struggled with expanding her notion of nursing to include the role of case manager. "It's a different job and it's not what you think nursing is going to be and it's not where you thought you would be as a nurse when you graduated from nursing school." Because of what she has experienced in her role as a case manager, and the type of problems she has faced in interactions with some WC claimants, Belinda feels a need to hold back on what she considered a characteristic nursing behavior, which is empathizing with and unconditionally supporting the patients she deals with. She also concedes, however, that she is enhancing knowledge and skills that she finds valuable.

Irene's difficulty is associated with the lower esteem she affords her role as case manager in comparison with her role as caregiver. At the same time, she feels that she is becoming more skilled and knowledgeable as a case manager, and that she is much more aligned with her identity as a pediatric nurse.

Although all participants reported that their professional identity is that of a nurse, some aspects of the case manager role seem to be in conflict with the unbiased and apolitical image they predominately hold of themselves as nurses. For some, clinical competence and unconditional nurturing care is held in higher esteem than the role they play as case managers.

To summarize, characteristic sources of role strain for new NCMs revolved around four themes: (a) time–task orientation, (b) interactions and relationships, (c) business culture and objectives, and (d) professional identity and self-image. Participants shared their experiences of confronting the need to accommodate their assumptions and approaches in several areas of their work. The process of this accommodation contributed to role strain, but also stimulated professional growth and eventually contributed to job satisfaction.

Job Satisfaction

Despite experiences of role strain in the transition from caregiver to case manager, participants reported sources of job satisfaction that they associate with their role as case manager. These sources fall into five categories: (a) facilitating recovery and impacting healthcare outcomes, (b) opportunities to expand knowledge and skill, (c) enhanced professional growth and confidence, (d) appreciation and respect from others, and (e) autonomy.

Nurse case managers involved in WC cases find satisfaction in facilitating the recovery and return to work process for injured workers. This process can be long and complicated. It involves getting to know the claimant as well as his or her treating physician(s) and employer. For new NCMs, it may involve research into an unfamiliar medical specialty to learn about treatment protocols and available resources. It involves determining claimants' ability to cope and follow through with the prescribed treatment plans. It can involve referring claimants to a more appropriate medical specialist, coordinating treatment goals and plans among multiple providers, providing patient education and encouragement, and arranging for work accommodations with employers. It very often involves twists and turns in the form of physical, emotional and interpersonal complications along the way that the NCM must address and try to problem-solve around to realize the long-term goal of recovery and return to work for the claimant.

Belinda explains that her satisfaction in facilitating recovery and return to work is often preceded by situations that also cause her a considerable amount of frustration. Being able to influence the outcome, however, provides her with a sense of accomplishment and competence. She also finds that difficult cases provide opportunities for her to expand her knowledge of various medical specialties and the WC claims process.

Cathy describes a sense of satisfaction she gets from producing outcomes that meet the needs of all stakeholders involved in the claim process. Her understanding of the dynamics of multiple stakeholders in the claim process is part of the expanded knowledge and skill she has realized in enacting her new role as case manager.

Nurse case managers who are employed by HMOs find satisfaction in their roles from their capacity to help members gain the most benefit from their health plan or find alternative sources for services or financial support. They have the capacity to identify members who are in need of special services and to access them, to influence coverage approval for extraordinary circumstances and to run interference for members in need of immediate assistance.

Fran states that her main source of job satisfaction is in assisting members to navigate through a complex healthcare system that often is over- or underutilized by patients because of the confusion it fosters. "I truly like navigating someone through this hideous horrible monstrosity called healthcare. . . . This is the corniest of all. When someone asked me why did you go into managed care and I said, 'You know why I went into managed care? I wanted to humanize managed care.'"

Evelyn finds the personal thanks she gets from families of the pediatric patient population she serves to be quite rewarding. Her capacity as a case manager to influence coverage decisions, and get questions answered for members, has also enhanced her confidence. In addition to facilitating recovery, and being appreciated by claimants who were helped, many participants find that their roles as case managers affords them more respect for their knowledge and judgment than they experienced in caregiving roles. Hannah explained how the patients, physicians, and adjusters respect the value of her involvement in the claim process, and that adds to her job satisfaction.

Participants identified autonomy as a source of job satisfaction. They explained that the case manager role allows them autonomy in working flexible schedules, in prioritizing and organizing tasks associated with their caseloads, and in addressing their own learning needs. Although there are specific policies and procedures that NCMs are required to comply with, they feel relatively free from constraints in how they go about the business of managing cases, compared with the rigid structure of hospital or clinic routines.

Donna finds satisfaction with the autonomy allowed in creating a work schedule that accommodated her family obligations. She also finds the opportunity this autonomy provides for professional growth and development to be satisfying.

Although the autonomy associated with the role of case manager offers the convenience of flexible schedules, the freedom to exercise personal preferences in work organization, and the challenge to develop professionally, it is also a source of role strain for new NCMs. Interview and focus group data suggest that autonomy can become problematic for nurses transitioning from caregiver roles who lack familiarity with effective practice strategies.

DISCUSSION

This study illuminated characteristic sources of role strain or tensions experienced by nurses in transition from caregiver to case manager.

Collectively, these tensions are associated with time–task orientation, interactions and relationships, business culture and objectives, and professional identity and self-image. Figure 1 illustrates this finding. Although participants experienced varying combinations and degrees of these tensions, data clearly demonstrate common experiences of role strain stemming from expectations and acquired expertise in past role contexts, and expectations and relative inexperience in new role contexts.

These tensions, associated with characteristic sources of role strain, have the potential for motivating growth and development on the one hand, or eroding self-confidence, delaying effective problem solving, and negatively affecting job satisfaction on the other. Preparing nurses for these tensions and structuring support for them during the transition process will possibly help them better understand their learning needs, take advantage of opportunities for professional growth and development, and expedite their achievement of new competencies.

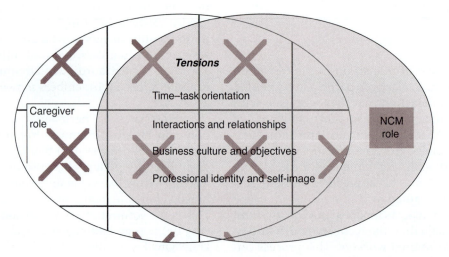

FIGURE 1   Tensions described by nurses in role transitions from caregiver to case manager.

Those with interests in the performance of NCMs should weave the following items into the fabric of education and training agendas: (a) assessing the differences in individuals' past and present performance expectations, (b) alerting new NCMs to tensions that may be created in moving from a caregiving context to a case management context, (c) informing them about relevant learning resources, (d) and guiding them in discovering the meaning of new experiences.

Facilitating a series of discussions between new and experienced NCMs can provide an effective venue for assessing, alerting, informing, and guiding new NCMs in their transition process. This type of forum lends itself to what Bruffee (1993) refers to as reacculturation, which is a learning process for individuals who leave one knowledge community and enter another. Nurses entering the role of case manager from the role of caregiver need to establish new allegiances, gain new perspectives, and attend to new priorities. Planning conversations about differences in experiences and expectations between past and present roles can expose new NCMs to the perspectives and wisdom of experienced NCMs, allowing them to voice their questions and concerns and assisting them with assigning meaning to their new experiences.

SUGGESTIONS FOR FUTURE RESEARCH

Some ideas for future research have emerged from studying the experience of role transition for nurses and other professionals. Specific to this professional population, expanding the sample to include a larger number of participants from various geographic areas and case management settings would certainly serve to validate or add new perspectives about this experience for nurses. Including male representation in the sample might demonstrate some variation in transition experiences between genders. It would also be interesting to examine how the stories of transition are similar or different among people of specific age groups or years of experience.

In addition, investigation into the assumptions that educators, trainers, and supervisors have about experienced nurses coming into the role of case manager and their expectations for how quickly they are expected to function independently would add to our understanding of the transition process from another perspective. It could also contribute to better training of the trainers, by identifying potential disconnects between the trainers' assumptions about the transition process and the actual experience of new NCMs.

CONCLUSION

This study demonstrates the experiences of nurses who have made transitions from a caregiver role to a case manager role. Common themes emerged from interview and focus group data that contribute to our knowledge about this transition. With enhanced awareness and insight about characteristic tensions and sources of job satisfaction, we can help nurses interested in the field of case management appropriately anticipate the challenges that may lie ahead, and develop plans for taking advantage of the learning potential in each of those experiences.

References

Allen, V. L., & van de Vliert, E. (1982). A role theoretical perspective on transitional processes. In V. L. Allen & E. Van de Vliert (Eds.), *Role transitions: explorations and explanations* (pp. 3–18). New York: Plenum.

American Healthcare Consultants. (2001). *Case management caseload data: Results of a national survey* (Executive Summary). Chicago, IL: Author.

Barefield, F. (2003). Working case managers' view of the profession. *The Case Manager, 14*(6), 69–71.

Bogdin, R., & Biklin, S. K. (1998). *Qualitative research in education* (3rd ed.). Boston: Allyn & Bacon.

Bruffee, K. A. (1993). *Collaborative learning: Higher education, interdependence and the authority of knowledge.* Baltimore: The Johns Hopkins University Press.

Case Management Society of America. (2004). Contemporary trends in case management. *The Case Manager, 15*(2), 45–47.

Chan, F., Leahy, M., McMahon, B., Mirch, M., & DeVinney, D. (1999). Foundational knowledge and major practice domains of case management. *The Journal of Care Management, 5*(1), 10–30.

Conti, R. (1996). Nurse case manager roles: Implications for practice and education. *Nursing Administration Quarterly, 21*(1), 67–80.

Creswell, J. W. (1994). Research design: Qualitative and quantitative approaches. Thousand Oaks, CA: Sage Publications.

Falter, E., Cesta, T., Concert, C., Mason, D. (1999). Development of a graduate nursing program in case management. *The Journal of Care Management, 5*(3), 50–78.

Merriam, S. (2001). *Qualitative research and case study applications in education.* San Francisco: Jossey-Bass.

What's in the future? More opportunities, fewer case managers. (2003). *Case Management Advisor, 14*(2), 13–15.

Nancy Schmitt, PhD, RN, CCM, is currently the co-ordinator of the URAC-accredited case management program at Citizens and Hanover Insurance Companies. In addition to case management, her work experience includes rehabilitation nursing, curriculum development for patient education and professional continuing education programs, and medical education administration.

Address correspondence to Nancy Schmitt, PhD, RN, CCM, 4142 Highcrest Dr, Brighton, MI 48116 (e-mail: nancys@ismi.net).

FAMILY MEDICINE AND THE HEALTH CARE SYSTEM

The Medical Home: Growing Evidence to Support a New Approach to Primary Care

Thomas C. Rosenthal, MD

Introduction: A medical home is a patient-centered, multifaceted source of personal primary health care. It is based on a relationship between the patient and physician, formed to improve the patient's health across a continuum of referrals and services. Primary care organizations, including the American Board of Family Medicine, have promoted the concept as an answer to government agencies seeking political solutions that make quality health care affordable and accessible to all Americans.

Methods: Standard literature databases, including PubMed, and Internet sites of numerous professional associations, government agencies, business groups, and private health organizations identified over 200 references, reports, and books evaluating the medical home and patient-centered primary care.

Findings: Evaluations of several patient-centered medical home models corroborate earlier findings of improved outcomes and satisfaction. The peer-reviewed literature documents improved quality, reduced errors, and increased satisfaction when patients identify with a primary care medical home. Patient autonomy and choice also contributes to satisfaction. Although industry has funded case management models demonstrating value superior to traditional fee-for-service reimbursement adoption of the medical home as a basis for medical care in the United States, delivery will require effort on the part of providers and incentives to support activities outside of the traditional face-to-face office visit.

Conclusions: Evidence from multiple settings and several countries supports the ability of medical homes to advance societal health. A combination of fee-for-service, case management fees, and quality outcome incentives effectively drive higher standards in patient experience and outcomes. Community/provider boards may be required to safeguard the public interest. (J Am Board Fam Med 2008;21: 427–440.)

This article was externally peer reviewed.

Submitted 31 December 2007; revised 18 May 2008; accepted 20 May 2008.

From the Department of Family Medicine, University of Buffalo, NY.

Funding: none.

Conflict of interest: none declared.

Corresponding author: Thomas C. Rosenthal, MD, Department of Family Medicine, University of Buffalo, 462 Grider Street, Buffalo, NY 14215 (E-mail: trosenth@acsu.buffalo.edu).

"The better the primary care, the greater the cost savings, the better the health outcomes, and the greater the reduction in health and health care disparities."[1]

The term "medical home" was first coined by the American Academy of Pediatrics in 1967.[2] The American Academy of Family Physicians embraced the model in its 2004 Future of Family Medicine project[3] and the American College of Physicians issued a primary care medical home report in 2006.[4] The concept of the medical home has recently received attention as a strategy to improve access to quality health care for more Americans at lower cost.

In the medical home, responsibility for care and care coordination resides with the patient's personal medical provider working with a health care team.[5] Teams form and reform according to patient needs and include specialists, midlevel providers, nurses, social workers, care managers, dietitians, pharmacists, physical and occupational therapists, family, and community.[4] Medical home models vary but their success depends on their ability to focus on the needs of a patient or family one case at a time, recruiting social services, specialty medical services, and patient capabilities to solve problems.[6] In the United States primary care has been viewed largely as a discrete hierarchical level of care. Recently, however, business organizations taking a systems approach to problem solving typical of industry have endorsed the concept of a personal primary care physician as an efficient strategy for delivering a broad range of services to consumers on an as-needed basis.[7,8] In its most mature form, a medical home may integrate medical and psychosocial services in a model more in concert with documented patient health beliefs.[9-11]

Most developed nations assure patient access to primary care physicians whose payments are, at least in part, based on guidelines and outcomes established by consumer/provider oversight. However, high utilization of technology and procedures in the United States have created the misperception that universal access to health care is too expensive, and some countries struggle to match Americans' access to procedures.[12] Unfortunately, the reliance on high technology and procedures has exposed Americans to adverse events and errors possibly related to overuse.[13,14]

Although many Americans are not certain about what constitutes primary care, they want a primary care physician.[15] They assume quality and appreciate technology but value relationship above all else.[16,17] Racial and ethnic disparities are significantly reduced for families who can identify a primary care provider who facilitates access to a range of health providers.[18] Urban and rural communities that have an adequate supply of primary care practitioners experience lower infant mortality, higher birth weights, and immunization rates at or above national standards despite social disparities.[19-22] This article reviews both the peer-reviewed literature and program evaluations of medical homes to assist primary care providers and health planners in assessing the usefulness of the model in their own communities and practices.

METHODS

The outline and subtitles for this article are from the 2006 Joint Principles of the Patient-Centered Medical Home issued by the American Academy of Family Physicians, the American College of Physicians, and the American Academy of Pediatrics.[4] They have been used to facilitate the application of findings presented in this paper to policy development at the medical office and government levels.

PubMed was searched using "medical home" and "patient-centered care" as search phrases. The Internet sites of the Commonwealth Fund, the Center for Health Care Strategies, the State of North Carolina, the National Health Service of the United Kingdom, and Web sites were searched. US Family Medicine Department Chairs were surveyed by e-mail in October 2007 to expand the list of medical home evaluation studies. The American Academy of Family Physicians' Graham Center supplied their growing bibliography on the medical home concept. These sources led to secondary searches of cited literature and reports. More than 200 publications and several books were reviewed by the author. Articles were selected for citation if they offered original research, meta-analyses, or evaluation of existing programs. The unique characteristics of programs and variations in methodologies made meta-analysis at this level inappropriate. An annotated bibliography of cited references was circulated to members of the New York State Primary Care Coalition, the New York State Health Department, and members of the Association of Departments of Family Medicine for response and reaction. Some key thought pieces are referenced to assist readers who may use this for policy development.

MEDICAL HOME PRINCIPLES

Table 1 summarizes several principles of medical homes and the quality of the literature supporting the principle.

Personal Physician

Each patient has an ongoing relationship with a personal physician trained to provide first contact and continuous and comprehensive care.[4]

TABLE 1   Support for Medical Home Features: Quality of Literature

Recommendation	Evidence Rating	References	Comments
Patients who have a continuity relationship with a personal care physician have better health process measures and outcomes.	1	23, 34, 41, 47, 52	Continuity is most commonly associated with primary care, but cancer care, dialysis, and diabetes care are examples of specialty continuity.
Multiple visits over time with the same provider create renewed opportunities to build management and teaching strategies tailored to individual progress and receptivity.	2	24, 25, 38, 39, 46, 49, 54, 55	Neither primary care nor specialty care can meet their full potential if provided in a vacuum. All studies are challenged to evaluate any piece of the system in isolation from the context of specialty or other community services.
Minorities become as likely as nonminorities to receive preventive screening and have their chronic conditions well managed in a medical home model.	2	19, 20, 22, 26, 27	Rigorous program evaluations, secondary population analyses, and observational comparison studies show consistent findings.
In primary care, patients present at most visits with multiple problems.	1	06, 64, 65	The use of each office visit to care for multiple problems is a property of primary care.
Specialists generate more diagnostic hypotheses within their domain than outside it and assign higher probabilities to diagnoses within that domain.	2	73, 74	The interface between primary care and specialty care needs further research.
The more attributes of the medical home demonstrated by a primary care practice, the more likely patients are to be up to date on screening, immunizations, and health habit counseling, and the less likely they are to use emergency rooms.	2	28, 29, 94, 95, 106, 107, 121	

Note: 1 = consistent, good quality evidence; 2 = limited quality, patient-oriented evidence; 3 = consensus, usual practice, expert opinion, or case series.[30]

SUPPORTING LITERATURE.   When people become sick, they use stories to describe their experience. Patient-oriented care is bound up in the physician's ability to accurately perceive the essence of a patient's story.[31,32] Perception, or empathy, is enhanced by a doctor–patient relationship which, like any relationship, develops incrementally.[33] Relationships do not replace technical expertise and patients accept that quality specialty care often means being cared for by providers with whom they have a limited relationship.[34]

In primary care, a longitudinal relationship is an important tool to enlighten a personalized application of strategies that will achieve incremental improvements in health sustainable through the ever challenging events of life.[35,36] Specialty care can often be judged by how well something is done to the patient. Primary care is often best judged by how well the patient changes behavior or complies with treat-ment, activities the patient must do themselves. This difference becomes blurred in areas of chronic kidney disease (nephrologist), cancer care (oncologist), and diabetic management (endocrinologist) because of the long-term management relationship with the patient.

A relationship over time between patient and generalist also modifies resource utilization. A survey of physicians in Colorado by Fryer et al.[37] demonstrated that in communities with high numbers of specialists or low numbers of generalists, specialists may spend 27% of patient contact time performing primary care services. Just as with anyone practicing outside of their area of comfort, this inevitability should raise concerns. Chart reviews of over 20,000 outpatient encounters by Greenfield[38] and 5,000 inpatient encounters by Weingarten[39] demonstrated that specialists practicing outside of their area of expertise order more tests and make more referrals than generalists.

Americans spend less time with a primary care physician than patients in countries with better health outcomes.[40] Yet, community-level studies indicate that availability of primary care lowers mortality.[41] The influence of primary care is second to socioeconomic conditions in lowering the frequency of strokes and cancer deaths.[42–45] In a study of 11 conditions, Starfield et al.[46] found that patients had more monitoring of more parameters for all their conditions if they received care within a continuous primary care physician relationship as opposed to disease-specific specialty care.

Quality care is not solely dependent on insurance coverage. An analysis of administrative data in a Midwestern Canadian city with universal coverage documented that patients who had a continuous relationship with a personal care provider were more likely to receive cancer screening, had higher vaccination rates, and had lower emergency department use.[47] In a critical review of the literature on continuity, Saultz and Lochner[34] analyzed 40 studies tracking 81 care outcomes, 41 of which were significantly improved by continuity. Of the 41 cost variables studied, expenditures were significantly lower for 35. Saultz and Lochner[34] concluded that the published literature could not reveal if patient satisfaction with a provider lead to continuity or if continuity lead to satisfaction, but findings were generally consistent with a positive impact on measured outcomes.

A Norwegian study determined that 4 visits with a provider were necessary for accumulated knowledge to impact use of laboratory tests, expectant management, prescriptions, and referrals.[48] Each visit in a continuous relationship renews an opportunity to build management and teaching strategies tailored to individual progress, receptivity, and capacity for compliance and change across the multiple medical conditions faced by many patients.[48] Gulbrandsen et al.'s[50] review of visits by 1401 adults attending 89 generalists demonstrated that continuity of care increased the likelihood that the provider was aware of psychosocial problems impacting health. Others[51–53] studied the impact of a primary care "gatekeeping" model's impact on Medicaid health management organization patients in Missouri and showed an increase of visits to primary care and fewer visits to emergency rooms, specialists, and nonphysician providers. Continuity has generally been shown to achieve quality at a lower cost.[54,55] In a qualitative analysis, Bayliss et al.[56] concluded that patients with multiple comorbidities experienced barriers to self care, such as medication problems, chronic disease interactions, and adverse social and emotional environments requiring coordination of strategies across the comorbidities. Patients attribute health care errors to the breakdown of the doctor–patient relationship 70% of the time.[57]

Team-Directed Medical Practice

A personal medical provider, usually a physician, leads a team of caregivers who take collective responsibility for ongoing patient care.

SUPPORTING LITERATURE. Eighty-seven percent of primary care physicians think an interdisciplinary team improves quality of care.[58] Separate studies of primary care offices in upstate New York and California, identified by their positive community reputation, found that all used a coordinated team model regardless of structure (private practice, community health center, hospital-owned). The practices either directly provided or coordinated a spectrum of services including social/behavioral services, rehabilitation, and coordinated specialty care.[10,59]

A team expands on the inherent limits in a 15-minute office visit during which demands for preventive care, chronic disease management, and new complaints compete.[60] Team care increases the contact points between patient and health care team and decreases the likelihood that acute complaints will distract providers from making appropriate adjustments in the care of chronic conditions.

Comprehensive patient management implies more than office visits. In one model a medical assistant measures vital signs and takes an interim history in the examination room then remains with the patient during the physician encounter and stays behind for a debriefing with the patient after the visit. The same assistant contacts the patient after the visit and before the next visit.[61] Phelan et al.[63] found that a interdisciplinary geriatric team model screened for more syndromes and improved care at 12 months, although there was little significant improvement thereafter. Disease-specific team models produce good results for the focal disease but are less successful with comorbidities.[45] Multidisciplinary team care of disabled adults in sheltered housing shifted expenditures from unproductive repeat hospitalizations to personal care and increased outpatient visits.[63]

Whole-Person Orientation

The personal physician or provider maintains responsibility for providing for all of the patient's health care needs and arranges care with other qualified professionals as needed. This includes care for all stages of life: acute care, chronic care, preventive services, and end-of-life care.[4]

SUPPORTING LITERATURE. Family physicians manage 3.05 problems per patient encounter. They chart 2.82 problems and bill for 1.97. Ninety percent of patients have at least 2 concerns.[64] Patients over the age of 65 average 3.88 problems per visit and diabetics average 4.6.[65] In a study of 211 patient encounters, Parchman et al.[66] found that the number of complaints raised by patients tended to decrease the likelihood that a diabetic would have an adjustment made to a needed medication. Providers compensated by shortening the time to next visit by an average of 8.6 days.

By way of illustration, headache is often a secondary complaint in primary care. Only 3% of patients seen in a primary care office with a headache will have a computed tomography scan, and of these only 5% will have significant findings.[67] If the history and physical fail to raise suspicion of an intracranial process, headache patients are often treated according to symptoms and encouraged to return if symptoms do not resolve as expected while still receiving care for the primary chronic condition. Tactical options include follow-up contact by a member of the health team or earlier recheck.

The recheck plan for nonurgent conditions is a critical element of primary care. Continuity in the relationship establishes the mutual confidence needed for a watchful waiting or recheck strategy.[68] Whereas an immediate diagnostic work-up may quickly arrive at a specific diagnosis, a measured wait and see approach in the absence of "red flags" often confirms the initial impression. "Wait and see" has become a legitimate focus of research in otitis media and some pain syndromes.[69,70]

Care Is Coordinated and/or Integrated Across All Domains of the Health Care System

Modern health care presents several effective strategies for any single complaint, creating important options for diagnosis and treatment but also increasing the potential for overuse and confusion.[4]

SUPPORTING LITERATURE. The integration of primary care as an overarching approach to population health management is perhaps best elucidated by a discussion of care integration in a robust modern health care system. Medical homes should not function as entry-level care providers but rather as strategic access managers.

Back pain is a frequent primary care complaint. Patients with "red flag" orthopedic or neurologic complications need to be identified and urgently referred for specialty care. Most will require supportive care including pain relief, exercise, stretching, and physical therapy. A minority of patients who fail to respond still need help selecting a surgeon or a rehabilitation program and need guided readjustment to their workplace.[8] Fears and misunderstandings are the greatest threat to recovery but receiving an magnetic resonance imaging scan early in the course of back pain is more strongly associated with eventual surgery than are clinical findings.[71] The challenge is to meet the patient's need for management and order additional tests at the precise point in the course of illness to be productive.

The skills associated with specialty care must be learned in centers that see preselected patients with a high likelihood of needing specialty procedures. An intense experience essential for training predisposes toward overestimation of the likelihood of severe or unusual conditions in the general population and contributes to an overuse of diagnostic and therapeutic modalities.[72–74] Care across the continuum is more than access to procedures.

When generalist physicians are less available than specialists, specialists often refer secondary problems to other specialists. For example, after a myocardial infarction a patient may be referred by the cardiologist to an endocrinologist, pulmonologist, and a rheumatologist to manage the patient's longstanding diabetes, cardiac obstructive pulmonary disorder, and osteoarthritis. Specialists who feel unsupported by primary care services schedule more follow-up appointments, many of which duplicate services provided by the primary care physician.[73,75]

However, even in universal coverage societies like the United Kingdom, patients report greater satisfaction when they are able to access specialty care directly.[76] The lesson here is that medical homes should not become barriers to specialty access. The personal care team should facilitate referral to the most appropriate specialist at the appropriate time, consistent with patient concerns.

There is evidence to suggest that primary care involvement in a referral to another physician may improve quality. Children with tonsillitis who are referred by primary care physicians to surgeons have fewer postoperative complications than do children whose parents bypassed the primary care provider.[77]

At Kaiser Permanente, primary care physician-facilitated referrals have lower hospitalization rates than do self referrals.[78] Primary care physicians who care for their hospitalized patients provide care that is as efficient as that provided by hospitalists.[76]

Mental health coordination is no different. Smith et al.[80] reviewed the literature on management of patients with unexplained symptoms and psychosocial distress, concluding that 80% of these patients accept management by primary care physicians but only 10% will attend a psychosocial referral. When a referral is made, the primary care physician plays an important role in outcome success.[81] Full integration of primary medical care with mental health care improves outcomes in both arenas.[82–84]

Quality and Safety

Clinical excellence is enhanced by integration of information technology into medical practice and tracking of quality measures.[4]

- *Evidence-based medicine* and clinical decision support tools should be incorporated into practice.

SUPPORTING LITERATURE. One challenge to medical home evaluation will be establishing outcome measures that truly affect patient wellness. Specialists are good at adhering to guidelines within their field of expertise.[85–87] However, Hartz and James[88] reviewed 42 published articles comparing cardiologist to generalist care of myocardial infarctions and found that none of the studies took into account patient preferences, severity of comorbid disease, general health status, or resource availability. Confounding comorbidities, physical or behavioral, frequently exclude patients from the clinical trials that generate disease specific guidelines.[89,90]

Yet when primary care group practices systematically organize themselves to meet guideline standards they achieve equivalent outcomes.[91–93] It is a challenge to primary care that generalists perform better at meeting patient-centered guidelines such as exercise, diet, breastfeeding, smoking cessation, and the use of seat belts and less well at meeting disease-specific guidelines. However, patients who report having a continuous relationship with a personal care provider are very likely to receive evidence-based care.[94,95]

- Physicians will accept *accountability for continuous quality* improvement through voluntary engagement in performance measurement.

SUPPORTING LITERATURE. Public reporting of health care measures encourages physicians to meet benchmarks. The conundrum is that reporting variations does little to *explain* variations.[96] Fifty-five percent of generalists agree that patients should have access to performance data although there is little consensus yet on parameters.[58] Whereas the Healthplan Employer Data Information Set has more than 60 different measures (including immunizations, women's health, maternity care, behavioral health, and asthma), accuracy has been limited because the data are based on billing records. Efforts to collect data directly from the patient's primary care record have been piloted by the Wisconsin Collaboration for Health Care Quality but the lack of standard interoperability of records is challenging.[97]

Because continuity is central to patient satisfaction with, and the function of, a medical home, quality should be trended over time and include aspects of care that reflects functions of the whole team.[98] One model incorporates all office personnel (assistants, nurses, and providers) in interviews that identify perceived challenges to quality. Together the office staff and physicians rank priorities, brainstorm solutions, implement action, and monitor results.[99] The science of quality measurement in primary care is evolving and more research is needed. However, waiting for perfect measures should not delay implementation of good measures.

- *Patients actively participate* in decision making, including seeking feedback to ensure that patients' expectations are being met.

SUPPORTING LITERATURE. Only 36% of generalists and 20% of specialists survey their patients.[58] A recent survey of all primary care and ambulatory specialty physicians in Florida showed only modest advances in the adoption of e-mail communication, and little adherence to recognized guidelines for e-mail correspondence.[100] A study of 200 patients with rheumatoid arthritis who initiated their own follow-up found patients were significantly more confident and satisfied with their care and used fewer specialty services, including fewer hospitalizations, and saw their primary care physician as frequently as a matched control group for whom specialty care was more limited.[76] These findings again suggest that the primary care physician's role as a gate opener and advisor may be more efficient than as a gatekeeper. Such a role requires effective communication.

- *Information technology* has potential to support optimal patient care, performance measurement, patient education, and communication.

SUPPORTING LITERATURE.   Primary care is at a tipping point for implementation of electronic medical records. Twenty-three percent of practices currently use electronic medical records; another 23% would like to implement electronic records within the next year.[58] Electronic records have not yet automated collection of consultant reports and test results for patient visits. Eventually a system of health information management will network electronic records in offices, hospitals, and ancillary care centers within a well-protected national grid capable of managing huge amounts of data.[101]

A qualitative study of family medicine practices suggests that approximately a year after implementation, practices with electronic records initiate but struggle with effective tracking of clinical outcomes data.[102] At 5 years, practices with electronic records document more frequent testing of glycosylated hemoglobins and lipid levels but do not achieve better control.[103] High quality primary care groups find having an electronic medical record a useful tool but not essential to meeting guidelines.[104]

- Practices go through a *voluntary recognition* process by an appropriate nongovernmental entity to demonstrate that they have the capabilities to provide patient centered services consistent with the medical home model.

Successful implementation of the medical home model will necessitate recruitment of early adopting, high-performing practices that wish to be measured against benchmarks. During this period measures that lead to improved patient management can be identified and actual costs of care and savings demonstrated. Realistically, it will take years to roll out an evolution in health care of this magnitude and early innovators may be more highly motivated and successful than later implementers.[105]

- *Enhanced access* to care through systems such as open scheduling, expanded hours, and new options for communication between patients, their personal physician, and office staff.

Medical homes should be challenged to assure that patients have access to the right care at the right time in the right place, including the right specialty care. Many of these strategies are focused on viewing services from the patient's perspective, including extended hours and open access.[106–108]

E-mail or Internet-based communication promises to increase patient/physician interaction and interfere less with the patient's work schedule. To be embraced in health care, electronic communication will need to be reimbursed. Kaiser Permanente of Colorado is paying 95% of the CPT 99213 office visit fee for virtual office visits.[109] Internet-based portals are also available to provide secure communication.[110]

DEMONSTRATION PROJECTS

Reorganization of primary health care in the United States may be reaching its own tipping point. In 2007 the UnitedHealth Group in Florida, CIGNA, Humana, Wellpoint, and Aetna began supporting primary care practices willing to incorporate quality improvement and active patient management in medical home systems.[111] North Carolina's Medicaid managed care program, North Carolina Community Care, offers a per-member/per-month management fee to physician networks that use evidence-based guidelines for at least 3 conditions, track patients, and report on performance.[112] By 2005 primary care practices realized $11 million in enhanced fees but generated savings of $231 million.[113] Erie County, NY, implemented a primary care partial capitation program in 1990 for Medicaid/Medicare patients with chronic disabilities, including substance abuse. A per-member/ per-month management fee improved quality of care, decreased duplication, lowered hospitalization rates, and improved patient satisfaction while saving $1 million for every 1000 enrollees.[114] The Veterans Affairs Administration integrated information technology with a primary care-based delivery system for qualified Veterans and improved quality of care. It now costs $6,000 less per year to care for a veteran over the age of 65 than for a Medicare recipient.[115]

The Netherlands offers physicians incentives for efficiency, outcomes, and quality in a universal coverage model originally proposed for the United States.[116] Everyone must purchase basic community-rated health insurance through private insurers. The plan has improved compensation for primary care services and has improved distribution of services into previously underserved communities.[117,118]

In 2001, the United Kingdom's National Health Service contracted with general practitioners to provide medical home services to patients. By 2005 these contracts had improved quality of care.[119] The rate of improvement further accelerated when financial incentives were added in 2005.[105,120]

LIMITATIONS OF THIS REVIEW

Primary care practices are very complex. Each practice has a philosophy, style, and culture within which physicians and staff deliver patient care.[121] Any review of the medical home should be balanced by a concern that many practices already feel burdened by existing work demands and perceive little capacity to accept new responsibilities in patient care. Measuring outcomes further adds to the workload and may not be successful in unmotivated practices.[122] It is possible that placing additional responsibilities on a primary care visit may actually interfere with secondary detection of conditions such as skin cancers or depression.[123–125]

Finally, there are limitations in the methods used in this review. The quality of each study was subjectively determined and could not be analyzed in the aggregate because most studies and evaluations used different interventions and approaches to data collection. Studies often reflect unique characteristics of providers and patients in incomparable settings. Generalizations are possible only in light of the consistency of the conclusions drawn by a large body of work.

REIMBURSING THE MEDICAL HOME

Institutionalizing the medical home as the foundational approach to health delivery strategy in the United States will require a reformulation of reimbursement policy. Overall, the average salary of American physicians is 7 times greater than that of the average American worker. Primary care physicians in the United States earn 3 times the average worker's income. In most of the industrialized world the overall physician-to-average worker income ratio is 3:1.[126] The Centers for Medicare and Medicaid Services' (CMS) Resource-Based Relative Value Scale, designed in 1992 to reduce inequality between fees for primary care and payment for procedures, has failed. As structured, the committee that advises CMS has 30 members, 23 of whom are appointed by medical specialty societies.[127] This group has tended to approve procedural services resulting in increased revenues for procedural specialties.[128] Between 2000 and 2004, primary care income increased 9.9% whereas specialty incomes rose 15.8%.[129] A 2007 effort to increase primary care reimbursement improved payments by 5%, not the 37% projected by Medicare.[130]

Compounding these salary discrepancies, 40% of the primary care work load (arranging referrals, completing forms, communicating with patients, emotional support, and encouragement) is not reimbursed by a face-to-face fee-for-service methodology.[131] A sophisticated payment system would support team care, health information technology, quality improvement, e-mail and telephone consultation, and be adjusted by case mix.[132]

Where Will the Money Come From?

The need for change in the reimbursement structure has even reached the popular press. Consumer Reports blames reimbursement policies for the overuse of 10 common procedures, concluding that the US payment system discourages counseling, care coordination, and evidence-based assessment.[133] A primary care-based system may cost 30% less[134] because patients experience fewer hospitalizations, less duplication, and more appropriate use of technology.[75,135] Case-adjusted rates of hospitalizations for heart disease and diabetes are 90% higher for cardiologists and 50% higher for endocrinologists than for primary care physicians.[38,136] Even acute illnesses, such as community-acquired pneumonia, cost less for equivalent outcomes when managed by a primary care physician.[137]

Federally funded Community health centers form the largest network of primary care medical homes in the United States. In 2005 the average cost of caring for a patient in a community health center was $2,569 compared with $4,379 for the general population.[138]

Variations in expenditures from one community to another also suggest opportunities for reducing expenditures while preserving quality. New York State and California spend over $38,000 per Medicare recipient in the last 2 years of life compared with Missouri, New Hampshire, and North Carolina, where expenditures are below $26,000.[139] If half of the expenditure variation could be captured, there would be adequate resources to provide uninsured Americans with a personal physician in a patient-centered medical home.[134]

Improved quality will also cut expenditures. An analysis by Bridges to Excellence estimated that maintaining the glycohemoglobin at 7 in a diabetic patient saves $279 a year in health costs per patient. Keeping a diabetic's low-density lipoprotein below 100 saves $369 per year, and keeping the blood pressure below 130/80 saves $494. Keeping all measures at target saves $1,059 per patient per year.[140]

Reimbursement Models

Medical practices are business entities. Rewards for change must exceed the cost of change.[141,142] A 3-component fee schedule considered by the American Academy of Family Physicians, the American Academy of Pediatrics, and the American College of Physicians would consist of (1) a fee for service (per visit); (2) a monthly management fee for practices contracting to provide medical home services; and (3) an additional bonus for reporting on quality performance goals.[143,144]

Maintaining *fee-for-service* reimbursement supports provision of essential face-to-face services. However fee-for-service reimbursement should be broadened to embrace e-mail or Web-based virtual office visits, perhaps pegging them to some proportion of a routine office visit.[109]

A *per-member/per-month management fee* for Medicaid patients with or without chronic disease was enough to trigger case management and quality reporting in the North Carolina Medicaid program.[112] In one upstate New York county the enhanced management fee for patients with both mental and physical health problems approximates $10 per member/per month.[114] Other models have paid fractional fees for specific activities such as chronic disease registries, guideline implementation, and outcomes tracking. A capitation of $5.50 per member/per month ($66 per year) is roughly half of the $110 per year savings projected by the Bridges to Excellence project for well persons enrolled in a medical home.[140] The fee would be expected to support physician management time, outcomes reporting, electronic record maintenance cost, and a full-time professionally trained case manager. Enhanced services include patient education, telephonic case management, and improved patient access.

The *quality incentive* is a pay-for-performance fee that recognizes achievement of standards of care. HMOs have traditionally relied on claims data for tracking billed procedures. The patient record is more accurate but will require new resources to harvest.[145] When paid at 3-month intervals, quality incentives are frequent enough to trigger continuous improvement efforts but spaced sufficiently to reflect impact of changes. Observation studies have confirmed that practices add staff, install electronic records, and network with community agencies to be eligible for incentives.[105,144] To be effective, criteria must be measurable, based on evidence, and amenable to medical management. Both the measures and incentives must be chosen and incentivized with care to assure providers do not simply deselect complex patients, for it is the complex patients who have the most to gain in a medical home environment.[146] Eventually, public reporting of physician data will facilitate greater patient participation and trust.[147] Studies for as long as 6 years show that appropriately selected incentives can maintain physician satisfaction, patient satisfaction, and long-term performance.[148] Incentives also reinforce the office team structure.[149]

Oversight is essential to the ultimate success of a patient centered medical home system of care. The United Kingdom established the National Institute for Health and Clinical Excellence to manage incentives and define objectives of their health system. Using full-time investigators, National Institute for Health and Clinical Excellence publishes and updates clinical appraisals on efficacy. Oversight of National Institute for Health and Clinical Excellence is provided by a board of health professionals, patients, and employers.[150]

References

1. Epstein AJ. The role of public clinics in preventable hospitalizations among vulnerable populations. Health Serv Res 2001;36:405–20.
2. Sia C, Tonniges TF, Osterhus E, Taba S. History of the medical home concept. Pediatrics 2004;113(5 Suppl): 1473–8.
3. Future of Family Medicine Project Leadership Committee. The Future of Family Medicine: a collaborative project of the family medicine community. Ann Fam Med 2004;2(Suppl 1):S3–32.
4. Barr M. The advanced medical home: a patient-centered, physician-guided model of health care. Philadelphia (PA): American College of Physicians; 2006.
5. Grumbach K, Bodenheimer T. A primary care home for Americans: putting the house in order. JAMA 2002; 288:889–93.
6. Lantz PM, Lichtenstein RL, Pollack HA. Health policy approaches to population health: the limits of medicalization. Health Aff (Millwood) 2007;26:1253–7.

7. Finch RA. An employer's guide to behavioral health services: a roadmap and recommendations for evaluating, designing, and implementing behavioral health services. Washington, DC: National Business Group on Health; 2005.

8. Enthoven AC, Crosson FJ, Shortell SM. 'Redefining health care': medical homes or archipelagos to navigate? Health Aff (Millwood) 2007;26:1366–72.

9. Engel GL. The need for a new medical model: a challenge for biomedicine. Science 1977;196:129–36.

10. Rosenthal T, Campbell-Heider N. The rural health care team. In: Geyman JP NT, Hart G, eds. Textbook of rural health care. New York: McGraw-Hill; 2001.

11. Bodenheimer T, Lorig K, Holman H, Grumbach K. Patient self-management of chronic disease in primary care. JAMA 2002; 288:2469–75.

12. Royal College of General Practitioners. The future direction of general practice: a roadmap. London, UK: Royal College of General Practitioners; 2007.

13. Schoen C, Osborn R, Huynh PT, et al. Primary care and health system performance: adults' experiences in five countries. Health Aff (Millwood) 2004;(Suppl Web Exclusives):W4–487–503.

14. Woolf SH, Johnson RE. The break-even point: when medical advances are less important than improving the fidelity with which they are delivered. Ann Fam Med 2005;3:545–52.

15. Green LA, Graham R, Bagley B, et al.. Task Force 1. Report of the Task Force on patient expectations, core values reintegration, and the new model of family medicine. Ann Fam Med 2004;2(Supp 1):S33–S50.

16. Main DS, Tressler C, Staudenmaier A, Nearing KA, Westfall JM, Silverstein M. Patient perspectives on the doctor of the future. Fam Med 2002; 34:251–7.

17. Coulter A. What do patients and the public want from primary care? BMJ 2005;331:1199–201.

18. Beal AC, Doty MM, Henandez SE, Shea KK, Davis K. Closing the divide: how medical homes promote equity in health care. Results from the Commonwealth Fund 2006 Health Care Quality Survey. New York, NY June 2007 2006.

19. Parchman ML, Culler S. Primary care physicians and avoidable hospitalizations. J Fam Pract 1994; 39:123–8.

20. Gadomski A, Jenkins P, Nichols M. Impact of a Medicaid primary care provider and preventive care on pediatric hospitalization. Pediatrics 1998;101: E1.

21. Shi L, Macinko J, Starfield B, et al.. Primary care, infant mortality, and low birth weight in the states of the USA. J Epidemiol Community Health 2004; 58:374–80.

22. Shi L, Macinko J, Starfield B, Politzer R, Wulu J, Xu J. Primary care, social inequalities, and all-cause, heart disease, and cancer mortality in US counties, 1990. Am J Public Health 2005;95:674–80.

23. Berry LL, Parish JT, Janakiraman R, et al.. Patients' commitment to their primary physician and why it matters. Ann Fam Med 2008;6:6–13.

24. Moscovice I, Rosenblatt R. Quality-of-care challenges for rural health. J Rural Health 2000;16: 168–76.

25. Moore LG. Escaping the tyranny of the urgent by delivering planned care. Fam Pract Manag 2006;13: 37–40.

26. Shi L, Macinko J, Starfield B, Politzer R, Wulu J, Xu J. Primary care, social inequalities and all-cause, heart disease and cancer mortality in US counties: a comparison between urban and non-urban areas. Public Health 2005;119:699–710.

27. Fiscella K, Holt K. Impact of primary care patient visits on racial and ethnic disparities in preventive care in the United States. J Am Board Fam Med 2007;20:587–97.

28. Flocke SA, Stange KC, Zyzanski SJ. The association of attributes of primary care with the delivery of clinical preventive services. Med Care 1998;36(8 Suppl): AS21–30.

29. Ryan S, Riley A, Kang M, Starfield B. The effects of regular source of care and health need on medical care use among rural adolescents. Arch Pediatr Adolesc Med 2001;155:184–90.

30. Ebell MH, Siwek J, Weiss BD, et al. Strength of Recommendation Taxonomy (SORT): a patient-centered approach to grading evidence in the medical literature. J Am Board Fam Pract 2004;17:59–67.

31. Brody H. Edmund D. Pellegrino's philosophy of family practice. Theor Med 1997;18:7–20.

32. Groopman J. How doctors think. New York (NY): Houghton Mifflin Co.; 2007.

33. Pink DH. A whole new mind: why right-brainers will rule the future. New York (NY): Riverhead Books; 2006.

34. Saultz JW, Lochner J. Interpersonal continuity of care and care outcomes: a critical review. Ann Fam Med 2005;3:159–66.

35. Charon R. Narrative medicine: a model for empathy, reflection, profession and trust. JAMA 2001; 286:1897–902.

36. Halpern J. From detached concern to empathy: humanizing medical practice. London: Oxford University Press; 2001.

37. Fryer GE, Jr., Consoli R, Miyoshi TJ, Dovey SM, Phillips RL Jr, Green LA. Specialist physicians providing primary care services in Colorado. J Am Board Fam Pract 2004;17:81–90.

38. Greenfield S, Nelson EC, Zubkoff M, et al.. Variations in resource utilization among medical specialties and systems of care. Results from the medical outcomes study. JAMA 1992;267:1624–30.

39. Weingarten SR, Lloyd L, Chiou CF, Braunstein GD. Do subspecialists working outside of their specialty provide less efficient and lower-quality care to hospitalized patients than do primary care physicians? Arch Intern Med 2002;162:527–32.

40. Bindman AB, Forrest CB, Britt H, Crampton P, Majeed A. Diagnostic scope of and exposure to primary care physicians in Australia, New Zealand, and the United States: cross sectional analysis of results from three national surveys. BMJ 2007;334: 1261.

41. Shi L. The relationship between primary care and life chances. J Health Care Poor Underserved 1992; 3:321–35.

42. Vogel RL, Ackermann RJ. Is primary care physician supply correlated with health outcomes? Int J Health Serv 1998;28:183–96.

43. Campbell RJ, Ramirez AM, Perez K, Roetzheim RG. Cervical cancer rates and the supply of primary care physicians in Florida. Fam Med 2003;35:60–4.

44. Shi L, Macinko J, Starfield B, Xu J, Politzer R. Primary care, income inequality, and stroke mortality in the United States: a longitudinal analysis, 1985–1995. Stroke 2003;34:1958–64.

45. Starfield B, Shi L, Macinko J. Contribution of primary care to health systems and health. Milbank Q 2005;83:457–502.

46. Starfield B, Lemke KW, Bernhardt T, Foldes SS, Forrest CB, Weiner JP. Comorbidity: implications for the importance of primary care in 'case' management. Ann Fam Med 2003;1:8–14.

47. Menec VH, Sirski M, Attawar D. Does continuity of care matter in a universally insured population? Health Serv Res 2005;40:389–400.

48. Hjortdahl P, Borchgrevink CF. Continuity of care: influence of general practitioners' knowledge about their patients on use of resources in consultations. BMJ 1991;303:1181–4.

49. Higashi T, Wenger NS, Adams JL, et al.. Relationship between number of medical conditions and quality of care. N Engl J Med 2007;356:2496–504.

50. Gulbrandsen P, Hjortdahl P, Fugelli P. General practitioners' knowledge of their patients' psychosocial problems: multipractice questionnaire survey. BMJ 1997;314:1014–8.

51. Hurley RE, Paul JE, Freund DA. Going into gatekeeping: an empirical assessment. QRB Qual Rev Bull 1989;15:306–14.

52. O'Malley AS, Forrest CB. Continuity of care and delivery of ambulatory services to children in community health clinics. J Community Health 1996; 21:159–73.

53. Richman IB, Clark S, Sullivan AF, Camargo CA Jr. National study of the relation of primary care shortages to emergency department utilization. Acad Emerg Med 2007;14:279–82.

54. Raddish M, Horn SD, Sharkey PD. Continuity of care: is it cost effective? Am J Manag Care 1999;5: 727–34.

55. De Maeseneer JM, De Prins L, Gosset C, Heyerick J. Provider continuity in family medicine: does it make a difference for total health care costs? Ann Fam Med 2003;1:144–8.

56. Bayliss EA, Steiner JF, Fernald DH, Crane LA, Main DS. Descriptions of barriers to self-care by persons with comorbid chronic diseases. Ann Fam Med 2003;1:15–21.

57. Kuzel AJ, Woolf SH, Gilchrist VJ, et al.. Patient reports of preventable problems and harms in primary health care. Ann Fam Med 2004;2:333–40.

58. Audet AM, Davis K, Schoenbaum SC. Adoption of patient-centered care practices by physicians: results from a national survey. Arch Intern Med 2006; 166:754–9.

59. Feifer C, Nemeth L, Nietert PJ, et al.. Different paths to high-quality care: three archetypes of top-performing practice sites. Ann Fam Med 2007;5: 233–41.

60. Jaen CR, Stange KC, Nutting PA. Competing demands of primary care: a model for the delivery of clinical preventive services. J Fam Pract 1994;38: 166–71.

61. Bodenheimer T, Laing BY. The teamlet model of primary care. Ann Fam Med 2007;5:457–61.

62. Phelan EA, Balderson B, Levine M, et al.. Delivering effective primary care to older adults: a randomized, controlled trial of the senior resource team at group health cooperative. J Am Geriatr Soc 2007; 55:1748–56.

63. Yaggy SD, Michener JL, Yaggy D, et al.. Just for us: an academic medical center-community partnership to maintain the health of a frail low-income senior population. Gerontologist 2006;46:271–6.

64. Fortin M, Bravo G, Hudon C, Vanasse A, Lapointe L. Prevalence of multimorbidity among adults seen in family practice. Ann Fam Med 2005;3:223–8.

65. Beasley JW, Hankey TH, Erickson R, et al.. How many problems do family physicians manage at each encounter? A WReN study. Ann Fam Med 2004;2:405–10.

66. Parchman ML, Pugh JA, Romero RL, Bowers KW. Competing demands or clinical inertia: the case of elevated glycosylated hemoglobin. Ann Fam Med 2007;5:196–201.

67. Becker LA, Green LA, Beaufait D, Kirk J, Froom J, Freeman WL. Use of CT scans for the investigation of headache: a report from ASPN, Part 1. J Fam Pract 1993;37:129–34.

68. Rosenthal TC, Riemenschneider TA, Feather J. Preserving the patient referral process in the managed care environment. Am J Med 1996;100:338–43.

69. Spiro DM, Tay KY, Arnold DH, Dziura JD, Baker MD, Shapiro ED. Wait-and-see prescription for the treatment of acute otitis media: a randomized controlled trial. JAMA 2006;296:1235–41.

70. Calnan M, Wainwright D, O'Neill C, Winterbottom A, Watkins C. Making sense of aches and pains. Fam Pract 2006;23:91–105.

71. Jarvik JG, Hollingworth W, Martin B, et al.. Rapid magnetic resonance imaging vs. radiographs for patients with low back pain: a randomized controlled trial. JAMA 2003;289:2810–8.

72. Mathers N, Hodgkin P. The gatekeeper and the wizard: a fairy tale. BMJ 1989;298:172–4.

73. Franks P, Clancy CM, Nutting PA. Gatekeeping revisited–protecting patients from overtreatment. N Engl J Med 1992;327:424–9.

74. Hashem A, Chi MT, Friedman CP. Medical errors as a result of specialization. J Biomed Inform 2003; 36:61–9.

75. Franks P, Fiscella K. Primary care physicians and specialists as personal physicians. Health care expenditures and mortality experience. J Fam Pract 1998;47:105–9.

76. Hewlett S, Kirwan J, Pollock J, et al.. Patient initiated outpatient follow up in rheumatoid arthritis: six year randomised controlled trial. BMJ 2005;330: 171.

77. Roos NP. Who should do the surgery? Tonsillectomy-adenoidectiomy in one Canadian Province. Inquiry 1979;16:73–83.

78. Feachem RG, Sekhri NK, White KL. Getting more for their dollar: a comparison of the NHS with California's Kaiser Permanente. BMJ 2002; 324:135–41.

79. Lindenauer PK, Rothberg MB, Pekow PS, Kenwood C, Benjamin EM, Auerbach AD. Outcomes of care by hospitalists, general internists, and family physicians. N Engl J Med 2007;357:2589–600.

80. Smith RC, Lein C, Collins C, et al.. Treating patients with medically unexplained symptoms in primary care. J Gen Intern Med 2003;18:478–89.

81. Rosenthal TC, Shiffner JM, Lucas C, DeMaggio M. Factors involved in successful psychotherapy referral in rural primary care. Fam Med 1991;23:527–30.

82. Blount A. Integrated primary care: the future of medical and mental health collaboration. New York (NY): W.W. Norton & Company; 1998.

83. Griswold KS, Greene B, Smith SJ, Behrens T, Blondell RD. Linkage to primary medical care following inpatient detoxification. Am J Addict 2007; 16:183–6.

84. Griswold KS, Servoss TJ, Leonard KE, et al.. Connections to primary medical care after psychiatric crisis. J Am Board Fam Pract 2005;18:166–72.

85. Bartter T, Pratter MR. Asthma: better outcome at lower cost? The role of the expert in the care system. Chest 1996;110:1589–96.

86. Hirth RA, Fendrick AM, Chernew ME. Specialist and generalist physicians' adoption of antibiotic therapy to eradicate Helicobacter pylori infection. Med Care 1996;34:1199–204.

87. Harrold LR, Field TS, Gurwitz JH. Knowledge, patterns of care, and outcomes of care for generalists and specialists. J Gen Intern Med 1999;14:499–511.

88. Hartz A, James PA. A systematic review of studies comparing myocardial infarction mortality for generalists and specialists: lessons for research and health policy. J Am Board Fam Med 2006;19:291–302.

89. Kravitz RL, Duan N, Braslow J. Evidence-based medicine, heterogeneity of treatment effects, and the trouble with averages. Milbank Q 2004;82:661–87.

90. Rothwell PM. External validity of randomised controlled trials: "to whom do the results of this trial apply?" Lancet 2005;365:82–93.

91. James PA, Cowan TM, Graham RP, Majeroni BA, Fox CH, Jaen CR. Using a clinical practice guideline to measure physician practice: translating a guideline for the management of heart failure. J Am Board Fam Pract 1997;10:206–12.

92. Donohoe MT. Comparing generalist and specialty care: discrepancies, deficiencies, and excesses. Arch Intern Med 1998;158:1596–608.

93. Grumbach K, Selby JV, Schmittdiel JA, Quesenberry CP Jr. Quality of primary care practice in a large HMO according to physician specialty. Health Serv Res 1999;34:485–502.

94. Bindman AB, Grumbach K, Osmond D, Vranizan K, Stewart AL. Primary care and receipt of preventive services. J Gen Intern Med 1996;11:269–76.

95. Villalbi JR, Guarga A, Pasarin MI, et al.. [An evaluation of the impact of primary care reform on health]. Aten Primaria 1999;24:468–74.

96. Berwick DM. Public performance reports and the will for change. JAMA 2002;288:1523–4.

97. Wisconsin Collaborative for Healthcare Quality. Wisconsin Collaborative for Healthcare Quality [Homepage]. Available from www.wchq.org. Accessed 7 May 2008.

98. Nutting PA, Goodwin MA, Flocke SA, Zyzanski SJ, Stange KC. Continuity of primary care: to whom does it matter and when? Ann Fam Med 2003;1: 149–55.

99. Singh R, Singh A, Taylor JS, Rosenthal TC, Singh S, Singh G. Building learning practices with self-empowered teams for improving patient safety. J Health Management 2006;8:91–118.

100. Brooks RG, Menachemi N. Physicians' use of email with patients: factors influencing electronic communication and adherence to best practices. J Med Internet Res 2006;8:e2.

101. Kaushal R, Blumenthal D, Poon EG, et al.. The costs of a national health information network. Ann Intern Med 2005;143:165–73.

102. Crosson JC, Stroebel C, Scott JG, Stello B, Crabtree BF. Implementing an electronic medical record in a family medicine practice: communication, decision making, and conflict. Ann Fam Med 2005;3:307–11.

103. O'Connor PJ, Crain AL, Rush WA, Sperl-Hillen JM, Gutenkauf JJ, Duncan JE. Impact of an electronic medical record on diabetes quality of care. Ann Fam Med 2005;3:300–6.

104. Mehrotra A, Epstein AM, Rosenthal MB. Do integrated medical groups provide higher-quality medical care than individual practice associations? Ann Intern Med 2006;145:826–33.

105. Campbell S, Reeves D, Kontopantelis E, Middleton E, Sibbald B, Roland M. Quality of primary care in England with the introduction of pay for performance. N Engl J Med 2007;357:181–90.

106. Parente DH, Pinto MB, Barber JC. A pre-post comparison of service operational efficiency and patient satisfaction under open access scheduling. Health Care Manage Rev 2005;30:220–8.

107. O'Connor ME, Matthews BS, Gao D. Effect of open access scheduling on missed appointments, immunizations, and continuity of care for infant well-child care visits. Arch Pediatr Adolesc Med 2006;160:889–93.

108. Kopach R, DeLaurentis PC, Lawley M, et al. Effects of clinical characteristics on successful open access scheduling. Health Care Manag Sci 2007;10: 111–24.

109. Eads M. Virtual office visits: a reachable and reimbursable innovation. Fam Pract Manag 2007;14: 20–2.

110. Medfusion, Inc. Medfusion [Homepage] Available from http://www.medfusion.net. Accessed 26 December 2007.

111. Backer L. The medical home: an idea whose time has come again. Fam Pract Manag 2007;14:38–41.

112. NC Foundation for Advanced Health Programs, Inc. Community Care of North Carolina. Program overview. Available from http://www.community-carenc.com/. Accessed 1 May 2008.

113. Arvantes J. Support for medical home to be focus of upcoming bill. AAFP NewsNow. September 9, 2007.

114. Rosenthal TC, Horwitz ME, Snyder G, O'Connor J. Medicaid primary care services in New York state: partial capitation vs. full capitation. J Fam Practice 1996;42:362–8.

115. Moran DW. Whence and whither health insurance? A revisionist history. Health Aff (Millwood) 2005;24:1415–25.

116. Enthoven AC. Consumer-choice health plan (second of two parts). A national-health-insurance proposal based on regulated competition in the private sector. N Engl J Med 1978;298:709–20.

117. Enthoven AC, van de Ven WP. Going Dutch–managed-competition health insurance in The Netherlands. N Engl J Med 2007;357:2421–3.

118. Knottnerus JA, ten Velden GH. Dutch doctors and their patients–effects of health care reform in The Netherlands. N Engl J Med 2007;357:2424–6.

119. Campbell S, Steiner A, Robison J, et al.. Do personal medical services contracts improve quality of care? A multi-method evaluation. J Health Serv Res Policy 2005;10:31–9.

120. Pollock AM, Price D, Viebrock E, Miller E, Watt G. The market in primary care. BMJ 2007;335: 475–7.

121. Crabtree BF, Miller WL, Aita VA, Flocke SA, Stange KC. Primary care practice organization and preventive services delivery: a qualitative analysis. J Fam Pract 1998;46:403–9.

122. Valderas JM, Kotzeva A, Espallargues M, et al.. The impact of measuring patient-reported outcomes in clinical practice: a systematic review of the literature. Qual Life Res 2008;17:179–93.

123. Aitken JF, Janda M, Elwood M, Youl PH, Ring IT, Lowe JB. Clinical outcomes from skin screening clinics within a community-based melanoma screening program. J Am Acad Dermato. 2006;54: 105–14.

124. Fraguas R Jr, Henriques SG Jr, De Lucia MS, et al.. The detection of depression in medical setting: a study with PRIME-MD. J Affect Disord 2006;91: 11–7.

125. Rodriguez GL, Ma F, Federman DG, et al.. Predictors of skin cancer screening practice and attitudes in primary care. J Am Acad Dermatol 2007;57:775–81.

126. Gawande A. Complications: a surgeon's notes on an imperfect science. New York (NY): Picador USA; 2003.

127. American Medical Association. RVS Update Committee (RUC). Available from http://www.amaassn.org/ama/pub/category/16401.html. Accessed 4 December 2007.

128. Goodson JD. Unintended consequences of resource-based relative value scale reimbursement. JAMA 2007;298:2308–10.

129. Bodenheimer T, Berenson RA, Rudolf P. The primary care-specialty income gap: why it matters. Ann Intern Med 2007;146:301–6.

130. Ginsburg PB, Berenson RA. Revising Medicare's physician fee schedule–much activity, little change. N Engl J Med 2007;356:1201–3.

131. Gottschalk A, Flocke SA. Time spent in face-to-face patient care and work outside the examination room. Ann Fam Med 2005;3:488–93.

132. Landon BE, Schneider EC, Normand ST. Quality of care in Medicaid managed care and commercial health plans. JAMA 2007;298:1674–81.

133. Reports C. Treatment traps to avoid: insured? You're money in the bank to the health care system. Consumer Reports 2007;72:12–7.

134. Mahar M. Money-driven medicine: the real reason health care costs so much. New York (NY): HarperCollins Publishers; 2006.

135. Mark DH, Gottlieb MS, Zellner BB, Chetty VK, Midtling JE. Medicare costs in urban areas and the supply of primary care physicians. J Fam Pract 1996;43:33–9.

136. Basu J, Clancy C. Racial disparity, primary care, and specialty referral. Health Serv Res 2001;36 (6 Pt 2):64–77.

137. Whittle J, Lin CJ, Lave JR, et al.. Relationship of provider characteristics to outcomes, process, and costs of care for community-acquired pneumonia. Med Care 1998;36:977–87.

138. National Association of Community Health Centers. [Homepage.] Available from www.nachc.com. Accessed 28 September 2007.

139. Dartmouth Atlas of Health Care. Performance report for chronically ill beneficiaries in traditional Medicare. Available from http://www.dartmouthat-las.org/data/download/perf_reports/STATE_per-f_report.pdf. Accessed 18 December 2007.

140. Bridges to Excellence. Diabetes care analysis-savings estimate. Available from http://www.bridgestoex-cellence.org. Accessed 2 August 2008.

141. Casalino LP, Devers KJ, Lake TK, Reed M, Stoddard JJ. Benefits of and barriers to large medical group practice in the United States. Arch Intern Med 2003;163:1958–64.

142. Pham HH, Ginsburg PB, McKenzie K, Milstein A. Redesigning care delivery in response to a high-performance network: the Virginia Mason Medical Center. Health Aff (Millwood) 2007;26:w532–44.

143. Davis K. Paying for care episodes and care coordination. N Engl J Med 2007;356:1166–8.

144. McDonald R, Harrison S, Checkland K, Campbell SM, Roland M. Impact of financial incentives on clinical autonomy and internal motivation in primary care: ethnographic study. BMJ 2007;334:1357.

145. Pawlson LG, Scholle SH, Powers A. Comparison of administrative-only versus administrative plus chart review data for reporting HEDIS hybrid measures. Am J Manag Care 2007;13:553–8.

146. Snyder L, Neubauer RL. Pay-for-performance principles that promote patient-centered care: an ethics manifesto. Ann Intern Med 2007;147:792–4.

147. Dunbar L, Hiza D, Hoffman J, et al.. Outcomes-based compensation: performance design principles. Paper presented at 4th Annual Disease Management Outcomes Summit, Rancho Mirage, California, 2004.

148. Gilmore AS, Zhao Y, Kang N, et al.. Patient outcomes and evidence-based medicine in a preferred provider organization setting: a six-year evaluation of a physician pay-for-performance program. Health Serv Res 2007;42(6 Part 1):2140–59.

149. Campbell SM, McDonald R, Lester H. The experience of pay for performance in English family practice: a qualitative study. Ann Fam Med 2008;6:228–34.

150. National Institute for Health and Clinical Excellence. [Homepage.] Available from www.nice.org.uk. Accessed 2 August 2008.

Professional Case Management
Vol. 12, No. 2, 70–80

Case Managers Optimize Patient Safety by Facilitating Effective Care Transitions

Dana Deravin Carr, RNC, CCM, MPH, MS

ABSTRACT

In this new era of patient safety, the case manager, as an advocate and facilitator of care, has a pivotal role on the front line of healthcare delivery. Effective communication and collaboration between disciplines is key to the promotion of patient safety, and ultimately the avoidance of life-threatening medical errors. Across the healthcare continuum and within hospitals in particular, patients are routinely transferred from one service to another, from one level of care to another, or from one provider to another. As patients are stabilized and transitioned through the hospital system, there are multiple hand-offs of care or care transitions that can often expose the patient to fragmented service and increase the risk of communication breakdown. Ineffective hand-offs can result in a disruption of continuity between one level of care and the next. In a culture that places a strong emphasis on patient safety, case managers can facilitate opportunities that ease care transitions whereby a change in venue is no longer perceived as a disruption in the flow of care but rather is viewed as a coordinated changeover where cautious and comprehensive communication sets the tone for the continued delivery of safe and effective healthcare.

Since the turn of the century, medical error and tort reform have increasingly taken center stage in the healthcare debate. Patients, politicians, policy makers, and healthcare professionals struggle with the striking prevalence and consequences of medical error, whether a "near miss" or one resulting in patient injury (Massachusetts Coalition for the Prevention of Medical Errors, 2006). The Institute of Medicine (IOM) defines medical error as, "the failure of a planned action to be completed as intended or the use of a wrong plan to achieve an aim" (IOM, 1999, p. 1).

In its 1999 report, "To Err Is Human," the IOM estimated that anywhere from 44,000 to 98,000 people die each year because of medical errors that could have been prevented. Among the problems that commonly occur during the course of providing healthcare are adverse drug events, improper blood transfusions, surgical injuries such as wrong site surgery, falls, burns, mistaken identity, and even death. Moreover, high error rates with more serious consequences are most likely to occur in intensive care units (ICUs), operating rooms, and the emergency department (ED). The Quality of Health Care in America Committee of the IOM has concluded that it is not acceptable for patients to be harmed by a healthcare system that is supposed to offer healing and comfort; a system that promises to "First, do no harm" (IOM, 1999). This increased proclivity toward medical errors both creates and fosters an environment of mistrust. It is because of concerns such as these that the matter of patient safety is now in the healthcare spotlight.

Patient safety is an important concern of many healthcare stakeholders, including patients, providers, employers, health plans, and insurers. According to the IOM, patient safety is: "Freedom from accidental injury; ensuring patient safety involves the establishment of operational systems and processes that minimize the likelihood of errors and maximizes the likelihood of intercepting them when they occur" (Greenberg, 2004, p. 223).

The consideration of "patient safety first" is central to every decision made and every action performed by healthcare professionals and other care providers at any level of the continuum, including in the patient's home. In great part, the patient safety movement is about being a team player (Peck, 2004). If the patient is at the center of our efforts, then case management is a cornerstone in the support system of patient care. With patient safety increasingly "under the microscope," the case manager's role as a multifunctional coordinator of care expands beyond the team and the patient/family members into the community and to other providers of care. Effective communication and enhanced decision making can reduce the fragmentation of care that places patients at risk for medical error.

There are five main areas of patient safety on which case managers exert their efforts on a daily basis. These areas center on:

- transitions or "hand-offs" of care;
- medication reconciliation;
- patient/caregiver education;
- access to the right services at the right time; and
- timely and effective communication. (Tahan, 2006)

This article addresses the particular area of patient safety related to matters of "Care transitions and hand-offs" and focuses on an essential responsibility of case managers to optimize patient safety by promoting the clear and concise transfer of information during transitions and hand-offs of care. The case study addresses different settings of inpatient acute care and preparation for a postacute care venue; areas where accuracy in the exchange of information is an important safeguard for patients whose clinically complex needs increase the likelihood for fragmentation of care, which can increase the risk of exposure to medical error. Throughout the article, the words "care transitions" and "hand-offs" are used interchangeably.

BACKGROUND

Across the healthcare continuum, patients are routinely transferred from one service to another, from one level of care to another, or from one provider to another. In large healthcare systems, patients can move through multiple levels of care during a single stay. There will likely be an interface with many providers such as physicians, case managers, and social workers. Often, there may be more than one specialty involved in the patients care at the same time. As patients are stabilized and transitioned through a hospital's system of care, there can be multiple hand-offs of care. Because patient care is often fragmented, duplicative, and sometimes disorganized and improperly planned, the risk of "life threatening" medical errors increases as the patients exposure within the healthcare system increases (Tahan, 2006).

Hand-offs or care transitions should not be an abrupt end of care previously provided, but rather considered to be a coordinated changeover for the patient to a new team of involved caregivers. With few mechanisms in place for coordinating care across settings, often no single provider or team assumes responsibility during transitions (HMO Workgroup on Care Management, 2004). If discharge planning truly begins at the time of admission, each care transition should ideally be a planned process, unless of course the transition is an emergent one. Collaboration and effective communication among team members, before, during, and after the "hand off" is crucial at each stage of the medical management process. These critical interactions offer opportunities for clinical interface that can promote patient safety and contribute optimally to the avoidance of "life threatening" medical errors.

Fortunately, there are mandated systems in place that help to ensure appropriate care transitions and hand-offs. These mechanisms were developed and implemented to ensure patient safety and regulatory compliance. Discharge planning is a component of various pieces of legislation at both the federal and state levels, and it is also the requirement of various accrediting bodies such as the Joint Commission on Accreditation of Healthcare Organizations (JCAHO).

FEDERAL CONDITIONS OF PARTICIPATIONS: DISCHARGE PLANNING

The Federal Conditions of Participations are rules that hospitals must follow in order to participate in the Medicare or Medicaid programs. Hospitals must

TABLE 1 Federal Conditions of Participations: Discharge Planning/Care Transitions

(b) *Standard: Discharge Planning Evaluation*

    (3) The discharge planning evaluation must include the likelihood of a patient needing posthospital services and of the availability of those services.

    (4) The discharge planning evaluation must include an evaluation of the likelihood of the patient's capacity for self-care or of the possibility of the patient being cared for in the environment from which he or she entered the hospital.

    (5) The hospital personnel must complete the evaluation on a timely basis so that appropriate arrangements for posthospital care are made before discharge, and to avoid unnecessary delays in discharge.

(c) *Standard: Discharge Plan*

    (4) The hospital must reassess the discharge plan if there are factors that may affect the continuing care needs or the appropriateness of the discharge plan.

    (5) The hospital must ensure that patients are provided with list of agencies and/or facilities that are appropriate to the identified care needs and are Medicare participating.

    (6) For patients enrolled in managed care organizations, the hospital must indicate the availability of home care agencies and extended care facilities through individuals or entities that are under contract with the managed care organization.

(d) *Standard: Transfer or Referral*

The hospital must transfer or refer patients along with necessary medical information to appropriate facilities, agencies, or outpatient services, as needed, for follow-up or ancillary care.

(e) *Standard: Reassessment*

The hospital must reassess its discharge planning process on an ongoing basis. The reassessment must include a review of the discharge plans to ensure that they are responsive to the discharge needs.

59 FR 64152, December 13, 1994, as amended at 69 FR 49268, August 11, 2004.

have in effect a discharge planning process that applies to all patients. The hospital's policies and procedures must be specified in writing and updated accordingly (Birmingham, 1998). Those conditions that relate to the discharge planning process were last published August 11, 2004, effective October 1, 2004, and can be found in Section 42 CFR 482.43 of the Social Security Act (Centers for Medicare & Medicaid Services, 2004). They are listed as standards in the Federal Conditions of Participations. Some of these relate directly to care transitions (see Table 1).

JCAHO: PROVISION OF CARE, TREATMENT, AND SERVICES

Care, treatment, and services are provided through the successful coordination and completion of several processes that include:

- appropriate initial assessment of needs;
- development of a plan for care, treatment, and services;
- provision of care, treatment, and services;
- ongoing assessment of whether the care, treatment, and services provided are meeting the patient's needs; and

- either the successful discharge of the patient or referral or transfer of the patient for continuing care, treatment, and services. (CAMH Update 2, Joint Commission for Accreditation of Healthcare Organizations, 2006b)

The goal of this function is to define, shape, and sequence the processes and activities related to care delivery along the illness to wellness continuum. Over time, the patient may receive a range of care in multiple settings from multiple providers. For this reason, it is important for the hospital to view the patient care it provides as part of an integrated system of settings, services, healthcare practitioners, and care levels that make up the continuum of care (Birmingham, 1998). Contained within the Table 2 are certain standards that relate to care transitions.

Although the presence of standards is crucial to establishing accountability, it is noteworthy that the standards primarily reflect the perspective of the sending institution, but not that of the receiving institution. For example, the JCAHO standards include language relating to the exchange of information during transfers; however, the language speaks globally to the sending facility. Clearly, both the sending and receiving teams have individual responsibilities as well as

TABLE 2   JCAHO Provision of Care, Treatment, and Services: Standards-Related Care Transitions

Discharge or Transfer

Patients may be discharged from the hospital entirely or discharged or transferred to another level of care, treatment, and services to different health professionals, or to settings for continued services. The hospitals processes for transfer are based on the patients assessed needs. To facilitate discharge or transfer, the hospital assesses the patient's needs, plans for discharge or transfer, facilitates the discharge or transfer process, and helps to ensure that continuity of care, treatment, and services is maintained.

Standard PC.15.10

A process addresses the needs for continuing care, treatment, and services after discharge or transfer.

Standard PC.15.20

The transfer or discharge of a patient to another level care, treatment, and services, different professionals, or different settings is based upon the patient's assessed needs and the hospitals capabilities.

Standard PC.15.30

When patients are transferred or discharged, appropriate information related to care, treatment, and services provided is exchanged with other service providers.

For further information regarding the rationales and elements of performance, refer to the *Comprehensive Accreditation Manual for Hospitals: The Official Handbook*, by the Joint Commission for Accreditation of Healthcare Organizations, 2006b, Chicago, IL: Author.

joint responsibilities. It is incumbent upon both to ensure, through effective collaboration and communication, that the patient's transition is safe. Enhancing accountability begins with setting expectations for both the sending and receiving healthcare teams (Table 3).

Transfers among care settings are common. Twenty-three percent of hospitalized patients aged older than 65 are discharged to another institution, that is, a skilled nursing facility (SNF), and 11.6% are discharged with home healthcare. Unfortunately, an estimated 19% of patients discharged from a hospital to an SNF are readmitted to the hospital within 30 days (HMO Workgroup on Care Management, 2004). While much of the literature addresses facility-to-facility transfers, or facility-to-home transfers, there is little written about intra-institutional care transitions, which is unit-to-unit, or from one level-of-care to another level-of-care within the hospital setting.

INPATIENT CARE TRANSITIONS

"Many hands" may typically touch a patient who enters the hospital through the ED during a single episode of care. A 58-year-old man, after a motor vehicle accident, who is emergently admitted to the trauma service with a closed head injury, multiple fractures, and internal injuries, may receive care from a variety of individuals including but not limited to:

• ED physicians, nurses, respiratory therapist, radiologists, and ancillary ED personnel;

• trauma surgeons, orthopedic surgeons, and anesthesiologists;

• various physician consultants from neurology, ortho-spine; psychiatry;

• critical care intensivists, critical care nurses, acute care nurses, rehabilitation nurses (if there is a facility-based rehabilitation unit), and discharge planners; and

• hospital-based case managers, case managers who represent car insurance companies, or if privately insured, case managers involved with the private health insurance provider.

The list of involved healthcare practitioners could lengthen on the basis of the patient's comorbidities. Accurate, clear, and concise communication is critical while this patient moves across the continuum. Poorly executed transitions between practitioners at each level of care can result in delays or duplication of tests/treatments, delays in surgical intervention, delays in obtaining consents and authorizations, and delayed or absent communication. The consequences of such could place a patient in serious jeopardy by increasing the risk of exposure to medical error and be injurious to the organization as well.

The ED case manager will often make the initial patient contact. At this time, patient demographic, social, and medical history is obtained either from the patient or significant other. Vital information can be shared with in-house case managers and/or social workers in order to anticipate

---

TABLE 3   Core Functions for Meeting the Needs of Patients in Transition

---

Both the sending and receiving care teams are expected to

- Shift their perspective from the concept of a patient discharge to that of a patient transfer with continuous management.
- Begin planning for a transfer to the next care setting upon or before the patient's admission.
- Elicit the preferences of the patient and caregivers and incorporate these preferences into the care plan, where appropriate.
- Identify a patients system of social support and baseline level of function (i.e., how will this patient care for himself or herself after discharge)
- Communicate and collaborate with practitioners across settings to formulate and execute a common care plan.
- Use the preferred mode of communication (i.e., telephone, fax, e-mail) of collaborators in the other settings.

The sending health care team is expected to ensure that

- The patient is stable enough to be transferred to the next care setting.
- The patient and caregiver understand the purpose of the transfer.
- The receiving institution is capable of and prepared to meet the patient's needs.
- All relevant forms and documents are completed with accuracy.
- The care plan, orders, and a clinical summary precede the patient's arrival to the next care setting. The discharge summary should include the patient baseline functional status (both physical and cognitive) and recommendations from the other professionals involved in the patients care, including social workers, physical therapist, and other ancillary services.
- The patient has timely follow-up with appropriate health care professionals.
- A member of the sending health care team is available to the patient, caregiver, and the receiving health care team is available for a reasonable length of time after the transfer to discuss any questions related to the care plan.
- The patient and family understand their health care benefits and coverage as they pertain to the transfer.

The receiving health care team is expected to ensure that

- The transfer forms, clinical summary, discharge summary, and physician's orders are reviewed prior to or upon the patient's arrival.
- The patient's goals and preferences are incorporated into the plan of care.
- Discrepancies or confusion regarding the plan of care, the patient's status, or the patient's medications are clarified with the sending health care team.

Adapted from *One Patient, Many Places: Managing Healthcare Transitions*, by HMO Workgroup on Care Management, 2004, Washington, DC: AAHP—HHIAA Foundation. Retrieved October 19, 2006, from http://www.ahip.org/content.default.aspx?bc-338/65/69/5743.

and plan for the patients needs (Bristow & Herrick, 2002). In the ED, nurse case managers often work as a dyad with social workers. While both are involved in interviewing and gathering information from family members, it is the case manager who often does the detective work related to insurance coverage, and in the case of Mr. DJ, facilitates the initial precertification for admission into the ICU (Gautney, Stanton, Crowe, & Zilkie, 2004). Patient advocacy is a key function, especially during the early stages of the admission.

CASE STUDY

Mr. DJ is a 58-year-old car salesman who is divorced and lives alone but has a close relationship with his younger sister and her children. As he was accompanying a perspective new car buyer on a "test drive," the car was broadsided and Mr. RJ sustained critical injuries. Mr. RJ was unconscious at the crash site and was emergently admitted to the local trauma center. He was intubated to protect his airway, and after much intervention in the ED—CAT scans, MRI, radiograms, and lab work, was diagnosed with a closed head injury with a small subdural hematoma, multiple fractures involving the cervical spine, pelvis, left femur, right tibial plateau, the right humerus, multiple rib fractures, and internal injuries involving a liver laceration and left hemothorax. A chest tube was inserted and Mr. RJ was taken to the OR to stabilize the most serious of his fractures.

The ED case manager was able to learn Mr. DJ's identity from the driver of the car. Although he too sustained injuries, he was able to provide relevant data, which assisted the team in obtaining additional critical information.

The social worker contacted Mr. DJ's employer, and from there was able to obtain family information and contact his sister. We were able to learn from her that Mr. DJ had a medical history of depression and was under the care of a psychiatrist; he had a healthcare proxy, a durable power of attorney, and managed healthcare insurance. This information was documented in the clinical record.

Mr. DJ underwent debridement of the right tibial fracture and was placed in skeletal traction; exploratory surgery to repair the liver laceration; stabilization of the right humeral fracture, and placement in a posterior splint. At a later time when he was found to be more stable, he would undergo surgery to repair the tibial plateau fracture with a plate and to repair the right femur. The fractures of the cervical spine and pelvis were nondisplaced, and therefore would not require surgical intervention

Postoperatively, Mr. DJ was transferred to the SICU; he was in and out of consciousness for 3 days' postoperatively. He was still intubated, had multiple tubes/drains exiting from his body; and a hard collar around his neck. His right lower leg was in skeletal traction and his right arm was in a posterior splint. On the fourth day, his arterial blood gases were stable enough for him to be extubated, and on Day 5, he was transferred to the surgical step-down unit. What became apparent soon after Mr. DJ's extubation was that he had no recall of the accident. He remembered reporting to work on the morning of the accident but nothing else. As the physician began to explain the extent of the injuries, Mr. DJ began to cry.

The treatment plan included the need for Mr. DJ to return to the OR to have his right tibial plateau fracture and his left femur fracture repaired. The swelling in the right tibia had decreased markedly and all clinical indications were for swift intervention and then to transfer Mr. DJ to acute rehabilitation. One by one, as his systems stabilized, the physician consultants were signing off his case. Mr. DJ was so overwhelmed by his injuries and loss of memory that he was unable to make any decisions regarding his care. He would not sign the consent for further treatment and he would start to cry at any discussion regarding his future care needs. He did agree, however, to allow his sister to continue in role as his healthcare proxy.

With Mr. DJ's sister at the helm, decisions for care, treatment, and discharge planning moved rapidly. At his sister's insistence, Mr. DJ reluctantly agreed to the psychiatric consult. He was able to acknowledge that the loss of memory was frightening to him and the recurrent nightmares were exhausting him. He underwent the additional surgeries to his right and left legs, and soon had a physiatrist consult

to begin to pave the way for his rehabilitation and subsequent transition to the next level of care. The initial therapy was hampered by pain, emotional outbursts, and tears. It became apparent from the physical therapist initial evaluation that Mr. DJ could in no way tolerate an aggressive restorative program. The cognitive evaluation confirmed the plan for a TBI facility. Mr. DJ was nonweight bearing on his right upper extremity, nonweight bearing on right lower extremity, and partial weight bearing on his left lower extremity. Mr. DJ's sister was becoming overwhelmed by her brother's tears and neediness. She expressed concern that he would never be able to come to her home to recuperate until he was much more functional and much less emotionally fragile.

The hospital case manager, in conjunction with the worker's compensation case manager, maintained close contact throughout the duration of Mr. DJ's stay in the medical center. In fact, the worker's compensation case manager made two visits to the medical center to meet with the team and Mr. DJ's sister to discuss options for Mr. DJ's care. Through diligent work efforts, they were able to locate a TBI facility that offered acute rehabilitation and had 25 subacute beds. The goal was to start Mr. DJ on a less-aggressive rehabilitation program, and as his pain improved and his strength and tolerance increased, he would be transitioned to the acute rehabilitation section of the facility.

As a next step in the care transition process, Mr. DJ's sister would visit the facility to obtain relevant information. In turn, the facility case manager would come to see Mr. DJ at the medical center to confer with his sister as well as assess his appropriateness for admission and obtain relevant clinical information.

All involved case managers would continue to communicate in order to ensure that when Mr. DJ was stable enough for transfer, his transition would be a smooth one.

This plan was appropriate for the patient and his family/proxy. It was also appropriate for the team, as it served to facilitate the plan of care. In the long term and with the continued support of case management, Mr. DJ would eventually be discharged home with services and a whole new team would accept responsibility and accountability for Mr. DJ's care.

***

Of critical importance here is the continued communication with the team to certify that the treatment plan is on track. The case manager in the ED will document and share vital information with the case manager and other team members on the acute care side. Open lines of communication will be established and maintained with the case manager from the insurance company to ensure that the patient care continues to be certified. The case manager in the SICU will use evidence-based criteria to support the necessary length of stay on the basis of the patient's clinical presentation (McKendry & Van Horn, 2004). As the patient begins to make his transition to the next level of care, in this case, the step-down unit, the case manager ensures that the physician has accurately and appropriately documented the patients care for the next team of physician caretakers. In addition, if the case is handed off to another case manager, the care process should be documented, report given, and vital information regarding insurance contacts will be shared.

In the step-down unit, the case manager's role as an advocate for the patient and his family/healthcare proxy is of critical importance. The patient is assisted by the case manager, in every way possible, to make informed choices on the basis of information and understanding of his or her medical condition. Accordingly, case managers advocate for the patient throughout every phase of the hospitalization. As an advocate, the case manager has the ability to impact the course of the patient's treatment by establishing trust through relationship building, fostering communication between the patient and the team, and affecting the healthcare system by seeking opportunities to enhance the quality of care delivery (Deravin, 2006).

Mr. DJ's care was successfully affected by:

- three case managers from the medical center;
- the ED case manager,
- the SICU case manager,
- the step-down unit case manager;
- two case manager's from outside of the organization;
- the disability case manager; and
- the case manager from the TBI facility.

The case of Mr. DJ demonstrated how teamwork, collaboration, and communication, from the initial patient contact and throughout the hospital stay, could help ensure a successful outcome and minimize patient risk. The availability and processing of significant data early in the admission, such as the healthcare proxy information, the medical history, and insurance information, enabled all caretakers to understand and plan effectively to manage Mr. DJ's current and future care needs. It is likely that these interventions served to not only reduce Mr. DJ's length of stay but also further minimize his risk of exposure to medical error.

PLANNING FOR POSTACUTE CARE TRANSITIONS

As the plan for transition is established, problems can often occur as the patient is transferred from one healthcare setting to another because each setting typically operates in its own silo, with little understanding of what transpires in other settings. Until recently, national attention to the problems of medial errors had largely focused on care delivered in individual settings. Yet, care delivered across settings can create even greater vulnerabilities (Coleman & Fox, 2004). Moreover, a lack of understanding of the patient's functional health status, including the physical and cognitive aspects, may result in a transfer to a care venue that does not meet the patient's needs.

The transfer of timely and accurate information across settings is critical to the execution of effective care transitions. Practitioners need an understanding of the patient's goals, baseline functional status, active medical and behavioral health problems, medication regimen, family or support resources, durable medical equipment needs, and ability for self-care; otherwise, they may duplicate services, overlook important aspects of the care plan, and, as a result, convey conflicting information to the patient and provider (HMO Workgroup on Care Management, 2004). Incomplete information can result in critical errors such as the patient transferring to an alternate care setting without vital equipment or medication ordered or the availability of an isolation room, if warranted.

Over time, patients may receive a range of care in multiple settings from multiple providers. For this reason, it is important for a hospital to view the patient care it provides as part of an integrated system of settings, services, healthcare practitioners, and care levels that make up a continuum of care (Birmingham, 1998). Practitioners need to shift their mindset from the concept of a patient discharge to that of a patient transfer for continued care management. This shift includes but is not limited to the formulation of a common care plan developed by the involved disciplines, evaluation of patient's social supports, baseline level of function, and potential for discharge. All of this must be initiated well before the transfer to the next setting (Table 4) (HMO Workgroup on Care Management, 2004).

TABLE 4 Core Data Elements Needed Across the Continuum of Care

Domains	Information Required	Short-term Goals[a]	Long-term Goals[a]
Functional status	Baseline (ADL and IADL) Current		
Medical status	Summary of admitting problems(s)		
	Most pressing medical problem and prognosis		
	Other medical problems complicating management		
	Comprehensive list of current medications (including prescribed and over the counter)		
	Current list of allergies and intolerances		
Self-care ability	Current ability		
	Educational training and needs		
Social support	Primary caregiver (name, relationship, phone number)		
	Ability/willingness to provide care		
	Community level support		
Disposition	Where was the patient residing prior to the episode?		
	Where is the patient going now?		
	Where will the patient go next?		
Communication	Language		
	Literacy		
	Health beliefs		
Advance directives— Healthcare proxy	Preferences for CPR, ventilator support, enteral/parenteral feeding, hydration, dialysis		
	Power of Attorney		
Durable medical equipment	Current needs		
	Vendors name/phone number		
Coverage/benefits	Provider network for SNFs, home health agencies, hospice, respite, and durable medical equipment		

ADL 3 activities of daily living; IADL 3 instrumental activities of daily living; and SNF = skilled nursing facility.

Adapted from *One Patient, Many Places: Managing Healthcare Transitions*, by HMO Workgroup on Care Management, 2004, Washington, DC: AAHP—HHIAA Foundation, Retrieved October 19, 2006, from http://www.ahip.org/content.default.aspx?bc338/65/69/5743
[a]Goals take into account the patient's values and preferences.

Table 4 summarizes the core data elements required to ensure effective and efficacious care delivery. The columns for short-term and long-term goals are purposely left blank because the goals of care are ever-changing and should therefore be re-evaluated and revised through out the care delivery process. In effect, the table should be considered a working document for the team.

CASE MANAGEMENT INTERVENTIONS

The goal of case management interventions is to enhance an individual's safety, productivity, satisfaction, and quality of life (Case Management Society of America, 2001). In this new era of patient safety, the case manager, as an advocate and facilitator of care,

has a pivotal role in the front line of healthcare delivery across the care continuum. The case management role is a multifunctional one whose interventions place strong emphasis upon assessment and assimilation of information, coordination, and planning for care transitions; education of the patient and family; and collaboration with other caregivers for the key purpose of facilitating and optimizing communication throughout the patient's hospital stay. These interventions enhance and ensure patient safety.

From the beginning of the admission and throughout the patient's stay, the performance of key primary functions such as assessment, planning, facilitation, and advocacy allows the case manager to anticipate, identify, and monitor crucial events and issues that may affect the patient's movement across

TABLE 5   Essential Skills for Practitioners

Establish long-term and short-term goals for medical care that take into account patient preferences and the natural history of the disease process.

Determine the specific care the patient will require to achieve these goals.

Assess the patient's ability to meet his or her self-care needs, as well as the caregiver's ability and willingness to participate in the care plan.

Be knowledgeable of the care continuum and each facility's capability for providing care.

Determine the care site where the patient's needs will be best served.

Actively engage the patient and caregiver in the decision to move to a new site of care.

Communicate with the patient and caregiver in their language of understanding and exercise sensitivity to their sociocultural and economic status.

Initiate the transfer plan as early as possible. Recognize that patient may have difficulty processing information and may require consistent information for all practitioners and continued reinforcement.

Incorporate knowledge of the patient healthcare benefits into the design and execution of the care plan.

Communicate the patient's goals and preferences to all healthcare professionals who participate in the design and/or execution of the care plan.

Communicate the patient's essential clinical and functional status information to the receiving team.

Remain available to the receiving team should posttransfer questions or concerns arise.

Direct the patient and caregiver to the appropriate person when questions arise about benefits.

the care continuum. Since the presence of case management extends to every point on the care continuum, case managers can be key facilitators of the care transition process. Healthcare errors can be minimized by ensuring the preparation and communication of appropriate, correct, and concise information. Case management reduces the fragmentation of care, which is too often experienced by patients who have multiple providers involved in their care.

Communication failures, particularly those occurring during the care transition process, can open the door to life-threatening diagnostic errors. Theses errors are often manifested in the following ways:

- inaccuracies or delays in diagnosis or failure to employ indicated tests;
- errors in treatment or delayed response to an abnormal test result or laboratory value; and/or
- inadequate monitoring or follow-up treatment. (IOM, 1999)

The case manager has an essential responsibility to ensure that each team member meets his or her obligation in engineering the transition process.

Advocacy, communication, education, and coordination of care become critically important as the case manager provides guidance to the team and the patient. It is clear that case managers want to work together to affect safe, smooth patient transitions; it is also clear that physicians want the same thing (Powell, 2006). However, most practitioners lack the training necessary to manage effective transfers and may not recognize their role in transitional planning. Moreover, most practitioners lack exposure to sites of care other than those where they practice and are unfamiliar with the ability of the receiving institution to manage clinically complex patients (Coleman & Fox, 2004). Table 5 is a guideline of essential skills that can be of particular benefit to the team when planning for care and coordinating transitions.

These essential skills for practitioners consider the needs of the patient and the needs of the team, and can be beneficial for any care venue along the continuum.

CONCLUSION

Reliably and consistently assessing patient safety is important and promotes quality of care, but doing so for a diverse set of organizations and communities is extraordinarily challenging. Hospitals are as diverse as the populations they serve. There are academic medical centers whose primary mission is the preparation and teaching of healthcare professionals and performing research. There are tertiary care hospitals that provide high-tech, leading-edge services for many previously untreatable conditions. There are community-based hospitals that primarily serve the local community's more "typical" inpatient needs (e.g., obstetrics, community acquired pneumonias). The populations served by these hospitals also differ widely. For example, there are publicly funded hospitals that serve as a safety net for those lacking private medical insurance, hospitals focusing on the elderly or children, rural hospitals that must meet all the needs of its population base, and hospitals specializing in cancer, joint diseases, or mental health (George, Emons, Uchida, & Kosecoff, 2002).

As the demographics continue to shift toward a more aged population with chronic illnesses, case managers can make a significant impact upon the patient safety movement, especially with regards to the issue of care transitions and hand-offs. Case managers will be challenged to strengthen their role in areas of advocacy and education. As advocates, they can help ensure that patients have access to the right resources for the right care at the right time. As educators, they will support the team by ensuring that the delivery of care continues to be patient centered, that the providers of care are educated and informed of their responsibility to protect the patient by communicating effectively with all caregivers. As patient educators, case managers will ensure that patients and (or family members are able to make informed decisions around care management issues, have their rights respected, and confidentiality maintained.

As organizations shift their perspective toward a "culture of patient safety," case management can play a key role in the development of specific safety indicators of case management. Each stage of the medical management process offers opportunities for data collection and clinical interface to promote patient safety.

NEXT STEPS

Although the healthcare industry is in its infancy with respect to safe transitions, the commitment to the delivery of efficient, efficacious quality care continues to be a recurrent theme in the promotion of patient safety, and to ensure success in that arena, many hospitals are developing and implementing programs around the Joint Commission National Patient Safety Goals (Joint Commission for Accreditation of Healthcare Organizations, 2005).

Among the National Patient Safety Goals, Goal 2E was developed to help organizations improve hand-off communication. It states, "Implement a standardized approach to hand-off communications, including an opportunity to ask and respond to questions."

Two techniques currently in practice that have shown degrees of success in their implementation are the SBAR (Situation-Background-Assessment-Recommendation) technique, which was developed and implemented by Kaiser Permanente, and the SHARED (Situation-History-Assessment Request-Evaluate-Document) methodology, which was developed and implemented at Northwest Community Hospital.

Briefly, the purpose of the SBAR technique is to improve communication effectiveness through standardization of the communication process (Joint Commission for Accreditation of Healthcare Organizations, 2006a). Through use of a communication flow sheet, vital information is shared among the members of the team. This document is integral to the care, treatment, and service plan. The SHARED methodology is a more refined version of the SBAR technique and is organization specific—tailored to the needs of Northwest Community Hospital. It utilizes much of the same strategies of standardizing communication. (For more detailed information regarding the SBAR technique and SHARED methodology, refer to Web sites www.jcipatientsafety.org/show.asp/durki=3152&print= yes and http://www.nch.org, respectively)

Case managers who are employed in organizations that utilize these or other similar techniques have an opportunity to not only actively employ these methods as part of their own hand-off communication strategy but also could track, trend, and evaluate institutionally the effectiveness of these techniques through the development of performance improvement monitoring tools. Case management can monitor the effectiveness and success of these strategies and make recommendations toward the refinement or enhancement of such initiatives. These are areas in which case management can exert leadership and affect change (Greenberg, 2004).

The patient safety initiative will remain a high priority for years to come, and case management will be in the forefront of any change that is on the horizon. Although no single activity or group can offer a total solution for dealing with medical errors, the combined actions of informed and progressive healthcare professionals and administrators can offer a roadmap toward a safer healthcare delivery system.

References

Birmingham, J. (1998). *Discharge planning: The rules and reality* (pp. 8–33). South Natick, MA: The Center for Case Management.

Bristow, D. P., & Herrick, C. A. (2002). Emergency department case management—The dyad team of nurse case manager and social worker improve discharge planning and patient and staff satisfaction while decreasing inappropriate admissions and cost: A literature review. *Lippincott's Case Management*, 7(6), 243–254.

Case Management Society of America. (2001). *Standards of practice for case management*. Little Rock, AR: Author.

Centers for Medicare & Medicaid Services. (2004). *Conditions for coverage and conditions of participation*. Washington, DC: U.S. Department of Health and Human Services. Retrieved November 24, 2006, from http://www.cms.hhs.gov/CFCsandCoPs/06_Hospitals.asp Coleman, E. A., & Fox, P. D. (2004). *Managing patient care transitions: A report to the HMO Workgroup on Care Management*. Washington, DC: AHIP. Retrieved October 19, 2006, from http://www.ahip.org/content/default.aspx?bc=331/130/136/271/276 Deravin, C. D. (2006). Implications for case management: Ensuring access and delivery of quality health care to undocumented immigrant populations. *Lippincott's Case Management*, 11(4), 195–204.

Gautney, L. J., Stanton, M. P., Crowe, C., & Zilkie, T. M. (2004). The emergency department case manager: Effect on selected outcomes. *Lippincott's Case Management*, 9(3), 121–129.

George, D. L., Emons, M. F., Uchida, K. M., & Kosecoff, J. M. (2002). *The challenge of assessing patient safety in America's hospitals*. Santa Monica, CA: Protocare Sciences. Retrieved October 19, 2006, from http://www.fahs.com/issues/studies/HospitalStandards.pdf

Greenberg, L. (2004). Patient safety systems for case management. *Lippincott's Case Management*, 9(5), 223–229.

HMO Workgroup on Care Management. (2004, February). *One patient, many places: Managing health care transitions*. Washington, DC: AAHP—HHIAA Foundation. Retrieved October 19, 2006, from http://www.ahip.org/content.default.aspx?bc = 38/65/69/5743

Institute of Medicine. (1999). *To err is human: Building a safer health system*. Washington, DC: National Academies Press. Retrieved October 19, 2006, from http://www.iom.edu/object.file/master/4/117/toerr-8pager.pdf

Joint Commission for Accreditation of Healthcare Organizations. (2005). *Joint Commission Perspectives on Patient Safety*. Chicago, IL: Author. Retrieved November 22, 2006, from http//www.jcipatientsafety.org/show.asp?durki=10293&print=yes

Joint Commission for Accreditation of Healthcare Organizations. (2006a). Implementing the SBAR technique. In *Joint Commission Perspectives on Patient Safety* (Vol. 6, pp. 8–12). Chicago, IL: Author. Retrieved October 19, 2006, from http://www.jcipatientsafety.org/show.asp?durki=13152&print=yes

Joint Commission for Accreditation of Healthcare Organizations. (2006b, September). *Comprehensive accreditation manual for hospitals. The official handbook. Provision of care, treatment, and services* (CAMH Update 2). Chicago, IL: Author.

Massachusetts Coalition for the Prevention of Medical Errors. (2006). *When things go wrong: Responding to adverse events*. Boston, MA: Author. Retrieved October 19, 2006, from http://www.macoalition.org.

McKendry, M. J., & Van Horn, J. (2004). Today's hospital-based case manager: How one hospital integrated/adopted evidence-based medicine using InterQual criteria. *Lippincott's Case Management*, 9(2), 61–71.

Peck, P. (2004). *Patient safety requires fundamental changes to medical systems*. Philadelphia: Medscape Medical News. Retrieved October 2, 2006, from www.medscape.com/viewarticle/475217

Powell, S. K. (2006). Handoffs and transitions of care: Where is the lone ranger's silver bullet? *Lippincott's Case Management*, 11(5), 235–237.

Tahan, H. A. (2006). Enhancing patient safety: The role of the case manager. *Care Management*, 11(5), 19–24.

Dana Deravin Carr, RNC, CCM, MPH, MS, is the principal Care Manager for Inpatient Physical Rehabilitation and the Stroke Team at Jacobi Medical Center, Bronx, NY. Ms. Carr brings to the field of case management a diverse clinical and administrative background, which includes home health and long-term care. The author has no conflict of interest.

Address correspondence to Dana Deravin Carr, RNC, CCM, MPH, MS, Jacobi Medical Center, Care Management Department–2 South 3, 1400 Pelham Pkwy South, Bronx, NY 10461 (dana.deravincarr@nbhn.net; dcpny@aol.com).

Professional Case Management
Vol. 12, No. 3, 132–146

ACUITY AND CASE MANAGEMENT

A Healthy Dose of Outcomes, Part I

Diane L. Huber, PhD, RN, FAAN, CNAA, BC, and Kathy Craig, MS, RN, CCM

ABSTRACT

Purpose of Study: This article presents acuity and dosage as two concepts that describe how the business case for case management (CM) can be made. Dosage and acuity concepts are explained as client need-severity, CM intervention-intensity, and CM activity-dose by amount, duration, extent, and timing. Concepts are related to the practice of CM using evidence-based knowledge and methods to develop instruments that measure and score pivotal CM actions. The purpose of this series of three articles is to introduce the two concepts of dosage and acuity, discuss their importance for making the business case for CM and for translation into evidence-based practice, and present a powerful example of how they can be used in everyday CM. The articles feature a specific exemplar, the CM Acuity Tools project, and explain how the melding of the acuity and dosage innovations will improve the capture of CM outcomes. Part I focuses on the CM Acuity Tool© instrument.

Primary Practice Setting(s): The article's information applies to all CM practice settings, and contains ideas and recommendations useful to CM generalists, specialists, supervisors, and outcomes managers. The Acuity Tools Project was developed from frontline CM practice in one large, national telephonic CM company.

Methodology and Sample: For dosage, the Huber-Hall Dosage Model and its testing are described and explained. The intersection of dosage and acuity is analyzed. For the Acuity Tools Project, a structured literature search and needs assessment launched the development of the suite of acuity tools. The resulting gap analysis identified that an instrument to assign and measure case acuity specific to CM activities was needed. Clinical experts, quality specialists, and business analysts ($n = 7$) monitored the development and testing of the tools, acuity concepts, scores, differentials, and their operating principles, and evaluated the validity of the acuity tools' content related to CM activities. During the pilot phase of development, interrater reliability testing of draft and final tools for evaluator concordance, beta (β) testing for content accuracy and appropriateness, and representative sample size testing were done. Expert panel reviews occurred at several junctures along the development pathway, including after initial tool draft and both before and after β-test ($n = 5$) and pilot tests ($n = 28$). The pilot testing body ($n = 33$) consisted of a team of case managers ($n = 28$) along with quality analysts ($n = 2$), supervisory personnel ($n = 2$), and the lead product analyst (the developer). Product evaluation included monitoring weekly reports of open cases for the 28 case managers for 3 months (June to August 2000).

Results: Positive results generated approval from the expert review panel to apply the suite of acuity tools beyond (1) the initial draft phase, (2) the test population phase, and then (3) at a national CM organization level.

Implications for Case Management Practice: This article defines and discusses acuity and dosage as two practical conceptual tools that successfully unite clinical quality and business practices and measure and analyze CM activities. The CM Acuity Tool© is a master conceptual framework in three dimensions that synthesizes key components of CM practice, organized into indicators, drivers, and subdrivers. To show value, case managers need to access the evidence base for practice, use tools to capture quantities of intervention-intensity, and specify the activities that produce better outcomes.

Leaders call for case managers to demonstrate positive results. Mastal (2000) noted that to prove value, case managers must report intervention outcomes and develop indicators specific to each practice environment. She challenged case managers to "define the indicators of our worth, select valid measurement tools and processes, and share the outcomes with colleagues and employers" (Mastal, 2000, p. 10). The outcomes quandary for case managers hinges on a persistent absence of one established way to best measure the worth of and to make the business case for case management (CM). Establishing a best method requires blending outcomes measures that feature service provision elements specific to the positive results that occur from actions case managers take on behalf of their clients with a configuration that can be translated into a financial formula.

Previous efforts to make the business case of CM employed one of two different strategies: showing positive cost savings or demonstrating cost avoidance. However, another approach exists. To make the business case for CM effectively, case managers need to move past the outcomes goal of the "absence of bad outcomes" (Powell, 2000, p. 59) and into the goal of applying evidence-based practice (EBP). EBP assists case managers to define terms of worth such as primary and secondary effects of illness severities; treatment appropriateness; efficient cost-saving management; and improvements for clients, providers, and payers. Going beyond the business case for CM means integrating financial measures into CM practice. The purpose of this series of two articles is to introduce the three concepts of dosage and acuity, discuss their importance for making the business case for CM and for translation into EBP, and present a powerful example of how they can be used in everyday CM. Part 1 presents the background on dosage and acuity, discusses the business case for CM, and introduces the Acuity Tools Project. Part 2 describes the Acuity Tools Project in greater depth and features the two measurement instruments, CM Acuity Tool© and AccuDiff©. Part III explains how to apply the concept of CM dosage and the outcomes instruments that measure CM acuity.

DOSAGE

The actual activities carried out by healthcare providers in the delivery of an intervention and the amount of time these activities take are two key variables that form the core of the specification of an intervention. Notwithstanding the call for dosage (Brooten & Naylor, 1995), little has been done to actually describe and test either nurse-sensitive or CM-sensitive dosage. Such specification is important in order to be able to measure, compare, and then evaluate interventions as to their effectiveness and cost. Practice improvement is dependent upon such measurement and evaluation. Researchers have identified the need to capture the dose of an intervention as an urgent problem (Lindsay, 2004). However, dose has been difficult to understand and measure in CM practice because it is not as intuitive as is the dose of a medication. Brooten and Youngblut (2006) noted that the dictionary definition of dose is a measured quantity of medicine or a therapeutic agent, and they conceptualized nurse dose as having three components: (1) dose (either the number of nurses or amount of care by nurses), (2) nurse (education, expertise, experience), and (3) host response (either patient or organizational receptiveness). Their measures included patient/staff ratios, amount of nurse time, and the nurse's education and expertise. They noted that the outcomes most commonly used to measure nurse dose are mortality, morbidity, patient satisfaction, and healthcare costs (Brooten & Youngblut, 2006). Unfortunately, these variables and measures do not capture the complexity of interventions, especially in CM; are not sensitive to the work that nurses or case managers do; nor do they generate ongoing process-level information needed to link dose to outcomes in a way that compares and evaluates for contemporaneous quality and cost management. A sound and tested dosage methodology will exhibit better matching capability or titration of interventions and associated activities. This is the wasteful "fire hose" effect where provider interventions such as CM are poured on without careful analysis. In the opposite undertreatment effect interventions and activities are restricted because of cost factors and then result in sequelae, such as occurred when the restriction of childbirth coverage to 24 hr in a hospital was legislatively reversed on the basis of unsafe patient care incidents.

Starting with questions from the scientific community and federal funding sources about how to address *dosage* of a provider's intervention, Huber and colleagues (Huber, Hall, & Vaughn, 2001; Huber, Sarrazin, Vaughn, & Hall, 2003) developed a definition and conceptual model of intervention dosage in CM based on the work of Ridgely and Willenbring (1992) and Sidani and Braden (1998) and then tested it in substance abuse treatment. In the Huber-Hall Dosage Model, the dosage of a provider intervention is defined as the amount, frequency, duration, and breadth of actual activities used in an intervention, as a unique combination of discrete provider actions, at a level of intensity (amount and frequency), over a duration of time (Huber et al., 2001). Dosage encompasses both intervention integrity (Did the provider actually deliver the intervention?) and client engagement (Did the client actually participate?). For dosage, it is imperative that the intervention be fully and clearly described (Huber et al., 2003). Huber et al. (2001, p. 122) identified and defined the four essential elements of intervention dose as:

1. *Amount:* The quantity of the target activity in one episode.
2. *Frequency:* The rate of occurrence or repetition.
3. *Duration:* How long the activity is available over time.
4. *Breadth:* The number and type of possible intervention components or activities.

CM is a healthcare provider intervention and process used to deliver services related to client education, monitoring, surveillance, and care coordination. CM is expensive because it entails the provision of services from experts, often as a one-on-one healthcare service. Human resources and time are needed to produce outcomes. Therefore, it is critical that case managers have methods that use EBP to

formulate the correct configurations and amounts of their intervention activities to ensure that targeted outcomes are achieved. Financial imperatives compel case managers to look at what activities they are doing or not doing: too little or too much of a "dose" of CM may go beyond a failure to produce the desired effects on outcomes, to wasting resources nonproductively, or even producing harmful outcomes (Huber et al., 2001). Indeed, case managers need to know "which intervention components, at which dosage, under what circumstances, and with which clients, result in which outcomes" (Sidani & Braden, 1998, p. vii).

The selection of the CM activities, as well as their sequencing and timing, is generally within the discretion of the individual case manager's judgment. While some activities occur early in the timing of interventions, others occur over time or late in the delivery of intervention activities. In addition, activities may vary both in amount and in frequency over time. Dosage determination is done to reveal both the array of specific CM activities and their timing. It goes beyond measuring CM as an hour of service delivery to become more precise and descriptive. By describing the dosage of a CM intervention, the activities actually delivered can be characterized more precisely and concretely, usually taking the form of provider actions combined in unique time-and-intensity sessions such as discrete doses of intensity over specific durations of time (Huber et al., 2001).

The dose of a CM intervention includes a variety of discrete, specific activities that may be delivered simultaneously, individually, or in sequence. The variety of actions that may be selected, plus the variation in how they may be timed, contributes to the complexity of measuring and formulating dosage. For example, the measurement of dosage starts with a description. Huber et al. (2001, 2003) first captured and analyzed the specific activities and interventions that were part of case managers' work in substance abuse treatment to more precisely describe what CM was. Next, researchers used the Huber-Hall Dosage framework, consisting of the four elements outlined earlier, to analyze activities and found that defining dosages by amount, frequency, duration, and breadth provided clarity and definition useful in both practice and outcomes analysis. In this population, CM needed to be "front loaded," meaning that cases required heavier dosages of CM activities at the start of treatment. However, the study results showed that the heavy dose did not need to be maintained over time. CM activity dosages were reduced in amount, frequency, duration, and breath as the cases neared the 1-year completion mark.

By measuring these four elements of interventions, case managers can construct profiles of their actual practice activities, anchor them to financial and other value-related measures through reproducible evidence trails, and connect these to predictable outcomes. This orientation differs from the typical CM process. Rather than a focus on achieving CM through a stepwise process, the dosage approach integrates activities with the processes of CM. The synchronization of activity with process into prescribed doses simplifies the complexity of the components of CM interventions and augments the evaluation of CM interventions toward clinical, functional, satisfaction, and financial outcomes.

ACUITY

Defined as severity of illness or client condition that indicates the need for the intensity of the subsequent CM intervention (Craig, 2005; Huber, 2006), *acuity* links duration, quality, quantity, and volume to constitute pivotal aspects of the service delivery platforms of healthcare providers, especially CMS. CMS need to measure their clients' needs for care provision and match these client requirements more precisely with the activities CMS subsequently perform. Serving as proxy for time and extent of activities that care CMS should plan to undertake, acuity scores have become integrated into workload systems to determine staffing (Prescott & Soeken, 1996). Acuity represents the level of complexity or difficulty of a CM case in its three primary domains of CM activity: client need-severity, CM intervention-intensity, and healthcare service delivery responsiveness.

Intensity is a term related to acuity that represents both the amount of care and the complexity of care needed by patients or clients. Prescott (1991) identified four major dimensions to intensity: severity of illness, client dependency, complexity, and time. CM acuity relates the intensity of CM interventions to the degree of severity of clients' needs for health-care services in three broad practice areas—situation, satisfaction, and service (Craig, 2005). Using one-dimensional counts or case numbers fails to portray complexity. Cases gain a second dimension of weight by assigning acuity values to elements of CM complexity within cases. Acuity distinctions set up means whereby CM can be measured in its spheres of activity, intensity of interventions, and extent of success.

Dosage and acuity concepts arose in two different CM practice settings; both prompted by the need to capture and measure CM practice complexity. They emerged as conceptual frameworks that promote greater precision in measuring evidence-based CM practice. One innovative CM practice project, the Acuity Tools initiative (Craig, 2005), is presented in these three articles to demonstrate the use of acuity and dosage concepts in an outcomes analysis format. Details of the project's conception and development phases are featured as a model of translating evidence into a CM business application.

ACUITY TOOLS PROJECT EXEMPLAR

Craig originated the Acuity Tools Project, including the CM Acuity Tool© and AccuDiff© instruments, in 1999 in response to the business imperative to more precisely capture the evidence base of CM activities and more reliably measure CM outcomes (Craig, 2005). These two tools and their accompanying processes were developed as user-friendly devices to monitor changes in four outcomes domains: clinical, functional, satisfaction, and financial. The CM Acuity Tool© was conceived of as a way to capture CM impact created through targeted interventions and then to relate CM interventions to improved outcomes. Arising from frontline CM practice in one large, national telephonic CM company, it was designed to validate CM effectiveness by first assigning complexity values, called *acuities*, and then by measuring changes in the complexity values as subsequent CM interventions were applied. Although reproducibly demonstrating measurable CM impact was the primary outcomes objective, the project sought to accomplish the following aims as well: incorporate core CM criteria, quantify and qualify care needs accurately, report interventions systematically, and evaluate performance objectively.

ACUITY TOOLS DEVELOPMENT

Development of the acuity tools began with a literature search to uncover available outcomes instruments. None were found that provided an integrated system to produce evidence of best clinical practice, product efficacy, and financial results. Through surveys internal to the CM practice environment, Craig discovered that there was a gap between available CM data and CM practice demands, including

TABLE 1 Gap Analysis

Practice Demands		Components of CM Outcomes Gap
Correct CM essentials	→	Accurate capture of CM core criteria
True portraits of clients and of CM	→	Augment best practice imperatives
Functional and reliable tool	→	Adapt to alternate functional paradigms
Quick, small effort; big payoff	→	Accommodate practice needs
Objective evaluation of CM impact	→	Advance objective outcomes measures

Note. Development of the acuity instruments for case management (CM) sought to fill the outcomes gaps related to the five practice demands. The demands were identified and pursued in initial investigations of literature sources and available tools.

demonstrating value. A need existed to develop an instrument to assign and measure case acuity specific to CM activities. The resulting gap analysis, displayed in Table 1, indicated that there were five practice demands to be addressed and revealed the corresponding gaps to be filled. Specifically, for a tool to be developed and successful for CM, it had to bridge the identified gaps by providing content that:

1. represented the core essentials of CM practice correctly;
2. portrayed features of both clients and CM accurately;
3. functioned reliably;
4. presented a large incentive (payoff) for use while remaining quick and easy to actually use; and,
5. evaluated the impact of CM interventions objectively.

Components of the Acuity Tools Project are described and displayed here in abbreviated form. Full description and permission to use are available from Craig.

CM ACUITY TOOL© DESIGN

The CM Acuity Tool© is a master conceptual framework in three dimensions that synthesizes key components of CM practice. One of the valuable aspects of the tool is that it categorizes the variables that drive CM complexity into three levels that are from global to discrete. Table 2 displays the CM Acuity Tool© as a map of three core elements that are identified as central to CM practice: (1) indicators, (2) drivers, and (3) subdrivers.

Indicators

The broadest, most inclusive category of the elements in the CM Acuity Tool© is indicators. Derived from the clinical, satisfaction, and business aspects that span all CM activities, the CM Acuity Tool© groups the items

that drive CM complexity, called *drivers* and *subdrivers*, into three broad indicator domains that synthesize the overarching CM aspects. As shown in Table 2, the three indicators take the form of CM Acuity Tool© column headings with the following domains:

1. Clinical/Nursing (CN) indicators—Symptom and situation severity assessment
2. Psychosocial/Caregiver (PS) indicators—Satisfaction with and adherence to plan
3. Quality/Cost (QC) indicators—Resource utility intensity and provider cooperation

Indicator categories were synthesized from two main sources. The first source is the 1997 American Nurses Association Nursing Practice Congress' list of seven categories of non–hospital practice (Mastal, 2000). These categories are symptom severity, level of functioning, therapeutic alliance, service utilization, client satisfaction, risk reduction, and protective factors. The second source is from the Commission for Case Manager Certification (CCMC). This CM certification body has identified essential CM activities and promulgated core CM principles. The CCMC (2006) outlined the essential activities of CM as assessment, planning, implementation, coordination, monitoring, and evaluation. Outcomes tracking is added to these well-known CM activities. The CCMC clustered core components of CM into six global categories:

1. CM concepts,
2. CM principles and strategies,
3. psychosocial and support systems,
4. healthcare management and delivery,
5. healthcare reimbursement, and
6. vocational concepts and strategies.

The core principles are stated in full in the CCMC Code of Professional Conduct for Case Managers (CCMC, 2005).

TABLE 2   The Case Management Acuity Tool©

Clinical/Nursing Indicators	Psychosocial Caregiver Indicators	Quality & Cost Indicators
CN1	**PS1**	**QC1**
1) Physical status [-or Consent pending]	*1) Patient status*	*1) Care delivery*
– Active; able to do all/most age-adjusted acts	– Fully cooperative & adherent to treatment plan	– Plan established/maintained with 1–5 calls & efforts
– Optimal capacity compared to baseline	– No delay in cooperation or in obtaining consent	– Very good cost range; no unnecessary care
2) Symptoms (primary)	*2) Family/Caregiver*	*2) Care environment*
– Absent or well-controlled; none problematic	– Functional, with coping mechanisms intact	– Setting & intensity very effective, appropriate
– No physician review required	– Supportive	– Safe and stable; CM minimal or no supervision needed
3) Symptoms (co-morbidity)	*3) Satisfaction*	*3) Facility/Provider/Customer*
– Absent or well-controlled	– Large degree of satisfaction with care solutions	– Par* [or non-par* with the following]
– No problematic symptoms	– Few dissatisfactions & readily solvable	– Fully cooperative with team management approach
– Uncomplicated death possible		– Prospective & proactive problem solving of needs
CN2	**PS2**	**QC2**
1) Physical status	*1) Patient status*	*1) Care delivery*
– Slight restriction to age-appropriate activities	– Mostly cooperative & adhering to plan well	– 6–10 calls & efforts to establish/maintain care plan
– Slight impairment compared to baseline	– Capable of cooperation & giving/getting consent	– Good cost range; little excessive or unnecessary
2) Symptoms (primary)	*2) Family/Caregiver*	*2) Care environment*
– Some signs & symptoms present	– Stressed capacity to function	– Setting & intensity mostly effective & appropriate
– Minor interventions	– Increasing demands on patient/support system	– Capable of improvement in acceptable times & ways
– Physician review required; care plans concur	– Coping mechanisms, potential for breakdown	– CM of safe setting but changed/changing within 7 days
	– Able to cope with minimal support augmentation	
3) Symptoms (co-morbidity)	*3) Satisfaction*	*3) Facility/Provider/Customer*
– Present but little consequence	– Moderate degree of satisfaction with solutions	– Non-par* [or par with the following]
– Prognosis-appropriate death possible; few interventions required	– Dissatisfactions, acceptable time-work to solve	– Mostly cooperative with team management
		– Good but mostly reactive problem solving
CN3	**PS3**	**QC3**
1) Physical status	*1) Patient status*	*1) Care delivery*
– Limited capability of age-adjusted self care	– Minimally cooperative or little plan adherence	– 11-15 calls & efforts to establish/maintain plan
– Moderate to significant limits versus baseline	– Difficulty in participating; delay getting consent	– Fair costs; high probability of unnecessary care

TABLE 2	The Case Management Acuity Tool© *(continued)*	
Clinical/Nursing Indicators	**Psychosocial Caregiver Indicators**	**Quality & Cost Indicators**
CN3	**PS3**	**QC3**
2) *Symptoms (primary)*	2) *Family/Caregiver*	2) *Care environment [can be 1st 2nd or 3rd one]*
– Impacts ability to perform life activities – Frequent clinical/nursing interventions needed – Physician review required; care plans differ	– Compromised capacity to function – Excessive demands on support system – Respite or change in caregivers may be needed – Coping mechanisms breaking down or worsening	– Setting & intensity fairly effective, appropriate – Much CM intervention required to improve conditions – Intervention within 3 days for safety &/or stability
3) *Symptoms (co-morbidity)* – Present with destabilizing consequence – Complicated death (re-hospitalization) possible	3) *Satisfaction* – Little degree of satisfaction with care solutions – Dissatisfactions, much time-work to improve	3) *Facility/Provider/Customer* – Non-par* [or par with the following] – Poor cooperation with team management approach – Poor problem-solving or accommodation of needs
CN4	**PS4**	**QC4**
1) *Physical status* – Very limited age-adjusted activity level – Unable to accomplish self-care compared to baseline	1) *Patient status* – Frankly uncooperative and nonadherent to plan – Unable to participate or to give/obtain consent	1) *Care delivery* – 16 or more calls & efforts to establish/maintain plan – Excessive costs; frankly unnecessary care
2) *Symptoms (primary)* – Very ill & severe disability; high-risk disorder – 1 hospitalization or intensive clinical/nursing – Physician review required; care plan problems	2) *Family/Caregiver* – Dysfunctional or no caregivers/placement found – Excessive demands on support system – Respite or change in caregivers required – Coping skills, ineffective; severe breakdown	2) *Care environment [can be 1st, 2nd, or 3rd one]* – Current setting & intensity ineffective/inappropriate – Many, immediate interventions -or- on-site required – Complex CM maintained to avoid unsafe/unstable
3) *Symptoms (co-morbidity)* – Present with significant consequence – Unanticipated or very complicated death – Dissatisfactions with few solutions & much time	3) *Satisfaction* – Frank dissatisfaction with care solutions	3) *Facility/Provider/Customer* – Non-par* [or par with the following] – Noncooperation with team management approach – Lacks problem solving or accommodation to needs

Note. The chart used to assign levels of acuity in case management (CM) cases contains three elements: indicators, drivers, and subdrivers. Indicators are arranged in three columns with four boxes per column. Drivers are specific to each indicator column (domain) and repeat within the boxes but remain static. From the top to the bottom of each column, subdriver elements increase in characteristics such as quality, quantity, frequency, duration, degree, severity, and intensity. The driver/subdriver combinations are used to relate client need-severity to CM intervention-intensity and signify the levels of complexity within CM cases in the form of acuity scores. Copyright acknowledgments: Intracorp 1999. Based on originator's (K. D. Craig, MS) and corporate copyright (1999). Address reprint requests to: CIGNA PR Dept; 2 Liberty Plaza, Chestnut Street; Philadelphia, PA 19201.

[a]Par/nonpar - provider, participating/not participating.

Drivers

The CM Acuity Tool© displayed in Table 2 is made up of indicators, drivers, and subdrivers. Under the column headings, called *indicators*, because they indicate the three large areas (domains) of CM activities, there are items known as drivers. *Drivers* (Table 2, italicized items) connect the broad indicator domains to the pinpoint items of CM interventions called subdrivers. The driver/subdriver combinations describe the combined severity of the client's needs and intensity of the case manager's interventions. As the complexity goes up or down, the acuity score rises or falls in a corresponding manner. Therefore, drivers and subdrivers "drive" the degree of CM acuity up or down (Pink & Bolley, 1994).

Drivers organize subdrivers into similar groups and form a bridge between the sets of subdrivers and the three columns of indicators. As the drivers repeat down each indicator column in the four boxes, they remain static and do not change. The three drivers that repeat in the *CN indicator* column are (1) physical status, (2) primary symptoms, and (3) secondary or comorbid symptoms. The column of *PS indicators* contains drivers relating to (1) patient status, (2) family/caregiver, and (3) satisfaction (client/caregiver adherence). The *QC indicator* column contains drivers pertaining to (1) care delivery (provider adherence), (2) care environment, and (3) facility/provider/customer elements.

DRIVERS: CASE EXAMPLE

As an illustration, a CM client comes to a case manager with many needs and several issues that are the most predominant problems to be resolved. For example, three main problems might be:

- uncontrolled pain issues resulting from a terminal illness and its end-of-life changes,
- unstable family and caregiver issues relating to palliative arrangements, and
- family doctor and oncologist disagreements about who is to take responsibility for writing orders and making care setting or placement referrals.

In this case, the case manager can use the CM Acuity Tool© to locate the highest and best match of subdrivers for this client's three main issues that are driving the acuity. To score the pain symptoms or death issues, the case manager would go to the CN indicators column where both comorbid symptoms and death issues can be found, specifically under Driver #3, "Symptoms (comorbidity)." Depending on the severity of the pain or death issues, the case manager would choose the most severe need that is driving the case's complexity, either box CN3 or box CN4. Regarding the caregiver issues, located under the PC indicators column, the case manager will find that Driver #2 "Family/caregiver" provides different degrees of coping success and should choose box PS2, PS3, or PS4, whichever best represents the most accurate and most severe conditions known to exist for this client. Doctor and facility issues reside in the QC indicators column. The case manager would choose the driver and sub-driver that best describes the most complex interventions needed to address the physician and setting difficulties, probably QC2, QC3, or QC4. Although Driver #1 "Care delivery" indicates the number of calls the case manager must make or cost issues, Driver #2 describes "care environment" and Driver #3 shows degrees of issues related to "facility/provider/customer." Customer in the original Acuity Project context relates to the corporate customer with whom the company contracts for service delivery.

Subdrivers

Subdrivers are the elements that most closely describe the specific factors that generate complexity within a CM case. Indeed, subdrivers pinpoint discrete factors of complexity within different CM cases. The complexity factors that subdrivers represent arise from several main spheres, such as CM activities to improve an individual client's clinical situation and the delivery environment of the care the client is receiving. Also, subdriver items characterize the specific model (type) of CM being practiced. For example, the practice model under which the CM Acuity Tool© began is CM delivered telephonically on a national scale under contract stipulations from corporate clients. Other CM delivery systems could be a regional community program with direct in-home client assessments or a military CM model with base-specific and facility-specific components. The QC indicators column would be adapted to capture the interventions specific to the type of delivery system used and the elements (subdrivers) that describe the degrees of severity, intensity, and complexity that exist within that system.

As seen in Table 2, subdrivers, like drivers, recur within the three columns of indicators. However, while drivers repeat and remain static, the

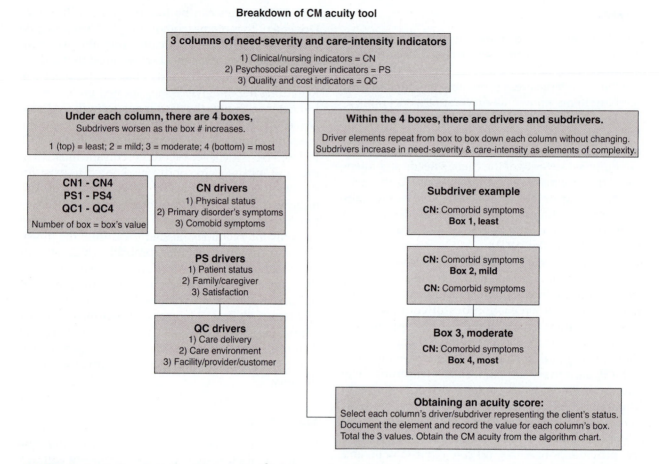

FIGURE 1 Acuity Flowchart. The CM Acuity Tool© has three columns of indicators with four boxes (cells) containing both drivers that remain constant for each column and subdrivers that increase in severity and intensity for each column.

content of the subdrivers changes within the four boxes. From top to bottom of each indicator column, the sub-drivers change in character and drive the level of complexity of a case. Subdriver elements increase in levels of difficulty, quality, quantity, satisfaction, adherence, or severity in the following grades:

1. Low complexity: CN1, PS1, QC1 (first cell, top of each column)
2. Mild complexity: CN2, PS2, QC2 (second cell)
3. Moderate complexity: CN3, PS3, QC3 (third cell)
4. Severe complexity: CN4, PS4, QC4 (fourth cell, bottom of each column).

Subdrivers in CN1, PS1, and QC1 are low in severity with respect to client baseline, in intensity of CM interventions required, and in overall case complexity. CN2, PS2, and QC2 subdrivers are incrementally more severe, intense, and complex, but still mild. CN3, PS3, and QC3 subdrivers are moderate in degree, frequency, quality, or quantity. CN4, PS4, and

QC4 subdrivers are the most pronounced in severity, intensity, and overall complexity. Figure 1 displays a flowchart that illustrates the architecture and inner layout of the CM Acuity Tool©.

ACUITY SCORING

An acuity score is calculated in five easy steps using the instrument displayed in Table 2 and the scoring algorithm presented in Table 3 (Craig, 2006). Under the directions for use of the CM Acuity Tool© presented in the table, the case manager documents three driver/subdriver selections, an interim sum, and the case acuity score.

When case managers apply the CM Acuity Tool© to different clients' cases, many combinations of driver/subdriver choices are possible, depending on the causes of complexity that are present in each client's situation. They vary by amount, time, and duration, that is, by dosage. Therefore, different

---

TABLE 3   Directions for Using the CM Acuity Tool©

Directions for using CM Acuity Tool© indicators, drivers, and subdrivers and how to use the algorithm to determine case acuity:

1. Select box's driver/subdriver combination that best fits from Columns 1, 2, and 3.

2. Add three values (one box value from each indicator column) to derive an acuity sum.

3. Locate the acuity sum in the algorithm chart below. Determine the "case acuity."

4. Record the case acuity value in specified numeric data field.* (*Specific to workflow.)

5. Document driver choices and case acuity in assessment narrative (i.e., A of SOAP).

6. Perform and date case acuity in each case at least twice—at commencing, at closing.

7. Revise, date, and document case acuity when significant change in health status occurs.

Acuity sum Alpha level	Case acuity	
3 or 4	Basic = B	1
5 or 6	Good = G	2
7 or 8	Fair = F	3
9 or 10	Poor = P	4
11 or 12	Worst = W	5

Note. Steps 1 through 3 direct case managers on how to use the CM Acuity Tool© to obtain an acuity sum and convert the sum to a case acuity score. Steps 4 and 5 indicate the mechanism for recording the score for reports to be run and documenting the acuity findings in the case narrative. Steps 6 and 7 discuss when to perform the acuity scoring.

driver/subdriver combinations represent the different elements that reflect complexity, and these combinations generate different interim sums and acuity values. An interim sum, which falls between 3 and 12, is mapped to a true acuity score that has values from 1 to 5, by using a custom-designed algorithm such as the one shown in Table 3.

The varying choices of severities afford case managers the ability to scale and score levels of care intensities at particular times in the course of CM service delivery. Scales based on elements of CM complexity, which have been tested for concordance (Fisher & van Belle, 1993), generate reproducible footprints of practice (evidence) and permit outcomes to be recorded, measured, and compared. The measurements facilitate comparisons of commonalities within and between case managers' cases and caseloads as well as across time, diagnoses, and geographic distances. Such data are useful for internal quality and cost evaluations and for meeting accreditation and regulation requirements.

SUBDRIVERS: CASE EXAMPLE

In the previous example where a CM client with uncontrolled pain issues resulting from a terminal illness, unstable caregiver issues relating to end-of-life arrangements, and physician disagreements about orders and placement referrals has come to a case manager, the CM Acuity Tool© can be used to score a case's acuity. As described earlier, the case manager would locate the different subdriver elements that best describe the most complex issues occurring in this case. The case manager should choose the sub-driver that is the most complex item she or he is dealing with on behalf of the client.

If the case manager were to choose CN4, Driver #3 "Comorbid" symptoms, the subdriver could be either "present with significant consequences" or "very complicated death." If PS3 and Driver #2 were chosen, the subdriver might best be "family/caregiver coping mechanisms breaking down or worsening." In QC4, the driver might be #1 "Care delivery" and "the number of calls the case manager needs to make" or Driver #3 "Facility/provider/customer" because of the subdriver "noncooperation" or "lack of accommodation to (client's) needs." When the decision is made, the case manager records the choices in the case narrative like this: CN4/3 complicated death; PS3/2 coping mechanisms breaking down; QC4/3 physician noncooperation = 4 + 3 + 4 = 11. Therefore, the acuity sum is 11. However, it is important to note that this score is not the case acuity. The case acuity score is found by using the conversion chart (algorithm) given in Table 3. Eleven as an acuity sum converts to a case acuity of 5, the highest case acuity. The completed chart notation would appear like this: CN4/3 complicated death; PS3/2 coping mechanisms breaking down; QC4/3 physician non-cooperation = 4 + 3 + 4 = 11.

ACUITIES: FROM EVIDENCE TO OUTCOMES

Case acuity measurement permits rigorous examination of CM practice and lends itself to systematic research (Davies & Logan, 1999) using evidence-based factors related to CM practice through research techniques such as blinding, cohort, retrospective, prospective, and longitudinal studies (Fisher & van Belle, 1993). The footprints of practice found in dosage and acuity data analysis provide traceable evidence of case severity and CM intensity in the form of complexity identification. Enrichment of CM intervention concepts is achieved as well by applying the dosage framework of CM activity prescription. Assigning complexity distinctions to cases based on core CM content sets up a pivotal source of outcomes tracking—the acuity differential—which is specific to the activities and actions of case managers.

THE BUSINESS CASE FOR CASE MANAGEMENT

CM is a more complex healthcare provider intervention than was originally thought. Multiple disciplines deliver CM services in a wide variety of service settings (Huber, 2000). As a result, the activities of CM practice vary and remain difficult to standardize (Tahan, Huber, & Downey, 2006). Attempts to measure and describe CM include the use of single outcomes variables such as a case count or service cost (e.g., 1 hr of a case manager's time) and mathematical projections such as the business parameter of return on investment (ROI). Inconsistent results across provider settings and focal populations have been reported regarding CM's ability, or inability, to save money. The quandary remains: What is the best way to capture, measure, and calculate the value of CM?

Although business decision makers recognize that CM is important to client satisfaction, some are tempted to say that CM is elusive and that its worth is ephemeral and not reducible to outcomes measurement. However, the educational psychologist Thorndike (1918, p. 16) said: "Whatever exists at all

exists in some amount," and therefore can be measured. Thus, case managers are challenged to "prove our worth," and part of the challenge is to discover how sophisticated the measurements of CM must be (Mastal, 2000). At this time, when it is important to make the business case for sustaining CM practice within healthcare organizations, the complexity of CM has so far impeded its accurate measurement.

CM was reinvented in the 1990s and attained its current position of importance as an advanced practice of healthcare providers using specialized interventions targeted to the coordination of care across the healthcare continuum. It has continued to evolve as a respected and essential professional healthcare service. Some have called CM the hope of the healthcare industry because of its ability to coordinate care and drive efficiency (Georgiou, 2005). In answering the call for clear, decisive, and demonstrative evidence of effectiveness, case managers have begun to produce strategies that verify the beneficial effects case managers have on their clients' healthcare experiences, on the broader healthcare system, and on the economic bottom line.

Differences of purpose exist between the business and practice aspects of healthcare. Business managers say, "show me the money"; healthcare providers focus on "achieve outcomes." Business proof refers to analyzing results with dollars attached, such as averted emergency department visits, reduced bed days, and money saved on treatments (Vann, 2006). From a business perspective, the CM outcomes portfolio includes metrics such as hours billed, savings realized, cost-benefit analysis (CBA) data, and ROI (Cesta & Tahan, 2003). Finance-based CBA connects short-term monetary outlay with longer term good. ROI involves a complicated equation of terms such as overt costs, hidden expenses, invested revenues, and side effect aversions (Goetzel, Ozminkowski, Villagra, & Duffy, 2005). However, in providing needed services and advocating for clients, healthcare providers, especially CMS, focus on outcome factors that are harder to tie to dollars, such as quality and satisfaction (Lurie & Sox, 1999).

Adapted from Aristotle's definition of ethical treatment (Ross, 1925), *case managers' five rights* encompass the practice obligations of accomplishing the *right* intervention in the *right* measure at the *right* time to the *right* person in the *right* setting. Acuity and dosage enhance the CM five rights by defining the right hash marks on the right scales, which then promotes the accurate assignment and assessment of CM interventions.

The evidence-based approach to making a business case for CM presented here takes a fresh look at proving worth by concentrating on dosage and acuity aspects of CM practice. These two concepts are measured at the discrete level, yielding greater specificity than do more global measures of provider interventions. Dosage assists CM providers to more fully describe the multidimensional characteristics of each healthcare intervention (Huber et al., 2001, 2003). After a healthcare intervention is fully described, it is then more easily evaluated from standpoints of both research and business outcomes. Description and specification of the dose of CM activities leads to more accurate measurement, which provides evidence that leads to a CM intervention being assessed for achievement of the results predicted, facilitates CM dosage analysis, and, ultimately, can lead to activity prescriptions designed to produce predictable results. A more precise description of the dosage of an intervention fleshes out the linkage of acuity to interventions.

CONCLUSION

In business language, CM interventions corresponding to prescribed dosages of CM practice result in outcomes that can be predicted and replicated. In practical application, the acuity concept associates severity of clients' illnesses (or situations) to intensity of CM interventions or responses (Craig, 2005). Together, dosage and acuity offer the CM outcomes portfolio useful and effective instruments for case managers to measure the worth of their practice. In Parts II and III of this series, the Acuity Tools Project is presented in greater depth. The two measurement instruments, CM Acuity Tool$^©$ and AccuDiff$^©$, are described and discussed. Their purposes of improving communications regarding the dimensions of CM practice and making the business case for CM practice by valid measurements of specific components of CM are explained. Part III explains how to apply the acuity instruments in CM practice to make comparisons between CM cases that enable quality improvements and outcomes tracking despite the complexity found in CM.

References

Brooten, D., & Naylor, M. D. (1995). Nurses' effect on changing patient outcomes. *Image, 27*(2), 95–99.

Brooten, D., & Youngblut, J. M. (2006). Nurse dose as a concept. *Journal of Nursing Scholarship, 38*(1), 94–99.

Cesta, T., & Tahan, H. (2003). *The case manager's survival guide: Winning strategies for clinical practice* (pp. 254–292). Philadelphia: CV Mosby.

Commission for Case Manager Certification. (2005). *Code of professional conduct for case managers with standards, rules, procedures, and penalties.* Schaumburg, IL: Author. Retrieved October 8, 2006, from http://www.ccmcertification.org/pages/13frame_set.html

Commission for Case Manager Certification. (2006). *CCM certification guide.* Schaumburg, IL: Author. Retrieved November 25, 2006, from http://www.ccmcertification.org/pages/4frame_set.html

Craig, K. (2005). *The Case Management Acuity Tool Kit$^©$.* Paper presented at the proceedings of Case Management Society of America, CMSA 15th National Symposium, Orlando, FL. Retrieved October 9, 2006, from http://www.cmsa.org/Portals/0/PDF/Conference/Attendees/2005%20Audio%20Recordings%20Order%20Form.pdf

Craig, K. (2006). *CM Acuity Tool$^©$ and AccuDiff$^©$ initiative.* (Available from Kathy Craig, MS, RN, CCM, Craig Research Continuum, Kingston, Ontario, Canada K7L 3Z2; 613.542.4554; kdcraigrn@earthlink.net)

Davies, B., & Logan, J. (1999). *Reading research: A user-friendly guide for nurses and other health professionals* (pp. 1–19). Ottawa: Canadian Nurses Association.

Fisher, L., & van Belle, G. (1993). *Biostatistics, a methodology for the health sciences* (pp. 897–901). New York: Wiley.

Georgiou, A. (2005). *Integrated care management: Moving from vision to reality.* Paper presented at the proceedings of Case Management Society of America, CMSA 16th Annual Symposium, Grapevine, TX. Retrieved October 9, 2006, from http://www.cmsa.org/Portals/0/PDF/Conference/2006/PostConference/KS01_PPT.pdf

Huber, D. L. (2000). The diversity of case management models. *Lippincott's Case Management, 5*(6), 248–255.

Huber, D. L. (2006). Staffing and scheduling. In D. L. Huber (Ed.), *Leadership and nursing care management* (3rd ed., pp. 713–732). St. Louis: Elsevier.

Huber, D. L., Hall, J. A., & Vaughn, T. (2001). The dose of case management interventions. *Lippincott's Case Management, 6*(3), 119–126.

Huber, D. L., Sarrazin, M. V., Vaughn, T., & Hall, J. A. (2003). Evaluating the impact of case management dosage. *Nursing Research, 52*(5), 276–288.

Lindsay, B. (2004). Randomized controlled trials of socially complex nursing interventions: Creating bias and unreliability? *Journal of Advanced Nursing, 45* (1), 84–94.

Lurie, J. D., & Sox, H. C. (1999). Principles of medical decision making. *Spine, 24*(5), 493–498.

Mastal, M. (2000). Nursing report cards. *Nursing Spectrum, 9*(3PA), 10.

Pink, G. H., & Bolley, H. B. (1994). Physicians in health care management. Part 3: Case mix groups and resource intensity weights: An overview for physicians. *Canadian Medical Association Journal, 150*(6), 889–894.

Powell, S. (2000). *Advanced CM, outcomes & beyond.* Philadelphia: Lippincott.

Prescott, P. (1991). Nursing intensity: Needed today for more than staffing. *Nursing Economics, 9*(6), 409–414.

Prescott, P. A., & Soeken, K. L. (1996). Measuring nursing intensity in ambulatory care. Part I: Approaches to and uses of patient classification systems. *Nursing Economics, 14*(1), 14–21, 33.

Ridgely, M. S., & Willenbring, M. C. (1992). Application of case management to drug abuse treatment: Overview of models and research issues. *NIDA Research Monograph, 127,* 12–33.

Ross, D. (1925). *The nicomachean ethics of Aristotle* (p. 45). London: Oxford University Press.

Sidani, S., & Braden, C. J. (1998). *Evaluating nursing interventions: A theory-driven approach.* Thousand Oakes, CA: Sage.

Tahan, H. A., Huber, D. L., & Downey, W. T. (2006). Case managers' roles and functions: Commission for Case Manager Certification's 2004 research, Part I. *Lippincott's Case Management, 11*(1), 4–22.

Thorndike, E. L. (1918). The nature, purposes, and general methods of measurement of educational products. In S. A. Courtis (Ed.), *The measurement of educational products: 17th yearbook of the National Society for the Study of Education* (pt. 2, pp. 16–24). Bloomington, IL: Public School Publishing Company.

Vann, J. (2006). Measuring community-based case management performance: Strategies for evaluation. *Lippincott's Case Management,* 11(3), 147–157.

Diane L. Huber, PhD, RN, FAAN, CNAA, BC, is Professor, Colleges of Nursing and Public Health, University of Iowa, Iowa City, teaching and doing research in case management and nursing administration. She is the author/editor of Leadership and Nursing Care Management and Disease Management: A Guide for Case Managers.

Kathy Craig, MS, RN, CCM, CRA, practices case management in 1000 Islands area, Ontario, Canada, and runs Craig Research Continuum for personal health research, biomedical writing, and innovative tool development. She serves as Business and Professional Women Canada vice president (Kingston), Canadian Hearing Society's Community Development Board member, and Cochrane Collaboration reviewer of evidence-based studies. She holds the originator copyrights for *CM Acuity Tool$^{©}$, Caseload Matrix$^{©}$,* and *AccuDiff$^{©}$.*

Appendix

Definitions Used in the Article

Term	Acuity Tool$^{©}$ Definition
Acuity, CM acuity	Measure of complexity in a CM case based on (1) severity (below) of illness or client condition (need-severity) and (2) intensity (below) of the subsequent CM response or intervention (intervention-intensity, below)
Acuity Tool$^{©}$, drivers	Factors that link the high-level indicators (below) to the discrete-level subdrivers that pinpoint the elements of CM activities. In the CM Acuity Tool$^{©}$ (Table 2), three sets of drivers are specific to each of the three columns of indicators and repeat in an unchanging way within the four boxes (cells) within each column.
Acuity Tool$^{©}$, indicators	Items that point to or indicate certain conditions. In the Acuity Tools Project, indicators are broad, high-level categories of influence derived from the clinical, satisfaction, and business aspects that span all CM activities. In the CM Acuity Tool$^{©}$ (Table 2), three broad domains of indicators are Clinical/Nursing indicators, Psychosocial/Caregiver indicators, and Quality (Cost indicators.
Acuity Tool$^{©}$, subdrivers	Elements that pinpoint the specific factors generating complexity in a CM case. In the CM Acuity Tool$^{©}$ (Table 2), subdrivers specific to each of the three columns of indicators (above) and grouped by drivers (above) repeat within the four boxes (cells) but change in degree, extent, amount, frequency, quality, or quantity from the top to the bottom of each column.
Complexity, CM	Characteristic representing the acuity (above) or level of difficulty of a CM case. Complexity involves several CM domains (below) including severity (below) of a client's needs, intensity (below) of CM interventions, dosage (below) of prescribed CM activities, as well as conditions of a healthcare delivery setting or those delivering the care.

Definitions Used in the Article (*continued*)

Term	Acuity Tool© Definition
Domain, CM	Scope, sphere, area, or extent of influence or activity of a unified or related field, topic, category, or subject. In CM Acuity Tool(©, three domains of CM influence are called indicators (below).
Dosage, CM intervention dose	Concept representing actual activities used in a CM intervention prescribed by amount, frequency, duration, and breadth (Huber-Hall Dosage Model). Unique combination of provider (case manager) actions at a specific level of intensity (below) over a discrete duration of time prescribed to achieve a known and predictable response.
Drivers	See acuity, CM, drivers, above.
Exemplar	Example serving as a concept or model worthy of imitation.
Intensity, CM intervention-intensity	Characteristic representing a level, degree, extent, amount, frequency, quality, or quantity of case manager's response to client need-severity (below) or appropriateness of healthcare delivery. Intensity of CM interventions (intervention-intensity) is a pivotal dimension of dosage (above) and the CM Acuity Tool©.
Isostatic differential	See acuity, isostatic acuity, isostatic differential, above.
Need-severity	See severity, CM, need-severity, below
Severity, CM need-severity	Characteristic representing the effects of a CM client's illness, degree of ability to function, or status of conditions that serve to alter the level of complexity of a CM case. Need-severity is one pivotal dimension of the CM Acuity Tool(c).
Subdrivers	See acuity, CM, subdrivers, above.
Tests and analyses definitions	
Beta (β) testing, β-test phase	Stage in the testing of a new process or product before release beyond the small group of initial testers. Phase when a new process or product is tested for real-world exposure by a small number of users, other than its developers. After a β-test, testing may advance to the "pilot-test phase" in which the process or product may be "piloted" or used by a "pilot group" that is larger and more diverse and usually of a longer duration than the β-test phase. In both phases, data are collected, reported, and analyzed and changes to the process or product are recorded and tracked systematically and diligently.
Concordance	Statistical evaluation that measures or ranks the amount of agreement among sets of items compared two at a time.
Cross-validation test	Statistical test that evaluates the ability of a test or model to accurately predict (validate) occurrences between uses within a test population (cross-validate) or from test samples to real-world applications (cross-validate).
Gap analysis	Organized study of the differences (gap) between what is desired and what exists in current or real-world practice.
Interrater reliability (IRR)	Statistical test that measures the amount of agreement between different users (raters) who do not
test, random, blinded	know the answers other raters are or have provided (blinded). If the IRR is high, the test can be
IRR tests	relied on to provide similar results (reliability), even though given to many different users in a disorganized (random) manner.

The dosage research discussed in these articles was supported by Grant #DA08733, National Institute on Drug Abuse (NIDA): Iowa Case Management Project for Rural Drug Abuse, PI = James A. Hall, PhD, LISW, Center for Addictions Research, M304 Oakdale Hall, University of Iowa, Iowa City, IA 52242 (james-a-hall@uiowa.edu). The Acuity Tools Project occurred at Intracorp's Center for Clinical Outcomes and Guidelines (1999–2000). CIGNA/Intracorp holds corporate copyrights and Kathy Craig, MS, RN, holds originator copyrights for Case

Management Acuity Tool©, Caseload Matrix©, and AccuDiff©. Send inquires to CIGNA PR Dept., Two Liberty Plaza, Chestnut Street, Philadelphia, PA 19201. Contact Craig via Craig Research Continuum, 313 Victoria St., Kingston, Ontario, Canada K7L 3Z2 (kdcraigrn@earthlink.net).

Address correspondence to Diane L. Huber, PhD, RN, FAAN, CNAA, BC, College of Nursing, University of Iowa, Iowa City, IA 52242 (diane-huber@uiowa.edu)

Professional Case Management
Vol. 12, No. 4, 199–210

ACUITY AND CASE MANAGEMENT
A Healthy Dose of Outcomes, Part II

Kathy Craig, MS, RN, CCM, and Diane L. Huber, PhD, RN, FAAN, CNAA, BC

ABSTRACT

Purpose: This is the second of a 3-part series presenting 2 effective applications—acuity and dosage—that describe how the business case for case management (CM) can be made. In Part I, dosage and acuity concepts were explained as client need-severity, CM intervention-intensity, and CM activity-dose prescribed by amount, frequency, duration, and breadth of activities. Part I also featured a specific exemplar, the CM Acuity Tool©, and described how to use acuity to identify and score the complexity of a CM case. Appropriate dosage prescription of CM activity was discussed. Part II further explains dosage and presents two acuity instruments, the Acuity Tool and AccuDiff©. Details are provided that show how these applications produce opportunities for better communication about CM cases and for more accurate measurement of the right content that genuinely reflects the essentials of CM practice.

Primary Practice Setting(s): The information contained in the 3-part series applies to all CM practice settings and contains ideas and recommendations useful to CM generalists, specialists, and supervisors, plus business and outcomes managers. The Acuity Tools Project was developed from frontline CM practice in one large, national telephonic CM company.

Methodology and Sample: Dosage: A literature search failed to find research into dosage of a behavioral intervention. The Huber-Hall model was developed and tested in a longitudinal study of CM models in substance abuse treatment and reported in the literature. *Acuity:* A structured literature search and needs assessment launched the development of the suite of acuity tools. A gap analysis identified that an instrument to assign and measure case acuity specific to CM activities was needed. Clinical experts, quality specialists, and business analysts ($n = 7$) monitored the development and testing of the tools, acuity concepts, scores, differentials, and their operating principles and evaluated the validity of the Acuity Tools' content related to CM activities. During the pilot phase of development, interrater reliability testing of draft and final tools for evaluator concordance, beta (β) testing for content accuracy and appropriateness, and representative sample size testing were done. Expert panel reviews occurred at multiple junctures along the development pathway, including the 5 critical points after initial tool draft and both before and after β-test ($n = 5$) and pilot-test ($n = 28$) evaluations. The pilot testing body ($n = 33$) consisted of a team of case managers ($n = 28$) along with quality analysts ($n = 2$), supervisory personnel ($n = 2$), and the lead product analyst (the developer). Product evaluation included monitoring weekly reports of open cases for the 28 case managers for 3 months (June–August 2000).

Results: The Acuity Tools suite was used to calculate individual case acuity, overall caseload acuity profiles, case length, and acuity differentials. Normal distributions and outliers were analyzed and the results used for internal quality improvement and outcomes monitoring.

Implications for Case Management Practice: To show value, case managers need to access the evidence base for practice, use tools to capture quantities of intervention intensity, and specify precisely the activities that produce better outcomes. Acuity and dosage can help case managers explore and fully describe their own practice in ways that can be measured. This data-driven evidence contributes to the accumulating body of definitive proof regarding the exceptional worth of CM. Proving business and professional worth in CM though evidence-based practice is a clarion call that case managers must heed and an innovation that all case managers can practice.

The dosage research discussed in these articles was supported by grant DA08733, National Institute on Drug Abuse (NIDA): Iowa Case Management Project for Rural Drug Abuse, PI 3 James A. Hall, PhD, LISW, Center for Addictions Research, M304 Oakdale Hall, University of Iowa, Iowa City, IA 52242, (phone: 319-3354922, fax: 319-335-4662, e-mail: james-a-hall@uiowa.edu).

The Acuity Tools Project occurred at Intracorp's Center for Clinical Outcomes and Guidelines (1999–2000). CIGNA/Intracorp holds corporate copyrights and Kathy

Craig, MS, RN, holds originator copyrights for Case Management Acuity Tool, Caseload Matrix, and AccuDiff. Send inquires to CIGNA PR Department, Two Liberty Plaza, Chestnut Street, Philadelphia, PA 19201. Contact Craig via Craig Research Continuum, 313 Victoria St., Kingston, Ontario, Canada K7L 3Z2; kdcraigrn@earthlink.net. The authors have no conflict of interest.

Address correspondence to Diane L. Huber, PhD, RN, FAAN, CNAA,BC, College of Nursing, University of Iowa, Iowa City, IA 52242 (mailto:diane-huber@uiowa.edu).

The purpose of this three-part series of articles is to present dosage and acuity as important innovations for establishing a business case for case management (CM) by using the right evidence and right measures. Dosage and acuity empower case managers to demonstrate the impact of their actions in concrete and concise ways. Often the task of demonstrating impact is difficult to do in CM because of its multidimensional complexity and its effects on intermediate outcomes such as client participation in therapy, transitions between healthcare disciplines and settings, and difficult-to-quantify outcomes such as soft savings, quality, and satisfaction. Part I featured the first major component of the Acuity Tools Project, the CM Acuity Tool©, which provides improved connections between the practice of CM and the business of CM by identifying elements specific to the complexity that resides in CM cases.

In Part II, the Acuity Tool and AccuDiff© instruments of the Acuity Tools Project are described in greater depth. Their theoretical potential is detailed regarding the instruments' abilities to capture reliably and measure accurately the right content that genuinely reflects the essence of CM practice. Also discussed is the evidence-based testing undertaken to demonstrate the ability of dosage and the acuity innovations to accomplish the dual goal of professional integrity and business worthiness.

BACKGROUND ON ACUITY AND DOSAGE: FOUR KEY BUILDING BLOCKS

Research in dosage and acuity reveals four key concepts that build the CM platform of practice. The first concept involves clients and the severity of their needs and circumstances. This building block is need-severity. The second building block is CM intervention-intensity, which is the corresponding level of intervention by which a case manager responds to client need-severity. Intervention-intensity is measured at the multiactivity level. The third building block is dosage (Huber, Hall, & Vaughn, 2001; Huber, Sarrazin, Vaughn, & Hall, 2003). Dosage measurement identifies the amount, duration, frequency, and breadth of activities for actual CM interventions and activities that case managers employ to achieve results. Dosage-prescription is measured at the discrete activity level. The fourth building block is complexity, a term that identifies the overall extent of difficulty existing in a CM case.

These four building blocks underpin acuity—the complexity characteristic of CM cases as identified by client need-severity, intervention-intensity, and dosage-prescription. The more involved and complicated the needs, interventions, and dosages are, the more complex the CM case is. The more complex a case is, the higher its acuity is. The Acuity Tool and how to use it to obtain a measure of the complexity of a CM case were presented in Part I (Huber & Craig, 2007).

ACUITY TOOL REPORTS

To gauge the tool's ability to deliver its potential, systematic reports were generated on a regular basis, as part of the Acuity Tools Project, a key ingredient for critical data analysis of an outcomes project. The reports profiled case managers' caseloads as snapshots covering each week of the 3-month pilot phase. One such report is the Acuity Tool Sample Report displayed in Table 1, which represents a descriptive data

TABLE 1   Acuity Tool Sample Report

														Caseload
Employee	**0**		**1**		**2**		**3**		**4**		**5**		**Cases**	**acuity**
Day	2	3%	8	14%	14	24%	24	42%	9	15%	0	0%	57	144
Page	9	18%	4	8%	27	55%	6	12%	3	6%	0	0%	49	88
Cecil	7	14%	8	17%	8	17%	16	34%	2	4%	6	12%	47	110
Dickey	9	15%	2	3%	12	20%	26	44%	7	11%	3	5%	59	147
Petty	4	8%	15	31%	22	45%	6	12%	1	2%	0	0%	48	81
Dobbins	2	3%	3	4%	23	35%	30	46%	6	9%	1	1%	65	168
Camp	3	5%	5	8%	28	50%	18	32%	2	3%	0	0%	56	123
Fenny	1	1%	0	0%	5	7%	37	55%	23	34%	1	1%	67	218
Pope	0	0%	31	52%	13	22%	11	18%	2	3%	2	3%	59	108
Decker	5	9%	9	16%	11	20%	7	12%	5	9%	17	31%	54	157
Napoli	3	11%	4	15%	7	26%	9	34%	3	11%	0	0%	26	57
Dunn	0	0%	6	11%	11	20%	16	29%	9	16%	12	22%	54	172
Circle	2	3%	8	14%	16	29%	16	29%	8	14%	4	7%	54	140
Colby	10	20%	2	4%	9	18%	11	22%	16	32%	1	2%	49	122
Dyson	4	6%	10	16%	7	11%	33	55%	5	8%	0	0%	59	143
Eaton	2	3%	1	1%	6	10%	26	44%	22	37%	1	1%	58	184
DaMond	0	0%	1	2%	5	10%	18	38%	11	23%	12	25%	47	169
Cybil	4	7%	0	0%	11	20%	28	51%	7	12%	3	5%	54	149
Newton	0	0%	4	14%	1	3%	5	17%	9	32%	9	32%	28	102
Fabian	1	1%	6	8%	7	10%	18	26%	27	39%	9	13%	68	227
Night	1	3%	1	3%	8	26%	14	46%	5	16%	1	3%	30	84
Purdy	2	4%	4	9%	15	36%	4	9%	5	12%	11	26%	41	121
Pickell	3	3%	9	10%	69	84%	1	1%	0	0%	0	0%	82	150
Ebony	1	1%	7	10%	15	22%	24	35%	20	29%	0	0%	67	189
DeWit	2	3%	1	1%	9	16%	28	50%	11	20%	4	7%	55	167
Novak	1	3%	1	3%	5	15%	2	6%	16	50%	7	21%	32	116
Currie	0	0%	0	0%	15	31%	23	48%	9	19%	0	0%	47	135
DiBardo	1	1%	14	21%	31	47%	18	27%	1	1%	0	0%	65	134
	79	**5%**	**164**	**11%**	**410**	**28%**	**475**	**32%**	**244**	**17%**	**104**	**7%**	**1698**	

[a]Weekly detailed reports showed case numbers and totals for the 28 case managers distributed by acuity scores 1 through 5 plus "0" acuity score placeholders, their respective percentages, and the caseload acuities (right column).

resource to monitor successes and expose problems. Table 1 shows that there were 1,088 open cases for the 28 case managers at the date of the report. It includes caseload numbers, case numbers distributed by acuity scores 1 through 5, and percentages for each group of acuity scores. Percentages indicate the number of cases in each acuity subgroup in relation to the total cases for each case manger. Also, Table 1 includes a column labeled "0," called "zero acuity." A "zero acuity" value acts as a placeholder for an actual acuity score and has important implications for caseload calculations and workflow issues.

CASELOAD ACUITIES

Caseload acuities, located in the right-most column of Table 1, are derived from the total case numbers and acuities in the cases for each case manager. They are calculated as weighted totals (Fisher & van Belle, 1993) of acuities scores. To determine a weighted caseload acuity, the acuity scores in a case manager's set of cases are added together as one caseload weight. This means that when the case manger scores all the cases in the caseload and adds them together, the resulting total of the individual cases' acuity scores is the caseload acuity. As the caseload acuity weight increases, the complexity for that set of CM cases increases (Figure 1).

Thus, by using the CM Acuity Tool$^©$, the case manager can profile the complexity of the cases in

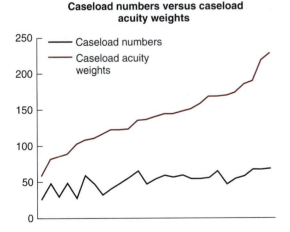

Caseload numbers versus caseload acuity weights

FIGURE 1 Caseload numbers compared to caseload acuity weights. This graph contrasts the numbers of cases versus their caseload acuity weights for the case managers involved in a 1-week period of the pilot test of the Acuity Tool. Although the numbers of cases (dark diamonds) range from about 25 to 70 cases, the caseload acuity weights (light squares) climb to almost 225. As the caseload acuity weight increases, the complexity for that set of CM cases increases.

the caseload and produce a caseload acuity for that set of cases. For example, Table 1 shows that while case manager DiBardo has 65 cases with a caseload acuity "weight" of 134, Fenny has 67 cases that "weigh" 218, about 60% more. Instead of stating a flat number of cases, case managers can use acuity scores to "volumize" the case count by identifying the difficulty of a set of cases. Through the use of acuity, caseloads move from a one-dimensional number, as Figure 1 demonstrates, by gaining the second dimension of weight as a proxy for the level of complexity.

During the Acuity Tools Project, Craig created the Caseload Matrix$^©$, an instrument that compares case numbers to caseload acuities and stratifies caseload into light, average, and heavy (Craig, 2006). (For more information on the Caseload Matrix$^©$ stratification feature, contact Craig.)

ANALYZING CASELOAD ACUITY

Table 1 can be used to study and contrast caseload differences, such as those of case managers Dobbins and Fabian (not their real names). The report indicates that Dobbins' 65 cases have a caseload acuity of 168 and Fabian's 68 cases have a caseload acuity of 227. It would appear that a difference of 3 cases makes a substantial difference (almost 25%) in the caseload acuity weights between the two case managers. Is it possible that a few high-acuity cases could demonstrate such a pronounced effect on caseload?

To analyze the actual differences between the two caseloads, the acuity distribution columns in Table 1 are studied. The distribution for case manager Dobbins' caseload reveals that this case manager scored the 65 cases for levels of complexity in this way: 3 cases with an acuity score of 1; 23 cases with acuity 2; 30 cases with acuity 3; 6 cases with acuity 4; and 1 case with acuity 5. Also, two of employee Dobbins' 65 cases are not yet scored for acuity; therefore, these 2 cases are registered in the acuity placeholder "0" column. When totaled, Dobbins' 65 cases carry a caseload acuity of 168 (median case acuity = 2.6). By contrast, case manager Fabian scored the 68 cases in that caseload with the following acuity distribution: 6 cases have acuity score of 1; 7 cases have acuity 2; 18 cases, acuity = ; 27 cases, acuity 4; 9 cases, acuity 5; and, 1 case has yet to be scored so it carries a "0" placeholder. Therefore, Fabian has 68 cases with a total caseload acuity of 227 (median case acuity = 3.3). While Dobbins is managing 7 complex cases, Fabian is managing 36 complex ones.

Acuity score information of this quality holds implications not only for structuring work processes but also for recognizing work distinctions. Acuity, with the added dimension of caseload weights, arms the case manager to prioritize and plan better and aids improved identification of CM activities and workloads. Through case acuities and caseload acuities, case managers can communicate more precisely about CM with their supervisors, and then the supervisors can communicate more comprehensively with quality and business managers.

"ZERO ACUITY" VALUES

A *zero acuity* in a systematic report is a placeholder for an actual acuity score. The placeholder indicates that a case manager was unable to assign the acuity score in the case before the report was run. Case managers who had less than 5% of their cases unrated for actual acuity scores are considered to have *low* percentages of "zero acuity" placeholders and those who had 5% or more of their cases unscored for acuities have *high* percentages.

It is important to realize that whether the caseload is large or small, having 5% or more of the cases in a caseload without acuity scores has the potential to affect the caseload acuity to a large extent. As the cases with "zero acuity" placeholders receive their actual acuity scores, the caseload acuity may increase substantially. Therefore, the need to score acuities quickly becomes an important work process step specific to CM.

ANALYZING "ZERO ACUITY" VALUES

In the data descriptions of the 28 case managers' caseloads in Table 1, the first column contains case manager employee names (not their real names). The two adjacent columns are the "zero acuity" case numbers and percentages, which ranged from 0% to 20% in this 1-week interval. One discovery made by analyzing a systematic report like Table 1 was that it is important to avoid "zero acuity" placeholders. Seeing reports with large numbers and percentages of cases with "zero acuity" placeholders often meant that case managers were too busy to assign acuities even though it was a high-priority task. Seeing large percentages of "zero acuity" placeholders week after week usually signaled work bottlenecks or backlogs.

Expert consensus established that, to ensure accurate calculations of caseload weights, the threshold was 95% of open cases per case manager that must have actual acuity scores assigned. The 95% threshold required that no more than 5% of open cases should lack actual acuity scores. If case managers had more than 5% of cases with "zero acuity" placeholder values, then the caseload acuities were skewed and the weighted caseload acuity calculations were incorrect. In addition to the measurement feature, the weekly detailed reports gave supervisors near real-time feedback about work slow-downs. This evidence-based, data-driven knowledge stimulated the discovery of timely and efficient work process solutions. The process insights facilitated practice improvements that were incorporated in the orientation of new users and influenced the direction of changes in the reporting of business outcomes.

For some case managers, the numbers of cases represented by the percentages are small even though the percentages themselves are high compared to the 5% threshold. For example, in Table 1, case manager Camp has 5% of the 56 cases with "zero acuity," which means that only 3 cases lack acuity scores. However, the caseload acuity has the potential to change from its current 123 to 126 if all 3 cases have acuity scores of 1, to 138 if all 3 cases are 5 acuities, or to a value between 126 and 138. Also, in Table 1, case manager Dickey, who has 59 cases with a caseload acuity of 147, exemplifies the important effect of a high "zero acuity" percentage. The accuracy of this level of caseload acuity is in doubt because 15% or 9 of Dickey's 59 cases do not have actual acuity scores. When these 9 cases are scored, the acuity distribution and caseload total may look very different from 147, depending on how many of the 9 cases have high-acuity scores and how many have low-acuity scores. It can be seen that the numbers of cases with "zero acuity" placeholders instead of actual acuity scores distort the real caseload acuity figures and totals for these case managers.

The Acuity Tool allows case managers to score the levels of complexity in the many different forms it takes in individual CM cases. Case acuities lead to calculations of caseload acuities, which add weight to the case numbers that individual case managers carry. Also, the use of acuity scores in CM cases leads to an outcomes measurement concerning the changes in acuity scores.

THE ACUITY DIFFERENTIAL: ACCUDIFF©

The fundamental instrument of the Acuity Tools suite is the CM Acuity Tool©. The second is called AccuDiff©, which is based on how acuity scores change. A major part of the business case for CM is the linkage of real-time CM interventions to finance-related outcomes. Little evidence has been available to guide practice and business managers about how to accomplish this linkage. As the primary outcomes instrument in the Acuity Tools Project, AccuDiff© presents differences in acuity scores as the means to join the actual practice of CM with the business of CM. An *acuity differential* is defined as the change or difference between two acuity scores in a CM case, usually the acuity score at the beginning of a case and the ending of a case (Craig, 2005).

This definition corresponds to the findings regarding studies of prescribed dosages of CM activity (Box 1; Huber et al., 2003). Huber and colleagues used the Huber-Hall model of dosage and found that the amount, frequency, duration, and types of interventional activities were higher at the beginning of CM cases and decreased or lessened as cases neared their case-life endings, although there were fluctuations within the case-life patterns. Furthermore, Huber et al. demonstrated that dosage can be modeled in three dimensions (Figure 2). The advantage of dosage is its ability to incorporate actual CM-provider activities that occur. Dosage analyses can lead to prescriptions of specific CM activities and interventions assigned to be made at identifiable times that are associated with predictable and desired outcomes.

In parallel ways, acuity differential and CM dosage prescriptions lead to outcomes that can be

BOX 1

Term	Definition
Acuity	Severity of illness or client condition that indicates the need for the intensity of the subsequent CM intervention
Acuity differential	The difference between two acuity scores in a CM case, usually the acuity score at the beginning of a case and at the ending of a case
Caseload acuity or caseload weight	Caseload acuities are weighted totals of the case acuities per case manager at any one time. Caseload acuity is found by multiplying the number of cases with an acuity level by that acuity level to obtain weighted subtotals and adding the subtotals together. Having a high numbers of cases lacking acuity scores can distort caseload weights.
Caseload complexity	The level of difficulty of cases in an individual case manager's portfolio of cases.
	Caseload complexity is found by stratifying the numbers of cases in a caseload by the acuity ranges per individual case manager. The Acuity Tools Project included such a stratification instrument called the Caseload Matrix (not presented in this article).
Drivers	Drivers are groups of CM practice intermediate factors that link the global-level indicators to the discrete-level subdrivers.
Indicators	The broadest, most inclusive category of the elements in the Acuity Tool. Indicators are derived from the clinical, satisfaction, and business aspects that span all CM activities.
Intensity	A term related to acuity that represents both the amount of care and the complexity of care needed by patients or clients. Prescott (1991) identified four major dimensions to intensity: severity of illness, client dependency, complexity, and time. Acuity includes the concept of CM intervention intensity that should match the need severity of the client.
Intervention dosage	The amount, frequency, duration, and breadth of actual activities used in an intervention, as a unique combination of discrete provider actions, at a level of intensity (amount and frequency), over a duration of time.
Isostatic differentials or Flat-line differentials	Refers to case acuity scores that were unchanged from commencement to closure. In this stagnant effect, unchanging acuities occurred in cases that had reached recovery plateau stages or in one-visit-only cases. In full, comprehensive CM cases, isostatic differentials occurred less often than the usual pattern (higher at opening than at closing) of acuity differentials.
Reverse acuity	The reverse pattern of acuities that scored higher at closure than at opening.
Subdrivers	The elements that most closely delineate the specific factors that generate complexity within a CM case. Subdrivers relate to times for tasks, numbers and complexity of interventions, levels of self-care and caregiver support systems, and appropriate setting and provider components that differ for individual clients at various times.

linked directly to the changes that case managers make in their clients' cases. Like the findings in dosage research, measuring acuity differentials through the AccuDiff© concept incorporates the principle that acuity is higher at case initiation than at case closure because complexity, severity, and intensity are usually higher at the commencement of a CM case. Also, in most cases, the case manager initially applies a higher concentration of activity to address the client's unmet needs. Therefore, the standard AccuDiff© formula subtracts the lower acuity (ending) from the higher one (beginning). Acuity differentials range in true value from 0 to 4. Zero emerges as a true acuity differential value because $5 - 5 = 0, 4 - 4 = 0, 3 - 3 = 0, 2 - 2 = 0$, and $1 = 1 - 0$, and represents cases in which the client does not improve from baseline. Table 2 presents a sample AccuDiff© report.

TABLE 2 AccuDiff© Sample Report (May 2000)[a]

| | Acuity differentials | | | | | | |
Dx group	0	1	2	3	4	Totals/diagnosis groups	Dx groups
A	53	8	11	4	2	78	A
B	8	7	3	1	0	19	B
C	18	6	2	2	1	29	C
D	2	0	1	0	0	3	D
E	0	0	0	0	0	0	E
F	2	2	1	0	0	5	F
G	11	1	1	0	0	13	G
H	4	3	4	0	0	11	H
I	1	0	2	0	0	3	I
J	2	1	0	0	0	3	J
K	0	0	0	0	0	0	K
L	11	3	0	0	0	14	L
Z	101	38	20	10	5	174	Z
May 2000 Totals	213	69	45	17	8	352	May 2000 Totals

| | Diagnosis[b] |
Groups	Descriptions
A	Oncology
B	HR infant
C	HR pregnancy
D	AIDS
E	Spinal cord injuries
F	Brain injuries traumatic
G	Trauma
H	CVA/strokes
I	Rehabilitation
J	COE-transplants
K	Psych
L	Transplants
Z	Other

[a]Monthly reports of acuity differentials presented aggregated groups of diagnosis codes tailored to the corporate specifications. Acuity differential values ranged from 0 through 4 found by subtracting the acuity scores at case closures from those at case beginnings. Higher differentials indicate that case managers made more impact in their cases to decrease case complexity from commencement to closing.
[b]The company's diagnosis groupings did not correspond strictly to the standard diagnosis-related groups (DRGs) and were found to be problematic.

For each CM case, the acuity differential measures two important elements: (1) the change in acuity indicator status based on elements stemming from the Acuity Tool, especially the driver/subdriver combinations (Huber & Craig, 2007) that identify client need-severity and CM intervention-intensity; and (2) a quantity of improvement created through the targeted, timed, and precisely triggered dosages of CM actions (Huber et al., 2003). *Larger* acuity differentials mean *greater* CM impact. The larger an acuity differential is in a case, the greater the CM impact is and the more successful the case manager's actions have been in reducing the severity of symptoms, intensity of interventions, and overall complexity through dosage prescriptions of CM activities. Therefore, by using the improvement (change) in complexity that is tethered to the essential elements of CM practice as an outcome, AccuDiff© measurements demonstrate both the clinical value and the business worth of CM in a valid and authentic manner and provide the potential for better human resources deployment and cost stabilization. For example, using

ANALYZING ACUITY DIFFERENTIALS

The analysis of acuity differentials provides an opportunity to demonstrate CM worth to business decision makers at two levels: by individual cases and by aggregated groups. Acuity differentials calculated for individual cases allow for the examination of single-case circumstances that drive acuity up or down. They also help determine the CM intervention dosages that will produce optimal efficiency and impact. After collecting and sorting differences in acuities in closed cases, aggregated acuity differentials can be grouped for outcomes analysis many ways, including into these four related categories:

1. *Corporate:* Corporate accounts; hospitals or hospital consortia; regions
2. *Diagnosis:* Standard or tailored diagnosis related groups (DRGs); related diagnosis codes (RDCs)
3. *Case managers per diagnosis:* Subspecialties (e.g., pediatrics, oncology); centers of excellence
4. *Investments:* Time per RDCs; resources per RDCs; return on investment (ROI) per RDCs

To demonstrate the evidence-based value of CM acuity differentials, data from one national telephonic CM company were analyzed using the AccuDiff© system (Table 2). Table 2 shows one AccuDiff© Monthly Summary Report of CM acuity differentials sorted by groups of selected RDCs that were chosen by the corporation where the study took place. In fact, this report revealed that business managers had based the groupings of diagnosis codes on old assumptions that proved to be problematic and ineffective.

The central concept of acuity differentials as an outcomes measure is reflected in the primary chart in Table 2. The AccuDiff© outcomes report lists three pivotal items: the total number of cases that were closed in the identified month, numbers of cases closed per each of the five acuity differential values, and subtotals for the RDC groupings. Across the header row of the AccuDiff© report in Table 2, the five acuity differential scores—0, 1, 2, 3, and 4—are listed. Cases with acuity scores that started and ended with the same acuity score (called flat-line or isostatic acuities) had 0 or no differences in acuity scores. These cases had virtually no reductions in complexity or no changes in acuity that could be shown through the acuity differential measurement. Some acuity levels changed by 1 or 2 measures of difference. The more pronounced changes in acuity levels, by 3 or 4 measures, occurred in cases in which the most dramatic improvements for clients occurred. Changes by three acuity measures occurred in two ways: in cases that started at acuity 5 and ended with acuities of 2 or in cases that began with 4 and fell to 1.

Complexity levels that changed by four acuity measures, the most change possible, represent cases that initially were scored with an acuity of 5 and then fell to an acuity of 1 at the time of closure. This emphasizes the claim that the larger the acuity differential is, the greater the CM impact has been to alleviate the client's severity of needs, and thus to reduce the intensity of interventions and dosages of prescribed activities.

ACCUDIFF© RESULTS

The information in the AccuDiff© Sample Report (Table 2) can be used to tell a business story of CM. Data in the report were collected and the reports were generated through the following manner. As a case manager closed a case during the 3-month pilot phase, the differences in the acuity scores from start to closure were obtained, recorded as acuity differential measurements, and stored electronically for outcomes reports. The acuity differential measurements were assigned to groups or categories of RDCs in reports according to the primary diagnosis codes identified in the cases.

In Table 2, the main body of the report lists acuity differentials, subtotals, and totals of closed cases. In the second part (Diagnosis) of Table 2, the company's RDC groupings are seen as categories A–L and Z and carry these description labels: oncology, high-risk infant, high-risk pregnancy, AIDS, spinal cord injuries, brain injuries (traumatic), trauma, CVA/strokes, rehabilitation, transplants/Centers of Excellence (COE), psych, transplants, and other. The company's business managers selected the 13 categories of RDC groupings before the AccuDiff© report was available, and these selections were based on assumptions established before the use of AccuDiff© system.

It can be seen in Table 2 that most acuity differentials were assigned to the other or "Z" category of RDC groupings and that for this interval many acuity differentials were 0. Examinations were undertaken for these two phenomena as well as the reasons for having no cases appearing in the E and K categories, specifically spinal cord injuries and psych, respectively. Also, the AccuDiff© report gave form and direction to both practice and business explorations aimed at determining the answers to important questions, such as "Why were there few case numbers in the higher acuity differentials?" Findings from these explorations would seek to drive more outcomes in genuine and authentic ways toward three and four acuity differentials.

Acuity differential measurements, or changes in acuity levels from commencement to closure, become powerful tools to reveal the impact case managers have in improving client circumstances and to leverage the business worth of CM into value-related dollars. From these outcomes, more correctly associated with the right indicators of CM activities, the business case for CM can be explored to link "soft" changes to hard currency.

Use of the AccuDiff© system uncovered information useful for clinical quality improvement and process improvement *internal* to the organization. In addition, acuity differential measurements held strong potential for outcomes predictions that were promoted *external* to the company, such as CM as a product in contracts and marketing initiatives. An important finding was that acuity differentials had a more direct relationship with actual CM activities than did the outcome measures, such as ROI, hours billed, case life, and savings that had been used be-

fore development of the AccuDiff© measurement. Furthermore, joining dosage and acuity to these common finance-driven outcomes presents an excellent opportunity for future evidence-based analyses and truth-in-advertising.

PRACTICE REFINEMENTS USING ACCUDIFF©

For acuity differentials to have optimal value as outcome indicators, better RDC groupings were needed that aligned business outcomes more closely with CM practice. This finding concerned this originating company's choice of RDCs. The use of acuity differentials revealed that the RDC groupings selected for reports should involve choices based on grounded analysis rather than on assumptions. The acuity reporting system also showed that choices should be tested for outcomes accuracy to ensure that poorly related diseases remained separated into discrete groups and that highly or well-related conditions are aggregated into like groups.

Because the decisions about sorting cases into RDC groupings made by the company's business managers before AccuDiff© used incorrect strategies and faulty reasoning, poor quality information about CM outcomes often was generated. Previous information caused erroneous assumptions to be made in business contracts when decisions stemmed from vague and ill-conceived beliefs about CM activities. It is postulated that borrowing a physician practice–driven financial model (e.g., DRG-related funding model) and assuming that it worked for CM without validating the assumptions contributed to the use of faulty outcomes strategies.

On the basis of the outcomes insights revealed by the AccuDiff© reporting system, the developer was able to advise the business managers on how to improve the RDC groupings and reporting methods they selected. The AccuDiff© outcomes measurement strategy presented an opportunity to refine the business case for

CM by providing improved analyses of CM work that was better matched to actual front-line practice. Acuity data from CM practice was of an advanced quality that enabled better business decisions. Acuity applications guided practice improvements by generating reliable data more connected to case managers' actions.

For this company, improved RDC grouping of cases was accomplished by mapping a case's primary diagnosis to one and only one group at a time, which helped eliminate ambiguity and overlap between RDC groups specific to the company. Recombining or reassigning cases by various RDC groups was scheduled to see the effects on improvements in business outcomes. Although this pursuit was not the primary thrust of the Acuity Tools Project, the pilot test of the AccuDiff© system allowed the correct data to be used to guide the appropriate regrouping of RDC taxonomies through planned experimental testing and systematic report analysis.

Informal observations revealed that sometimes common components of CM cases resided within the standard DRG classes and that sometimes CM commonalities were seen to cross between DRG classes. Identifying both commonly conjoined components and usually divergent components of CM in practice applications is an important step necessary to construct dosage configurations of the elements of CM activities.

Can allocations from specifically tailored RDC groupings accurately and appropriately capture CM practice? This question must be addressed in future investigations. For example, important findings in future studies could be the discovery of the best linkages between common CM practices, efficient CM interventions, hours billed, and high ROI. It is believed that the identification of the common CM elements will provide the foundation for evidence-based intervention protocols relating acuity and dosage to specific diagnoses or groups of diagnoses (RDCs) with the strong probability of precise linkages of intervention protocols to business outcomes.

IMPORTANT INSIGHTS FROM ACCUDIFF© ANALYSES

Studies of AccuDiff© outcomes made visible previously hidden information that needed to be explored. Analysis revealed that in the majority of cases of full and comprehensive CM, acuity *was* higher at case commencement than at case closure. Therefore, in most full-fledged CM cases, an acuity differential showed the decrease in complexity from the start to the end of the CM case. However, there were two striking exceptions to the usual difference in acuity scores, which came to be known as *reverse differentials* and *isostatic differentials*. These two exceptions provided valuable evidence for practice and for more precise tailoring of CM interventions using the dosage–demand principle. The discovery of reverse

and isostatic patterns in acuity differentials was a significant serendipitous finding.

REVERSE DIFFERENTIALS

Reverse acuity differentials occurred under two scenarios: (1) when case acuities were higher at closure than at the beginning of the cases and (2) when cases rose in complexity but were closed for contract or non-CM reasons. *Reverse differentials* were seen most often in cases that involved chronic debilitating diseases, for example, amyotrophic lateral sclerosis. The reverse pattern of acuities (scoring higher at closure than at opening) signaled that case complexity rose despite the case manager's actions to relieve clients' high or severe needs through matched doses of intense or frequent interventions. Cases in which complexity worsened over time represented a small percentage of the possible CM case scenarios. Could discovering the causes and occurrences of reverse acuity differentials help practice analysts and business managers anticipate the cases in which they might occur in the future?

Clearly identifying in which cases reverse acuity differentials might occur or cluster was seen as valuable information to have for protocol determinations. One application postulated was that case managers and other population health managers could use reverse acuity information in areas such as disease management paradigms to customize CM intervention dosages more effectively and proactively to benefit individuals in these populations. Disciplined investigations to identify and categorize situations paradoxical to standard acuity differentials would aid CM researchers and business managers to understand the number and dynamics of the acuity pattern reversals. Perhaps specific subsets of case populations did not respond to standard CM interventions because the subsets contained characteristics that were too uniquely specific to have their needs met by the usual CM intervention dosages.

For example, the cases may have contained dimensions that required specialized dosages pertaining to malignant or terminal pathologies. If these hypothesized conditions were confirmed and the subsets of cases that have high likelihoods of displaying reverse acuity patterns were known, then outcomes investigators could exclude the unique subpopulations from generalized acuity and dosage trials, and frontline case managers could custom-design their practice intervention protocols stemming from evidence-based knowledge to increase effectiveness. Studies of the subpopulations of cases shown to exhibit reverse acuity differentials would need to occur as distinct groups that are analyzed together but separated from the usual or typical CM cases. On the business side, business decision-makers might ask, "Could distinct costing strategies be devised for CM cases from these unique sub-populations?"

ISOSTATIC DIFFERENTIALS

Isostatic acuity differentials were associated with case acuity scores that did not change from commencement to closure. *Isostatic differentials* showed a characteristic stagnant effect in which acuities remained unchanged from start to end and occurred in cases in which clients had reached recovery plateau stages. Clinical plateaus meant that clients had achieved their fullest capacity to improve from the CM perspective of continuing management; however, CM cases remained open because the clients remained debilitated with ongoing care needs. The potential to reduce complexity (specifically, client need severity, intervention intensity, dosage prescription, and high service utilization) was absent or unlikely. It was found that cases were kept active (nonclosing) despite acuity stagnation for two main reasons: continued need for CM or for contract reasons. In these cases, acuity scores stagnated or became isostatic (flat-lined) and CM interventions continued but were unable to create changes in acuity levels.

An example of cases with isostatic differentials was clients with severe and persistent cerebral vascular accidents (strokes). Another example of a flat-line acuity differential arose in cases involving clients who retained permanent impairment to body systems and who also had technical or mechanical requirements that were not able to be taught to the clients or their caregivers, such as ventilator dependence. A third source of flat-line acuity differentials was observed in cases found to be inappropriate for true and full CM. Examples were one-visit-only cases that were required to be opened for CM by corporate contracts. An example is well-baby visits. One-visit-only cases were numerous and had a large effect on outcomes. Their effects can be seen in the column of zero acuity differentials in Table 2. Exploring and removing these inappropriate cases from outcomes studies would improve the business case of CM by including the right cases in the outcomes reporting process. Simultaneously, removing the cases that

are inappropriate for traditional CM would free case managers to concentrate their activities on cases, and therefore clients, more likely to benefit from comprehensive CM interventions.

RECOMMENDATIONS

What have reverse and isostatic acuity differential outcomes revealed? Reverse and isostatic acuity differentials indicated that further analyses are required to identify and manage the cases, courses, and outcomes of situations that created these paradoxical outcomes. Analyses could aim to identify the characteristics or hallmarks of cases that are likely to display reverse or isostatic (flat-line) acuity patterns. Once identified, more effective and efficient CM interventions, such as prevention-only monitoring or disease-state CM with subtle improvements as the only expected outcomes, should be investigated to determine which different interventions work successfully or whether comprehensive CM is appropriate at all. The changes in effects made by altering acuity through CM interventions, CM workload, and organizational financial performance need to be analyzed. The goals of research investigations would be to refine the acuity differential criteria using the dosage framework (of specific CM amount, frequency, duration, and breadth of activities) and to apply a merged acuity-dosage practice format to the management of these unique subpopulations.

One strategy for future refinement to diminish the deleterious dampening effects of isostatic and reverse differentials on the value of acuity differentials as outcomes tools is the removal of certain kinds of cases from the analysis pool of traditional, comprehensive CM cases. Appropriately removing these dampeners would act to improve the integrity of the data. As outliers, or nonhomogenous cases, full CM effects could not be realized in these cases.

A further recommendation is to identify case subpopulations that were numerous enough to warrant specific handling. Redesigned dosage specifications and custom-designed acuity tools would use drivers and subdrivers tested specifically to capture the CM components that drive complexity and acuity in subpopulations, for example, in mental health diagnoses. The business and practice appropriateness of removing these subsets of cases from standard CM outcomes studies would need to be examined.

CONCLUSION

Acuity and dosage can help case managers explore and fully describe their own practice in ways that can be measured. The cornerstone concepts of client need-severity, CM intervention-intensity, dosage activity-prescription, and complexity that underpin acuity aid case managers in this endeavor. Measurements of dosage, acuity, and changes in acuity, which are based in authentic CM practice, provide data and evidence that contribute to the accumulating body of definitive proof regarding the exceptional worth of CM. Proving business and professional worth in CM though EBP is a clarion call that case managers must heed and an innovation that all case managers can practice.

References

Craig, K. (2005). The case management Acuity Tool Kit[©]. Paper presented at the proceedings of Case Management Society of America, CMSA 15th National Symposium, Orlando, FL. Retrieved October 9, 2006, from http://www.cmsa.org/Portals/0/PDF/Conference/Attendees/2005%20Audio%20Recordings%20Order%20Form.pdf.

Craig, K. (2006). *CM Acuity Tool[©] and AccuDiff[©] initiative.* Available from Kathy Craig, MS, RN, CCM, Craig Research Continuum, Kingston, Ontario, Canada K7L 3Z2; 613.542.4554; kdcraigrn@ earthlink.net.

Fisher, L., & van Belle, G. (1993). *Biostatistics, A methodology for the health sciences* (pp. 897–901). New York: Wiley & Sons.

Huber, D. L., & Craig, K. (2007). Acuity and case management: A healthy dose of outcomes, part I. *Professional Case Management, 12*(3), 132–144.

Huber, D. L., Sarrazin, M. V., Vaughn, T., & Hall, J. A. (2003). Evaluating the impact of case management dosage. *Nursing Research, 52*(5), 276–288.

Diane L. Huber, PhD, RN, FAAN, CNAA,BC is Professor, Colleges of Nursing and Public Health, University of Iowa, Iowa City, Iowa, teaching and doing research in case management and nursing administration. She is the author/editor of Leadership and Nursing Care Management and Disease Management: A Guide for Case Managers. She holds copyright to dosage concept and visuals.

Kathy Craig, MS, RN, CCM, CRA, practices case management in 1,000 Islands area, Ontario, Canada, and runs Craig Research Continuum for personal health research, biomedical writing, and innovative tool development. She serves as Business and Professional Women vice president (Kingston), Canadian Hearing Society's Community Development Board member, and Cochrane Collaboration reviewer of evidence-based studies. She holds originator copyrights for *CM Acuity Tool[©]*, *Caseload Matrix[©]*, and *AccuDiff[©]*.

Professional Case Management
Vol. 12, No. 5, 254–269

ACUITY AND CASE MANAGEMENT
A Healthy Dose of Outcomes, Part III

Diane L. Huber, PhD, RN, FAAN, CNAA, BC,
and Kathy Craig, MS, RN, CCM

ABSTRACT

Purpose of Study: This is the third of a 3-part series presenting 2 effective applications—acuity and dosage—that describe how the business case for case management (CM) can be made. In Part I, dosage and acuity concepts were explained as client need-severity, CM intervention-intensity, and CM activity-dose prescribed by amount, frequency, duration, and breadth of activities. Concepts were presented that related the practice of CM to the use of evidence-based practice (EBP), knowledge, and methods and the development of instruments that measure and score pivotal CM actions. Part I also featured a specific exemplar, the CM Acuity Tool©, and described how to use acuity to identify and score the complexity of a CM case. Part II further explained dosage and 2 acuity instruments, the Acuity Tool and AccuDiff©. Part III presents linkage to EBP and practical applications.

Primary Practice Setting(s): The information contained in the 3-part series applies to all CM practice settings and contains ideas and recommendations useful to CM generalists, specialists, supervisors, and business and outcomes managers. The Acuity Tools Project was developed from frontline CM practice in one large, national telephonic CM company.

Methodology and Sample:
Dosage: A literature search failed to find research into dosage of a behavioral intervention. The Huber-Hall model was developed and tested in a longitudinal study of CM models in substance abuse treatment and reported in the literature.

Acuity: A structured literature search and needs assessment launched the development of the suite of acuity tools. A gap analysis identified that an instrument to assign and measure case acuity specific to CM activities was needed. Clinical experts, quality specialists, and business analysts ($n = 7$) monitored the development and testing of the tools, acuity concepts, scores, differentials, and their operating principles and evaluated the validity of the acuity tools' content related to CM activities. During the pilot phase of development, interrater reliability testing of draft and final tools for evaluator concordance, β testing for content accuracy and appropriateness, and representative sample size testing were done. Expert panel reviews occurred at multiple junctures along the development pathway, including the 5 critical points after initial tool draft and both before and after β-test ($n = 5$) and pilot-test ($n = 28$) evaluations. The pilot testing body ($n = 33$) consisted of a team of case managers ($n = 28$) along with quality analysts ($n = 2$), supervisory personnel ($n = 2$), and the lead product analyst (the developer). Product evaluation included monitoring weekly reports of open cases for the 28 case managers for 3 months (June–August 2000).

Results: The Acuity Tools Suite was used to calculate individual case acuity, overall caseload acuity profiles, case length, and acuity differentials. Normal distributions and outliers were analyzed and the results were used for internal quality improvement and outcomes monitoring.

Implications for CM Practice: To show value, case managers need to access the evidence base for practice, use tools to capture quantities of intervention intensity, and precisely specify the activities that produce better outcomes.

Acuity and dosage can help case managers explore and fully describe their own practice in ways that can be measured, and thus provide data and evidence that contributes to the accumulating body of definitive proof regarding the exceptional worth of CM. Proving business and professional worth in CM through EBP is a clarion call that case managers must heed and an innovation that all case managers can practice.

Key words: *acuity, caseload, caseload acuity, complexity, differentials, dosage, evidence-based practice, intervention-intensity, need-severity, outcomes*

The dosage research discussed in this article was supported by grant DA08733, National Institute on Drug Abuse: Iowa Case Management Project for Rural Drug Abuse, PI = James A. Hall, PhD, LISW, Center for Addictions Research, M304 Oakdale Hall, University of Iowa, Iowa City, IA 52242 (phone: 319–335-4922; fax: 319–335-4662; e-mail: james-a-hall@uiowa.edu).

The Acuity Tools Project occurred at Intracorp's Center for Clinical Outcomes and Guidelines (1999–2000). CIGNA/Intracorp holds corporate copyrights and Kathy Craig, MS, RN, holds originator copyrights for Case Management Acuity Tool©, Caseload Matrix©, and AccuDiff©. Send inquires to CIGNA PR Department, Two Liberty Plaza, Chestnut Street, Philadelphia, PA 19201. Contact Ms Craig via Craig Research Continuum, 313 Victoria St, Kingston, Ontario, Canada K7L 3Z2 (kdcraigrn@earthlink.net). The authors have no conflict of interest.

Address correspondence to Diane L. Huber, PhD, RN, FAAN, CNAA, BC, College of Nursing, University of Iowa, Iowa City, IA 52242 (diane-huber@uiowa.edu).

The purpose of this three-part series of articles is to present dosage and acuity as important for establishing a business case for case management (CM) by using the right measures to make the case. Not all CM cases are created equal. However, all CM cases need to be documented and evaluated for quality and cost improvements. Previously, the methods and measurements needed to do this have not been well developed. To meet this challenge, Craig developed the CM Acuity Tool© to quantify and display a profile of real-time CM activities (Craig, 2005).

In Part I of this series, the first major component of the Acuity Tools Project, the CM Acuity Tool© was presented with directions about how to calculate an acuity score in a CM case (Huber & Craig, 2007). This tool offers case managers, supervisors, quality specialists, and business managers alike an improved means to communicate with each other about the differences between and among CM cases. In Part II, the Acuity Tools Project was described in greater depth (Craig & Huber, 2007). It detailed the potential for accurate measurement of the right content that genuinely reflects the essence of CM practice. Part II also featured caseload analysis and the AccuDiff© tool. Part III presents the development of and the testing for reliability and validity of the two featured instruments, CM Acuity Tool© and AccuDiff©, as a basis for judging the rigor of the evidence base. Part III also discusses practical applications of the CM acuity instruments.

How do case managers measure a concept such as acuity, which offers sophisticated methods for measuring CM, when previous methods relied on intuition and expert judgment? Is it better to persist in the standard measures of practice even though the measures fail to present the true impact of CM? Clearly, the answer is no; however, until the Acuity Tools Suite, no innovative solution was available. Case managers need measurement tools that are valid and highly specific to their actual CM practice. Moreover, case managers need knowledge and skills to evaluate whether measurement tools live up to their claims of being evidence based and whether they are the right ones to use. Part III aims to help case managers, CM supervisors, and business managers look critically at the application of the Acuity Tool©, the AccuDiff © instrument, and the dosage-prescription construct to judge for themselves about the reliability and usefulness of the acuity and dosage tools for their practice paradigms.

Dosage and acuity empower case managers to demonstrate the impact of their activity in concrete and concise ways. Often the task of demonstrating impact is difficult to do in CM because of its multidimensional complexity and its effects on intermediate outcomes such as client participation in therapy, transitions between healthcare disciplines and settings, and difficult-to-quantify outcomes such as soft savings, quality, and satisfaction. Part III, the final installment of the *Acuity and Case Management* series, presents the evidence base behind the acuity tools innovation and features selected practical applications of the dosage and acuity concepts for case managers and business managers to use.

BACKGROUND ON ACUITY AND DOSAGE: FOUR KEY ACUITY BUILDING BLOCKS

From the research on dosage and acuity, four building blocks emerged as the foundations that underpin acuity: complexity, client need-severity, intervention-intensity, and dosage-prescription of providers' activities (Huber & Craig, 2007). Figure 1 displays the Craig-Huber CM acuity building blocks conceptual model. *Acuity*, defined as the severity of illness or client condition that indicates the need for the intensity of the subsequent CM intervention (Craig, 2005), is driven by the inherent complexity that is specific to CM cases. Dosage measurement in the Huber-Hall model (see dosage figure in Part II; Craig & Huber, 2007) includes the amount, frequency, duration, and type of activities done as a part of providers' interventions that case managers employ and activate to achieve results for their clients (Huber, Hall, & Vaughn, 2001; Huber, Sarrazin, Vaughn, & Hall, 2003).

In the Huber-Hall model, activity dosage is derived from its multidimensional factors. Specific and discrete CM provider activities, such as making a referral for a client, are identified and counted, and then displayed and analyzed by types of activity. The dosage of CM activity types includes identification of activities by what amount, what frequency, and over what duration they occur in different instances and for different purposes. Measurement issues relate to identifying how discrete an action is and whether it truly is a discrete activity or is an intervention instead.

Many provider disciplines are interested in dosage, yet little research has been done to measure it. In nursing, Brooten and Youngblut (2006) conceptualized a *nurse dose* as composed of dose (the number of nurses or an amount of care provided by nurses), the nurse, and the host response. *Nurse activity dose*, as conceptualized by Huber (2007), focuses on providers' specific activities and uses the more specific and measurable dimensions of amount, frequency, duration, and type to define a dose. At the next higher level of aggregation, the *nurse intervention dosage* concept has been studied using data captured within the Nursing Interventions Classification, a standardized language framework of the nursing process (Dochterman & Bulechek, 2004).

Although dosage is measured at the discrete activity level, complexity occurs at a global level as the overall extent of difficulty existing in a CM case. The more involved and complicated the client's needs, CM interventions, and activity dosages are in a CM case, the more complex the CM case is. The more complex a case is, the higher its acuity is and the more intense its interventions and dosages are. Measuring acuity means objectively and reliably identifying the level of complexity arising from a client's set of circumstances and specifying the degrees of need-severity, intervention-intensity, and dosage-prescriptions.

EVIDENCE FOR PRACTICE: RELIABILITY AND VALIDITY TESTING OF ACUITY TOOLS

The Acuity Tools Project grew out of recommendations and feedback from case managers and was developed using rigorous psychometric analyses. A review board ($n = 20$) of clinical experts, quality specialists, and business analysts internal to the originating CM company monitored the development and testing of the Acuity Tools Project's tools, including the acuity concepts, scores, and differentials, plus their operating principles and outcomes premises. Expert panel members ($n = 7$) evaluated the authenticity of the outcomes tools (CM Acuity Tool© and AccuDiff©) and presented their recommendations to the review board. The board oversight occurred at multiple junctures along the development pathway, including the five critical points—after the tools were drafted initially, before β tests and pilot tests were begun, and after β tests and pilot tests were completed (Figure 2). The review board consented at each juncture to commit company resources to obtain evidence of operational and outcomes validity.

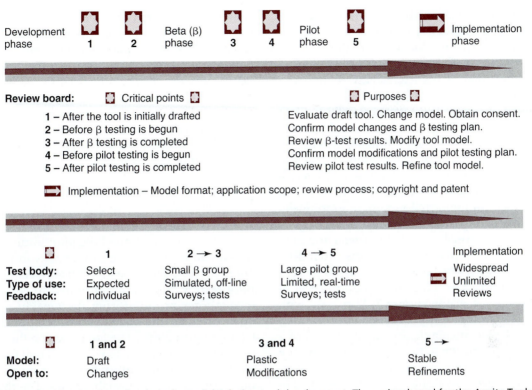

FIGURE 2 Five critical points in review board oversight during tool development. The review board for the Acuity Tools Project provided oversight at the five critical points in development: after the initial tool drafting, before and after beta testing, and, before and after pilot testing. The purposes of the board reviews are provided along with the testing groups, uses, feedback methods, and effects on the tool model.

The soundness of the acuity tools was tested through systematic reporting and multilevel analysis. Reviewers reached agreement, called reviewer consensus, about the merits of the acuity tools in a two-phase progression, after a small test sample (β test, $n = 5$) and after a larger test group (pilot test, $n = 28$). The progression had a two-fold purpose: (1) to evaluate content *validity* related to CM activities, and (2) to measure the *reliability* of the CM Acuity Tool© and AccuDiff© instruments. The operational question was: Does the CM Acuity Tool© faithfully capture activities to produce a clear and useful measure of the unique and specific elements that professional case managers contribute? The outcomes question was: Does the acuity concept produce a measurement of the effects of the CM work process that is real and reliable?

Beta Phase

Two CM supervisors and two quality specialists joined the developer (K. C.) to form the initial small-sized team of beta (β) testers ($n = 5$). During the β phase of the development of acuity tools, interrater reliability (IRR) evaluations of draft and final tools

for evaluator concordance (Fisher & van Belle, 1993, pp. 897–901) and user discussions for content accuracy and appropriateness were conducted. Refinements in and additions to the subdriver content of the Acuity Tool© were made on the basis of quality assessment feedback and mismatched IRR scores from the β testers. Special attention was paid to eliminating areas of interpretation discrepancies that caused raters, blinded to each other's work, to assign different acuity scores to the same case. The β team tested the Acuity Tool© by assigning acuity scores to about 50 cases per week for 4 weeks (5 cases per day, 5 days per week, 2 IRR pairs per week), which reached about 200 applications. Seven cases in total were found to be inappropriate for assigning acuity scores (such as cases closed at assessment), which slightly lowered the number of cases in the β phase. To ensure adequate variation in pairing associations, the five team members rotated through IRR pairs. The paired IRR testers were blinded to the other team member in the IRR pair as well as to the acuity scores the mirror had assigned. That week's unpaired (fifth) team member randomly selected cases from each week's active case log and sent them electronically to the paired IRR testers to review. The paired IRR testers separately reviewed the CM cases, assigned acuity scores, documented their choice rationale per the standard instructions, and electronically returned the results exclusively to the fifth β-team member.

The data from the IRR tests were collected into informal reports showing the numbers and frequencies of exact matches between IRR pairs, matches off by 1 acuity score, and matches missed by 2 acuity scores. There were no matches that missed by 3 or 4 acuity score differences. Also, acuity scores ($n = 193$) were collected into informal reports to graphically visualize the acuity distribution results. Statistical patterns called "normal" distributions were found to be present in the graphical spread of case quantities in the β-test phase. The "normal" statistical pattern meant that most cases showed a medium level of complexity with an acuity score of 3. Also, cases with lower levels of complexity (acuity scores of 1 and 2) and higher levels of complexity (acuity scores of 4 and 5) occurred, but these two "tails" were roughly equal to each other in the numbers of cases they contained (numbers not available) and were each less in comparison with the quantity of medium-complexity (acuity score 3) cases. This characteristic pattern of distribution, called a "bell-shaped" curve, held statistical importance for predicting behavior from one test sample to another.

Because these likely or "normal" percentages of acuity scores per number of cases were demonstrated in the β-test phase, they could be anticipated to occur during the pilot phase. Deviations from the normal distributions would be detected in the weekly detailed reports to be run in the pilot phase as quantities or percentages of unexpectedly low or high acuity scores called outliers. These outlier scores prompted rapid investigative analyses by the team of evaluators in the β phase (and in the pilot phase). Analyses included continuous quality improvement, content review, IRR score validations, and CM supervisory interactions.

When matched acuity scores were achieved consistently through multiple IRR pairings, the Acuity Tool© was considered ready for testing by a larger sample of users under stressed, live conditions (pilot testing). On behalf of the team of five reviewers in the β-test phase, the developer presented to the expert panel and the review board: (1) the positive results of concurrence in the IRR tests (*reliability*); and (2) the favorable findings from the quality assessment discussions confirming that the CM core

content was reflected accurately as levels of complexity in the acuity components of the Acuity Tool© (*validity*). The expert panel's unanimous recommendation to the review board was that the Acuity Tool© testing was ready to be advanced to a larger sample of frontline case managers. The review board assessed the β team's results and agreed with the expert panel's recommendation to dedicate more extensive company resources and personnel to test the acuity tools in the pilot phase.

Pilot Test

A team of case managers ($n = 28$) in one service delivery location constituted the pilot testing body for real-world testing of the instruments in the Acuity Tools Project. The β team of reviewers joined the pilot testing body and continued to conduct tool evaluations by monitoring the weekly reports of open cases for the 28 case managers for 3 months (June–August 2000). The focus was on the ability of the acuity instruments to capture actual CM impact accurately and reliably when used by many case managers on highly variable cases. The total number of cases handled by the case managers during the pilot phase of test trials of the acuity instruments was about 3,000. This estimate included many types of cases, including ones that were opened, scored, and closed during the 3-month pilot phase; ones opened but closed at assessment (unneeded or inappropriate cases); and cases that were opened, scored (and a few that awaited scoring), but which remained open and active at the end of the 3-month interval.

Because the acuity tool was used about 3,000 times to score CM cases, a large sample size was accrued to judge the features of the Acuity Tool©. Using this large database, three important analyses were conducted over the 3 months of the trial. First, the applicability (content *validity*) of the elements of the Acuity Tool© were verified, improved, or slated for improvement in later versions. Second, crosschecks of acuity scores for accuracy (*reliability*) were conducted. These crosschecks were *of users*, meaning how different case managers used the tools at roughly the same time, or *over time*, meaning how the tools were used by the same case managers at different points in time. Third, the ability (*veracity*) of the Acuity Tool© to capture, measure, and communicate salient information about the severity, intensity, dosage, and complexity of a wide variety of CM cases was examined.

Psychometric testing for scientific rigor included quality reviews, cross-validation scrutiny, and random, blinded IRR tests of the acuity scoring system. Both reviews and tests revealed high degrees of concordance (Fisher & van Belle, 1993, pp. 897–901) among case managers. Concordance examines whether case managers used the Acuity Tool© to assign acuity scores similarly in cases that were similar in complexity, a critical test for reliability in widespread application. In the representative sample batch ($n = 1{,}110$) extracted for testing, a combined total of 93% ($n = 1{,}032$) of reviews reached IRR concordance between the acuity scores from blinded, independent reviewers (other members on the pilot team) and the acuity scores from frontline case managers at their initial acuity assessments. Of the 93% reviews, 63% ($n = 710$) agreed exactly in the acuity scores they assigned, and 29% ($n = 322$) differed by 1 acuity score. Only 7% ($n = 78$) of IRR tests performed in the sample batch were shown to be matches that differed by 2 or 3 acuity scores. Such matches were labeled as outliers. No matches were found to differ by 4 acuity scores.

Cases with outlier matches (mismatched by 2 or 3 acuity scores [$n = 78$ in the sample batch]) were sent for immediate in-depth case audits by the quality review specialists involved in the pilot test to examine causes for the mismatch. In-depth case-by-case scrutiny determined that errors occurred for several reasons, chief among them were transfer, addition, and reading errors. Acuity score mismatches caused by *transfer* errors occurred when frontline case managers transferred acuity scores from the case narrative notes to the 1-digit numeric field used for drawing weekly reports. This copy error accounted for the largest source of error. Other discrepancies were *addition* errors caused by incorrect adding of acuity sums and *reading* errors caused by misreading or miss-assigning acuity subdrivers. As case managers became more familiar with acuity and complexity content, as well as the use of the tools, trends showed that assignment discrepancies decreased over time.

Postpilot survey responses from the 28 case managers yielded the following results:

- 73% [20 ± 2] found the Acuity Tool© to accurately capture core CM issues;
- 86% [24 ± 1] expressed certainty in ability of Acuity Tool© to reflect complexity;
- 94% [26 ± 1] reported it took less than 10 minutes to apply the Acuity Tool©; and
- 100% [28 ± 0] described the Acuity Tool© as easy to use.

Favorable results from the weekly detailed reports, IRR tests, and cross-validation checks showed that the Acuity Tool© was comprehensive in its content and valid in its measurement of acuity. Also, as seen in Figure 3, data analysis reports showed normal distributions of acuity scores, which are the specific graphic patterns obtained (inverted "U" appearance called "bell-shaped" curve) when the scores were plotted as data points. Normal distribution was a positive finding because results obtained *during* the 3-month pilot testing phase matched the expectations of the developer and review team *before* the pilot testing phase that acuity scores would display certain statistical behaviors. Normal behavior of the acuity data meant inferential statistics, probability statements, and predictions could be applied, which confirmed the developer's premise and delighted the business thinkers.

Finding normal statistical behavior patterns was important in establishing the CM business case because the company's business decision makers wanted to know whether specific occurrences could be counted on to happen. If data and statistical evidence were reliable, then marketing statements could be claimed and service results expected to be delivered

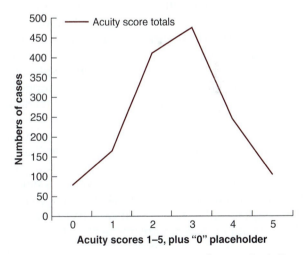

FIGURE 3 Total acuity score distributions for 1 week of pilot phase. This chart demonstrates the "normal" distribution of acuity scores for all the open cases for 1 week of the pilot phase of testing of the Acuity Tool. The acuity scores 1–5 derive from the weekly report. The "zero" placeholder indicates cases that were awaiting acuity scoring at the time the weekly report was generated. The total numbers of cases were for the 28 case managers engaged in the pilot study. This graph approaches the inverted "U" shape of a normal statistical distribution of data that allows projections to be made on the basis of the reliability of assumptions that underlie the data world and that represent behavior of events in the real world.

with high degrees of certainty. Indeed, the strength of the evidence from reliability and validity testing led the review board to call for an early cessation of the pilot testing and sped to the decision to implement the acuity concepts and tools nationwide within the company, to copyright the materials, and to pursue patent application.

PRACTICAL APPLICATION: HOW TO USE THE CM ACUITY TOOL

Because not all CM cases are created equal, all CM cases need documentation and evaluation for quality and cost improvements through a method of measurement that uses common indicators based on core CM components. Craig (2005) developed the CM Acuity Tool$^{©}$ to quantify and display a profile of real-time CM activities and to improve communications between case managers, supervisors, quality specialists, and business managers about the differences between and among CM cases. The following example uses the CM Acuity Tool$^{©}$ as explained in Part I (Huber & Craig, 2007) to measure a CM case's level of acuity.

To illustrate how a case manager would apply the Acuity Tool$^{©}$, consider a CM case in which a client who is a brittle diabetic and who has recently been diagnosed with a 60% vision loss has returned home after hip repair surgery complicated by prolonged hospitalization because of a 7-day bout of pneumonia. Circumstances are further complicated by both a mildly demented but friendly and supportive spouse and a physician who has not yet referred the client to an inpatient or outpatient rehabilitation admission. The case manager might choose the three indicators Clinical/Nursing CN4, Psycho/Social PS2, and Quality/Cost QC4 and record the driver–subdriver combinations in the case's narrative documentation such as: "CN4/3 (severe comorbid symptoms); PS2/2 (stressed caregiver capacity); QC4/2 (inappropriate care environment) = 4 + 2 + 4 = 10, acuity = 4". [*Note:* Although 10 is the sum of the drivers from the acuity instrument, the acuity score is 4, which is acquired using the transformation algorithm that accompanies the Acuity Tool$^{©}$ in Part I.] Therefore, at the time this case is assessed, it is considered to have an above-average complexity level as measured by an acuity score of 4. Acuity 4 is the second highest level of acuity, or complexity, obtainable through application of the Acuity Tool$^{©}$.

The Acuity Tools Project resulted in findings that revolutionized CM communications while remaining true to the fundamental elements of CM practice. The data and information proved to be useful both for quality and for outcome management within an individual case manager's caseload and for helping to guide decisions about the allocation of scarce resources across a group of case managers' caseloads.

PRACTICE APPLICATIONS: CASELOAD ANALYSES

Examinations of the systematic acuity reports based on the Acuity Tool$^{©}$ demonstrated the well-known adage that all CM *cases* are not created equal. Accordingly, caseload acuity analyses also revealed the ways in which CM *caseloads* are unequal. Insights derived from the use of the Acuity Tools Project yielded powerful information to better manage both an individual case manager's caseload and a CM unit's array of caseloads. As noted in Part II (Craig & Huber, 2007), caseload analyses using the scoring of acuity through the CM Acuity Tool$^{©}$ transformed a one-dimensional case count into a two-dimensional quantity: case numbers stratified by caseload acuity weights. Acuity scores provided an easily understood method to communicate about complicated cases and about the expertise of the case managers who manage these cases. By identifying the degrees of complexity in CM cases, the acuity scores carry implications about resource utilization by clients and work investments by case managers. Also, systematic reports, such as the one in Table 1, uncovered the sensitivity and ability to detect caseload distortion problems such as those generated by "zero acuity" values. "Zero acuity" values served as the placeholders for actual acuity scores in the cases that lacked them when reports were generated. The more "zero acuity" values a case manager had, especially in a continuing week-after-week pattern, the more distorted and inaccurate that case manager's caseload acuity weight was. This explicit, data-informed content was useful to CM and quality supervisors.

The CM-customized acuity scores opened many avenues of improved communication, like the exchange of information between frontline case managers and CM supervisors. For instance, a CM supervisor could use the acuity data to inform assignment decisions regarding new cases by considering the weights of case managers' caseloads, not just the numbers of their cases. Data-informed decision making could make the difference between simply assigning 9 new cases in comparison with assigning 9 new cases with knowledge about the levels of

TABLE 1   Acuity Tool© Sample Report[a]

Employee	0		1		2		3		4		5		Cases	Caseload acuity
Day	2	3%	8	14%	14	24%	24	42%	9	15%	0	0%	57	144
Page	9	18%	4	8%	27	55%	6	12%	3	6%	0	0%	49	88
Cecil	7	14%	8	17%	8	17%	16	34%	2	4%	6	12%	47	110
Dickey	9	15%	2	3%	12	20%	26	44%	7	11%	3	5%	59	147
Petty	4	8%	15	31%	22	45%	6	12%	1	2%	0	0%	48	81
Dobbins	2	3%	3	4%	23	35%	30	46%	6	9%	1	1%	65	168
Camp	3	5%	5	8%	28	50%	18	32%	2	3%	0	0%	56	123
Fenny	1	1%	0	0%	5	7%	37	55%	23	34%	1	1%	67	218
Pope	0	0%	31	52%	13	22%	11	18%	2	3%	2	3%	59	108
Decker	5	9%	9	16%	11	20%	7	12%	5	9%	17	31%	54	157
Napoli	3	11%	4	15%	7	26%	9	34%	3	11%	0	0%	26	57
Dunn	0	0%	6	11%	11	20%	16	29%	9	16%	12	22%	54	172
Circle	2	3%	8	14%	16	29%	16	29%	8	14%	4	7%	54	140
Colby	10	20%	2	4%	9	18%	11	22%	16	32%	1	2%	49	122
Dyson	4	6%	10	16%	7	11%	33	55%	5	8%	0	0%	59	143
Eaton	2	3%	1	1%	6	10%	26	44%	22	37%	1	1%	58	184
DaMond	0	0%	1	2%	5	10%	18	38%	11	23%	12	25%	47	169
Cybil	4	7%	0	0%	11	20%	28	51%	7	12%	3	5%	54	149
Newton	0	0%	4	14%	1	3%	5	17%	9	32%	9	32%	28	102
Fabian	1	1%	6	8%	7	10%	18	26%	27	39%	9	13%	68	227
Night	1	3%	1	3%	8	26%	14	46%	5	16%	1	3%	30	84
Purdy	2	4%	4	9%	15	36%	4	9%	5	12%	11	26%	41	121
Pickell	3	3%	9	10%	69	84%	1	1%	0	0%	0	0%	82	150
Ebony	1	1%	7	10%	15	22%	24	35%	20	29%	0	0%	67	189
DeWit	2	3%	1	1%	9	16%	28	50%	11	20%	4	7%	55	167
Novak	1	3%	1	3%	5	15%	2	6%	16	50%	7	21%	32	116
Currie	0	0%	0	0%	15	31%	23	48%	9	19%	0	0%	47	135
DiBardo	1	1%	14	21%	31	47%	18	27%	1	1%	0	0%	65	134
	79	5%	164	11%	410	28%	475	32%	244	17%	104	7%	1698	

[a] Weekly detailed reports showed case numbers and totals for the 28 case managers distributed by acuity scores 1 through 5 plus "0" acuity score placeholders, their respective percentages, and the caseload acuities (right column).

complexity inherent within each case. [Included in the Acuity Tools Project is an intake tool that sorts new cases into four levels of projected complexity based on numbers of expected service providers and strata of apparent difficulty. For more information on the CM Intake Tool©, contact Craig.]

Caseload Example 1

From Table 1, consider the caseload data for case manager Dickey (names in the table are not the case managers' real names) who has 59 cases with a caseload weight of 147 and now 9 new cases need to be assigned. Perhaps, the 9 cases have acuity scores in this configuration: 3 cases have acuity scores of 1; 3 cases have acuity 2; 1 has acuity 3; 1 has acuity 4; and 1 has acuity 5. If Dickey were to receive all 9 new cases, then the caseload acuity would rise by 21 [$(3 \times 1) + (3 \times 2) + (1 \times 3) + (1 \times 4) + (1 \times 5) = 3 + 6 + 3 + 4 + 5 = 21$], and Dickey's caseload acuity weight would increase from 147 to 168. However, if the 9 cases have the following acuity scores: 1 case with acuity 1; 1 case with acuity 2; 1 with acuity 3; 1 with acuity 4; and 5 with acuity 5, then the caseload acuity increases by 35 [(1 × 1) + (1 × 2) + (1 ×3) + (1 × 4) + (5 × 5) = 1 + 2 + 3 + 4 + 25 = 35]. In this scenario, Dickey's caseload weight increases from 147 to 182. (The Acuity Tools Project included a Caseload Matrix©, Craig, 2005, that stratifies case numbers by caseload weights and sorts CM caseloads into light, medium, and heavy. For information on the Caseload Matrix©, contact Craig.) Using the caseload acuity concept, it is easy to visualize how a jump in a caseload weight from 147 to 168 (a 14% increase) is sizeable and that a leap from 147 to 182 (a 24% increase) could be oppressive.

Because acuity scores directly relate to time for task, numbers of interventions, levels of self-care, robustness of caregiver support systems, and appropriate setting and provider components, a caseload acuity weight of 182 for Dickey's 59 cases can be much more complex and demanding than a caseload acuity of 168 for 59 cases. Rather than making assignments using intuition and guesswork that may turn out unbalanced results, a CM supervisor could use the Acuity Tool© as a valid alternative for assigning cases. CM supervisors (plus case managers and clients) would benefit by using the acuity data to look at the case managers' caseloads and distribute the new cases in an equitable way on the basis of evidence-based knowledge.

Instead of assigning case manager Dickey several new cases, the CM supervisor could use the content in the Acuity Tool© report (specifically the "0" columns in Figure 1) as a starting point to discover why this case manager has so many cases that are unscored for acuity. When a high number of "zero acuity" cases occur in a caseload as placeholders for actual acuity scores, the caseload acuity weight is rendered falsely low. The report shows that Dickey had 9 (15%) of the 59 cases in the caseload that lacked actual acuity scores; therefore, only 50 of Dickey's 59 cases had actual acuity scores. According to the consensus discussion about acuity assignment thresholds from Part II (Huber & Craig, 2007), for a caseload acuity weight to be reliable and trustworthy, at least 95% of the cases in a caseload should contain actual acuity scores. This threshold means that if 5% or more of the cases in a caseload at any point in time lack actual acuity scores, then the caseload weight is erroneous and unreliable. Part II presented the work analysis results that high "zero acuity" values in the weekly reports signaled work bottlenecks and backlogs or struggling case managers in need of

managerial coaching or staffing relief. Reasons why Dickey has a high percentage of cases without acuity scores in them could include employee illness, temporary reallocation away from normal CM duties, a high admission backlog, or work absorption in managing a crisis case. However, the evidence-informed CM supervisor can see that loading 9 new cases on to a case manager with a large percentage of "zero acuity" cases may be unwise and counterproductive for work achievement and for client satisfaction. More importantly, the advantage of the Acuity Tool© is its ability to capture and display visually the detailed information that provides a clear and precise language for communication between case manager and supervisor and for problem solving and quality improvement actions.

Caseload Example 2

Another example of the power of caseload critique afforded by use of the Acuity Tool© involves caseload comparison based on the equity of a common and valid tool of measurement. In Figure 1, case managers Fenny and DiBardo have vastly divergent caseload acuities, although they carry about the same number of cases: 67 cases with a caseload acuity weight of 218 (Fenny) and 65 cases with a caseload weight of 134 (DiBardo). Since each case manager has 1 case (1%) in the "zero acuity" column, the difference in caseload weights does not arise from DiBardo's having a large number of cases that lack acuity scores. Such a wide disparity made explicit through caseload acuity weights provides solid ground for in-depth work process examinations that keep client improvement foremost. Equitable caseloads permit case managers to apply their energies in the right directions—the right dosages in the right cases to achieve the best outcomes possible for the clients.

Caseload Example 3

In addition, because of its caseload equalizing capacity, the Acuity Tool© is useful for monitoring the work of both new and part-time case managers. Figure 1 displays how the work capacity of new employees Napolie, Newton, Night, and Novak can be tracked to better gauge when they are ready for the next steps in levels of difficulty or when to coach a case manager to progress if a static level has persisted. Also, the Acuity Tool© report in the table includes information about the caseload distributions of part-time personnel such as employees Page, Petty, Pope, Purdy, and Pickell. Caseloads of part-time employees can be equally as complex and demanding as those of full-time employees. In the caseload acuity research, which was a component of the Acuity Tools Project, a conversion equation was developed to translate the caseload numbers for new and part-time employees to full-time equivalencies. Placing less than full-time caseloads on par with full-time caseloads allows comparisons to be made from a platform of equity and aids in recognizing and rewarding part-time employees in the same way as full-time employees.

Carrying a high case volume with a higher overall caseload complexity was one of several hallmarks of CM practice at advanced levels that case managers reported the acuity tools were able to illustrate. Quality improvement and supervisory personnel undertook plans to structure the recognition of exceptional work and sustained excellence that was illuminated through the acuity instruments' abilities to assign acuity scores and obtain acuity differentials.

These examples demonstrate that acuity and dosage data provide facts open to verification when case managers claim high workload or assignment inequity. However, the caseload distinctions by weighted acuity measurements reach beyond case assignments. Caseload weights can be applied to decisions about expertise, mentoring, and rewards. Moreover, acuity analyses extend into explorations about quality and business outcomes. Examples of business outcomes involve caseload size, complexity, and diagnosis compositions and how changes in these dimensions relate to changes in satisfaction, resource uptake, and savings, as the needs of clients are met more effectively because the workloads of case managers are consistently analyzed and thoughtfully managed.

PRACTICAL APPLICATION: ACUITY TOOL© RESULTS USED FOR SYSTEMS IMPROVEMENTS

Analyses of bottlenecks and barriers encountered during the acuity assignment in the pilot phase led to important serendipitous findings. One of the many revelations that came from acuity tool usage was that it yielded rich data to guide CM practice, especially when strategies tailored to CM principles and workflows were applied. For example, the originating CM company's policy was that new cases should have acuity scores assessed, calculated, and assigned within 3 business days of receipt of the case by the case manager. Analysis of the causes of acuity scores' not being

assigned in new cases brought systems-related disconnects to light. Uncovered by data-driven analysis, disconnects highlighted the intersections where productivity became caught in process cracks. These discontinuities between the reporting systems for business outcomes and the realities and challenges of frontline CM practice were capable of impeding or disrupting organizational effectiveness.

As discussed in Part II, one specific disconnect involved the interaction between the company's timing for generating routine organizational reports *versus* the reality of complying with the work directive that cases should have acuity scores assigned within 3 business days of receipt by the case manager. This timing disconnect caused many cases to show an absence of acuity scoring ("zero acuity" values) when a routine report was generated. If the organizational reports were run before the close of the 3-business-day window but the acuity scores were in the process of being assessed and recorded, then the acuity scores appeared in the next week's report. This meant a delay of only 1 week, which caused no detrimental effects.

However, when case managers were unable to complete acuity assignments beyond 1 week, then high "zero acuity" placeholder percentages for these case managers repeated in the weekly detailed reports (see Part II for more detail on "zero acuity" values). Although it may have appeared that a case manager was behind only in superficial documentation, it was learned that the "zero acuity" percentages persisting beyond 1 to 2 weeks indicated organizational problem areas such as short staffing or struggling case managers. Examples of persistent "zero acuity" scenarios included return-to-work backlog circumstances, inefficient work processes by individual case managers, and transient intervals when high admission rates occurred.

Supervisory reviews were initiated to evaluate the causes, to make quality and process decisions, and to institute changes to relieve the backlog burdens or alter the causative factors identified by individual case managers. These supervisory reviews also triggered quality reports and process decision-based investigations about the events. The findings were used for systems-wide evaluations and, when appropriate, for development of proactive prevention or alleviation strategies. Alleviation strategies included "rapid response teams" of per diem case managers who were deployed for coverage fortification to address periods of temporary backlogs and high admissions. In this way, the Acuity Tool© served to capture CM practice better and to enhance internal work processes for greater internal quality, sense of fairness, and CM satisfaction.

The pilot-test phase uncovered the importance of evaluating the components of the various CM practices by the right factors. Process steps used for evaluation and change decisions in CM need to be true and relevant to the actual architecture of that specific CM paradigm of service delivery. Because CM is a distinct and advanced multidisciplinary provider intervention, it is best evaluated by measures derived from actual practice. However, it is common for CM to be measured and judged by a diagnosis-related group (DRG) funding scheme borrowed from financial models based on physician practices without appropriate validation to CM practice.

The Acuity Tool$^©$, AccuDiff$^©$ instrument, and the CM dosage-prescription construct have remarkable capacities for valid adaptation to different CM practice paradigms that are readily achievable and highly reliable. Therefore, acuity and dosage deliver the data- and evidence-based testing instruments that business, quality, and case managers need to demonstrate that CM has a unique skill set and distinct knowledge base with predictable best practice outcomes open to investigation and measurement. The Acuity Tools Project provides measurement methods to deliver the evidence-based practice (EBP) data and instruments to demonstrate the unique contribution of CM.

ACUITY, DOSAGE, AND OUTCOMES: HOW ACUITY DIFFERENTIALS DEMONSTRATE CM VALUE

The difference between the two acuity measurements—initial acuity score minus final acuity score—is called the *acuity differential*. An acuity differential reflects the CM outcome of reduction in complexity of core CM factors due to case managers' interventions. Reduction in complexity, and thus acuity, corresponds directly to reductions in client symptoms, inappropriate case environment, and ineffective provider use.

In Part II (Craig & Huber, 2007), it was noted that *larger acuity differentials mean greater CM impact*. This principle needs to be emphasized and explained. The imperative to establish the business case for CM means that case managers must demonstrate the worth of CM by clearly indicating the improvements they make to the healthcare circumstances, symptoms, and needs of clients under their stewardship. These improvements, which are made through the applica-

tions of activities common across the spectrum of CM, should be grounded in well-recognized CM interventions and based on the continuity of CM principles. The concepts of acuity scoring and dosage prescription capture the true effects that case managers create in their clients' cases represented by the changes in acuities. The changes in acuities, or acuity differentials, serve as indices of complexity (identified through the driver–subdriver combinations in the Acuity Tool$^©$), which become less severe and intense as case managers intervene successfully to the benefit of their clients. Because CM is the application of expertise to the process of care coordination and advocacy, it is used to address clients' needs for care and care-need changes over time. Therefore, the healthcare circumstances of clients engaged in the process of CM should exhibit improvement over time through reductions in complexity and acuity.

Case managers continue to need a method to indicate the true complexity levels of the cases that come to them in their original states at intake and the degree of improvement in the clients' circumstances at the close of these cases. Acuity and dosage provide the right tools that empower case managers and business decision makers to create and demonstrate an upward spiral of improvement. The more times that case managers can show large changes between the acuities at the beginning of cases than acuities at case closures, the greater the impact case managers show from the interventions they executed to help their clients. Simultaneously, the more clearly case managers demonstrate to supervisors and business directors the extent of improvement related to expenditure of dollars, which is return on investment (ROI) in business language, the better the business case for CM becomes. The more precisely case managers are able to manage the right cases (those cases in which acuity can be improved), the better the business return on investment outcomes can become. As case managers see evidence of the improvements they make, they are reinforced positively to achieve similar results in more cases for more clients. The positive reinforcement of this feedback cycle means case managers, supervisors, and directors alike are becoming better at targeting the right cases for CM and that the right activities are being highlighted for CM outcomes.

Illustrating CM impact through this concrete and concise method useful to business decision makers involves using the measurement tools of dosage, acuity scores, and acuity differentials. Thus, the measurement of acuity and dosage constructs a bridge that unites the actual practice of CM to the business case for CM. Because acuity differentials are based on the real effects of actual CM interventions, they offer quality and business managers the data needed to build the case for the exceptional worth of CM and its value in affecting both the soft-savings and hard-currency outcomes.

CASE LENGTH AND TIME: CALCULATIONS AND LIMITATIONS

In the telephonic CM organization where the Acuity Tools Project was initiated and tested, proving value in CM related in part to the length of time over which CM occurred. Shorter case-life appeared better for aggregate cost calculations, meaning that the quicker the case started and stopped, the easier it was to attach costs and expenses to the outcomes. During the pilot study in this telephonic CM practice, analyses of the amount of time that cases remained open and active revealed that case-life averaged 4.5 months. Acuity differentials may prove to be better outcomes indicators in cases that remain open longer than the average 4.5-month duration. However, the 3-month pilot time frame was too short to use the acuity differential concept to study and determine an optimal upper limit of a CM case-life by primary diagnoses, DRG codes, or other valid taxonomies.

The optimal case-life duration that accurately reflects the effects of CM interventions for subpopulations is unknown and largely untested. Studies to clarify the optimal case-life durations for best CM effects are needed in the future.

ACUITY TOOL© CHALLENGES

Challenges that arose during Acuity Tool© development and pilot testing involved errors, competing priorities, and perceptions. Challenges related to *errors* concerned fears of cheating by supplying false data or gaming the system. Supplying false data jeopardizes accuracy in measurements that are largely self-reported. In this setting, gaming would result when case managers falsified acuity scores by intentionally inflating them. However, diligent oversight during the pilot phase failed to detect any acuity score contamination through gaming.

The majority of case managers whose data were analyzed during the pilot phase held licenses in nursing or social work, and a growing minority held CM certifications. It was assumed that professional case managers were dedicated to high standards of ethics and practice integrity, including nonfalsification of

clinical data, motivation to correct errors once discovered, and acting to prevent error repetition. In IRR assessments and case reviews, it was found that, instead of inflating acuity scores, case managers tended to undervalue the complexity of clients' cases, and thus were more likely to report lower (undervalued) acuity scores rather than inflated ones. CM supervisors and quality specialists routinely conducted randomized and blinded IRR testing to evaluate both Acuity Tool© usage and scoring accuracy. Case audits were performed to analyze cases with mismatched acuity scores between raters who were primary (frontline case managers) and secondary (reviewers) to discover sources of variation in scoring results.

The team of five evaluators consisting of the project's developer, quality specialists, and CM supervisors reviewed weekly reports for outlier acuity scores. Case audits were done on these outlier cases, also. The five evaluators engaged in quality assessment discussions regarding acuity scores considered outliers, either too low or too high, in order to obtain consensus on the most appropriate scores. Supervisors conducted in-depth case reviews with the frontline case managers to gain insights into the assessment and scoring of acuity values. It was found that case manager coaching was provided more often to upgrade low acuity scores to match the levels of complexity decided through consensus rather than to downgrade high acuity scores. Overvalued scores were estimated in the pilot phase to be less than 1.3% ($n < 39$). The number of intentional inflation instances was not tracked in the original trial owing to the difficulty of identifying this type of action.

The second challenge involved *competing priorities* that vied for case managers' time. Competing priorities meant that pressures on case managers' available time and efforts to prioritize work created inefficiencies and impeded their effectiveness. Competing obligations and responsibilities caused lapses in timely assessments of initial acuity levels done by applying the Acuity Tool©. In some instances, the case manager's ability to effect changes in complexity was tempered or even truncated because of decisions based on contract constraints created at the company's business management level.

In the third area, *perception challenges* manifested as hesitancies to change. Hesitancy referred to the doubts, resistance, or reluctance expressed by some frontline case managers who initially felt that using instruments to rank acuity benefited their supervisors more than it benefited them. However, the more frontline case managers used the suite of acuity tools, the more they expressed acceptance and enthusiasm for the improved communications and caseloads and for the improved CM they felt they were able to accomplish on behalf of their clients.

GOING FORWARD: FUTURE RESEARCH FOR EBP

Future research using CM dosage prescriptions and the instruments of the Acuity Tools Project encompasses both pure research and applied development. Randomized controlled trials, the premier method to generate proof (Davies & Logan, 1999, pp. 1–19), should be undertaken to establish and frame the dosage–acuity synergy. Studies that incorporate the CM dosage concepts into the acuity instruments could show the ways dosage improves the acuity drivers, heightens specificity in CM outcomes, and adds clarity to the business case for CM.

Researchers could replicate and validate the suite of acuity tools and CM dosage for various case subsets and adaptations to alternate practice settings. Areas of investigation could target refinement of the elements used in determining acuity and further validate acuity scores. Developing tools with an improved range of core content to encompass the diversity of CM practice environments is an ambitious task, but an essential area of investigation.

Experiments could evaluate the optimal and effective resource control by case managers. Mapping resource intensity weights (Pink & Bolley, 1994) to the acuity tools would be valuable for resource management and outcomes improvement. *Resource intensity weights* refer to rating various healthcare providers or services that the providers submit in order to measure their levels of complexity, difficulty, effectiveness, and expense. This information would tie well into the dosage and acuity concepts. An avenue of sociological research could be to study the associations between acuity score inflation as an indication of possible gaming and the licensures and credentialing of frontline case managers. Locating a funding source for electronic formatting of the acuity measurement instruments is a first-order priority.

Large medical databases that contain DRG codes linked to CM cases could be analyzed to explore how core CM interventions relate to standard DRG classifications and to nonstandard (company-selected) DRG code groupings. The purpose would be to discover which CM activities are clustered in only a few DRG classes and which occur between and across diagnosis groupings, especially ones that associate in tightly or loosely related combinations. Similarly, in nursing, databases that contain nursing diagnoses, interventions, and outcomes formulated using standardized nursing language can be analyzed for common activities across interventions. The focus of investigations into the associations between diagnoses and dosages of CM interventions could be to refine the definitions of core CM components, explore the links of core components to common CM actions and acuities, and discover what drives these various connections.

Several important research topics for CM outcomes are tied to the acuity differential concepts. One example is studying optimal case-life durations for best outcomes through acuity differential measurements. Examining nonclosing (plateau, isostatic, or "flat-lined") case acuities discussed in Part II (Craig & Huber, 2007) and deriving criteria that best sort cases into most representative diagnosis groupings or provider intervention activities are two topics for outcomes research. Discovering valid ways to drive CM outcomes authentically toward improved differential results (obtaining larger acuity differences between acuities at opening and closing) represents an essential and critical avenue of outcomes research. Clearer examples and knowledge about CM cases that generate large differences in acuity will enrich the evidence base for CM practice and the business case for CM.

These examples are suggestions for research that the dosage and acuity concepts offer to academic researchers and applied developers. Use of the Acuity Tool©, AccuDiff©, and the acuity–dosage synergy will stimulate ideas about how CM functions to save money, avert inappropriate utilization, and, most importantly, improve CM practice to benefit CM clients.

CONCLUSIONS

Case managers are the right people in the right settings to generate correct and reproducible evidence on the basis of measurement of the right indicators and the right interventions. These rights facilitate accurate decision making about which aspects of CM practice are the right ones to establish the business case for CM while proving the worth of CM. Right indicators are the measurement concepts and tools such as CM acuity and dosage that accurately reflect CM complexity, client need-severity, and CM intervention-intensity. Right interventions include techniques such as acuity differentials that illuminate the improvements that case managers make in clients' cases and dosage prescriptions that encompass CM activity, quantity, and timing.

Acuity and dosage constitute important innovations that translate indicators of EBP into the measurable outcomes of CM interventions that business managers eagerly seek. Moreover, prescribed dosages of CM, plus the CM Acuity Tool© and AccuDiff© applications, provide concrete examples of how case managers can apply evidence-based knowledge in everyday practice to demonstrate the outstanding value of their interpractitioner contributions to healthcare delivery. The critical importance of this work is generated from the rigorous and detailed capture of the depth and range of CM practice, with all of its complexities, in real time. Using CM expertise to identify, measure, and analyze actual CM practice is recommended without reservation. Such CM self-determination stands in stark comparison to strategies that have happened in the past such as borrowing a physician practice-driven financial model (e.g., a DRG funding model) and assuming that it works for CM without appropriate validation.

In the present, case managers can call for the use of dosage and acuity principles in their own practice settings to better understand and communicate the unique components that generate complexity in CM cases. Case managers can encourage the use of the acuity tools to articulate the outcomes measures that signify improvements in soft currencies such as satisfaction and value. CM supervisors and quality specialists can educate business managers about the advantages of the Acuity Tools Suite of valid measurement and outcomes instruments that accurately and reliably reflect the elements specific to CM practice and impact.

Acuity and dosage help case managers explore and fully describe their own advanced, interdisciplinary practice in ways that can be measured to show the exceptional worth of CM. Proving business and professional worth in CM through EBP is a clarion call that case managers must heed and an innovation that all case managers can practice.

References

Brooten, D., & Youngblut, J. M. (2006). Nurse dose as a concept. *Journal of Nursing Scholarship, 38*(1), 94–99.

Craig, K. (2005). *The Case Management Acuity Tool Kit©* [Presentation]. Proceedings of Case Management Society of America, CMSA 15th National Symposium, Orlando, FL. Retrieved October 9, 2006, from http://www.cmsa.org/Portals/0/PDF/Conference/Attendees/2005%20Audio%20Recordings%20Order%20Form.pdf

Craig, K. (2006). CM Acuity Tool© and AccuDiff© initiative. Available from Kathy Craig, MS, RN, CCM, Craig Research Continuum, Kingston, Ontario, Canada K7L 3Z2; 613-542-4554; kdcraigrn@earthlink.net

Craig, K., & Huber, D. L. (2007). Acuity and case management: A healthy dose of outcomes, Part II. *Professional Case Management, 12*(4), 199–210.

Davies, B., & Logan, J. (1999). *Reading research: A user-friendly guide for nurses and other health professionals.* Ottawa, Ontario, Canada: Canadian Nurses Association.

Dochterman, J. M., & Bulechek, G. M. (2004). *Nursing Interventions Classification (NIC)* (4th ed.). St. Louis: Mosby.

Fisher, L., & van Belle, G. (1993). *Biostatistics: A methodology for the health sciences.* New York: Wiley.

Huber, D. L. (2007). *Nurse activity dose.* Unpublished manuscript, University of Iowa.

Huber, D. L., & Craig, K. (2007). Acuity and case management: A healthy dose of outcomes, Part I. *Professional Case Management, 12*(3), 132–146.

Huber, D. L., Hall, J. A., & Vaughn, T. (2001). The dose of case management interventions. *Lippincott's Case Management, 6*(3), 119–126.

Huber, D. L., Sarrazin, M. V., Vaughn, T., & Hall, J. A. (2003). Evaluating the impact of case management dosage. *Nursing Research, 52*(5), 276–288.

Pink, G. H., & Bolley, H. B. (1994). Physicians in health care management 3. Case mix groups and resource intensity weights: An overview for physicians. *Canadian Medical Association Journal, 150*(6), 889–894.

Prescott, P. (1991). Nursing intensity: Needed today for more than staffing. *Nursing Economics, 9*(6), 409–414.

Diane L. Huber, PhD, RN, FAAN, CNAA, BC, is Professor, Colleges of Nursing and Public Health, University of Iowa, Iowa City, teaching and doing research in case management and nursing administration. She is the author/editor of *Leadership and Nursing Care Management* and *Disease Management: A Guide for Case Managers.* She holds copyright to dosage concept and visuals.

Kathy Craig, MS, RN, CCM, CRA, practices case management in 1000 Islands area, Ontario, Canada, and runs Craig Research Continuum for personal health research, biomedical writing, and innovative tool development. She serves as Business and Professional Women President (Kingston), Canadian Hearing Society's Community Development Board member, and Cochrane Collaboration reviewer of evidence-based studies. She holds originator copyrights for *CM Acuity Tool©, Caseload Matrix©,* and *AccuDiff©.*

APPENDIX

Term	Definition
Acuity	Severity of illness or client condition that indicates the need for the intensity of the subsequent CM intervention. Represents a CM case's degree of inherent complexity based on the client need-severity, CM intervention-intensity, and CM dosage-prescription (below).
Acuity differential	The difference between two acuity scores in a CM case, usually the acuity score at the beginning and the ending of a case.
"Bell-shaped" or normal distribution	The pattern for the frequency distribution of a set of data that can be graphed as a bell-shaped curve. Many natural phenomena follow this normal statistical behavior pattern. Normal behavior, a positive finding, means inferential statistics, probability statements, and predictions can be applied.
Beta (β) testing	The stage in the testing of a new product or concept usually in a smaller test population before it is tested in a larger population sample or before commercial release. β testing can involve sending the product to β-test sites outside the vendor or real-world exposure and testing conducted by users, other than its developers, for real-world exposure.
Caseload acuity or caseload acuity weight	Weighted totals of the case acuities per case manager at any one time. Caseload acuity weight is obtained by multiplying the number of cases with an acuity level by that acuity level to obtain weighted subtotals and adding the subtotals together. Having high numbers of cases lacking acuity scores can distort caseload weights.
Caseload complexity	The level of difficulty of cases in an individual case manager's portfolio of cases. Caseload complexity is found by stratifying the numbers of cases in a caseload by the acuity ranges per individual case manager. The Acuity Tools Project included such a stratification instrument called the Caseload Matrix© (not presented in this article). (For information, contact Craig.)
Concordance	Agreement; a statistical calculation that measures the agreement among sets of rankings by two. Interrater reliability (below) tests seek high concordance or levels of agreement between ratings done by different users at the same or different times of use.
Dosage-prescription; CM intervention dosage	The amount, frequency, duration, and breadth of actual activities used in an intervention, as a unique combination of discrete provider actions, at a level of intensity (amount and frequency), over a duration of time. A prescribed dosage of CM includes the quantity, activity, and timing of an intervention or a set of interventions with a known effect or predictable outcome.
Drivers	Groups of CM practice factors in the Acuity Tool© that link the three indicator categories to the discrete-level subdrivers. The driver–subdriver combinations "drive" acuity up or down by indicating elements that make each CM case complicated.
Cross-validation tests	Statistical tests that assess the predictive accuracy of a model in a test sample. Assessment scrutiny that confirms a test or measurement works the same or generates the same results when applied in different situations.
Indicators	The broadest, most inclusive category of the elements in the Acuity Tool©. Indicators appear as the three column headers in the tool: Clinical/Nursing, Psychosocial/ Caregiver, and Quality/Cost. Derived from the clinical, satisfaction, and business aspects that span all CM activities.
Intensity	A term related to acuity that represents both the amount of care and the complexity of care needed by patients or clients. Prescott (1991) identified four major dimensions to intensity: severity of illness, client dependency, complexity, and time. Acuity includes the concept of CM intervention-intensity that should match the need-severity of the client.
Isostatic differentials or flat-line differentials	Refers to case acuity scores that were unchanged from commencement to closure. A stagnant effect in which acuities failed to change from opening to closing. "Flat-lined" differences in acuity scores usually occurred in cases that had reached recovery plateau stages. Isostatic differentials occurred less often in comparison with the usual pattern (higher at opening than closing) of acuity differentials.

Term	Definition
Outliers	Data that lie an abnormal distance from centric values in a random sample from a population. Any value that is markedly smaller or larger than other values.
Reverse acuity	The reverse pattern of acuities that scored higher at closure than at opening. Standard acuity differential patterns are higher at commencement than closure.
Interrater reliability (IRR) tests (random and blinded)	A statistical measure of agreement between raters at the same ("of raters") or between one rate measured at different times ("over time"). *Blinding* refers to performing the IRR test without knowledge of the responses of other raters. Answers were provided solely on the blinded and random presentation of the samples to those being tested without bias from knowledge of how other testers responded to the samples. *Random* refers to the process of mixing that shields identifiers that would provide foreknowledge, clues, or bias about the answers that others have given or about the subject under consideration.
Subdrivers	The elements that most closely identify the specific factors generating complexity in a CM case. Subdrivers relate to times for tasks, numbers and complexity of interventions, levels of self-care and caregiver support systems, and appropriate setting and provider components that differ for individual clients at various times. The driver–subdriver combinations "drive" the acuity score up or down by indicating elements that make each CM case complicated.

Professional Case Management
Vol. 13, No. 5, 253–261

FASTER THAN A SPEEDING BULLET

Changes in Medicare Rules for the Hospital Case Manager

Stefani Daniels, MSNA, RN, ACM, CMAC, and Marianne Ramey, RN, ACM, CPUR

ABSTRACT

Purpose/objectives: Compliance with the various Centers for Medicare & Medicaid Services rules and regulations is rapidly becoming a challenge in hospitals as the frequency and complexity of the new mandates have increased. Although compliance officers may oversee major elements emanating from the regulatory agencies, practical application during routine work activities requires current information and peer-to-peer reinforcement. This article addresses some of the more recent changes—or proposed changes—that may impact hospital case management practice and the case managers' role as patient advocate.

Primary practice setting(s): The settings include acute care hospitals, short-stay hospitals, long-term acute care hospitals, and critical access hospitals.

Findings/conclusions: The more information hospital case managers have about the regulatory changes that affect the hospital, its patients, physicians, and associates, the better they can serve as sources of information, resources, and advocates.

Implications for case management practice:
- Direct interactions between the case manager and the physician are the best opportunities to share information.
- Influencing medical documentation at the point of service will be dependent upon the case managers' ability to link documentation improvements with benefits for the physician.
- Hospital-Issued Notice of Noncoverage letters are tools that warrant the case managers' attention to protect the patient and the hospital against financial risk.

Key words: case management, CMS, HINN, HAC, Medicare, OIG, POA, ABN

Address correspondence to Stefani Daniels, MSNA, RN, ACM, CMAC, Phoenix Medical Management, Inc, 1401 S Ocean Blvd, Pompano Beach, FL 33062 (daniels@ phoenixmed.net). staying current with CMS requirements presents the greatest challenge to HCMs.

Nothing changes as fast as healthcare. Just when you thought you knew everything you had to know to do your job well, someone goes and changes the rules. Hospital case managers (HCMs), whose scope of practice straddles both the clinical and financial worlds of healthcare, confront changes on a daily basis. Internally, initiatives to strengthen work efficiencies, leverage economies of scale, and moderate costs are underway whereas staff shortages, physician practices, and new consumer expectations thwart the case managers' efforts to swiftly move the patient through the acute continuum. Externally, sponsoring agencies propose strategies to advance quality and access, modify payer policies, switch preferred providers, introduce new reimbursement rules, and revise regulatory demands, all of which require the mind of an Einstein to keep current.

In 2006, the Centers for Medicare & Medicaid Services (CMS) was the payer for 55.9% of inpatient hospital stays. As the primary payer, the CMS places heavy burdens on the financial performance of hospitals and CMS endorsement as a Medicare provider, vis-à-vis The Joint Commission accreditation, can make or break a hospital. Compounding the CMS influence is the Office of Inspector General (OIG), which serves as the investigatory arm of the CMS and is charged with making sure that Medicare and Medicaid service providers comply with all regulatory requirements. To get an idea of the scope of the OIG's scrutiny, log onto http://www.oig.hhs.gov/publica tions/docs/workplan/2008/Work_Plan_FY_2008.pdf for a copy of the 2008 OIG work plan. Single-handedly, the CMS accounts for the vast majority of "changes" hospitals must comply with. From rules relating to coding and billing procedures, new or changing beneficiary benefits, or additions and revisions to the Conditions of Participation,

For those of you who are trying to keep up with the changes initiated by the CMS, consider this to be a survival guide of sorts. We will try to help you navigate through the morass of new regulations and new procedures, which directly impact many case management programs and the customers they serve. Note that the nature and intensity of the impact will be in direct proportion to each hospital's case management program purpose, model, and scope of practice, and remember, by the time this gets published, the rules may change again!

MEDICARE SEVERITY ADJUSTED DIAGNOSTIC RELATED GROUPS

Medicare Severity Adjusted Diagnostic Related Groups (MS-DRG) is the grand-daddy of all the recent changes and in its potential impact on the hospital, the most dramatic. The CMS has restructured the current 538 DRGs to 745 MS-DRGs to better recognize severity of patient illness. It is thought that MS-DRGs will more accurately capture resource utilization by splitting a large number of current DRGs into three different categories based on the presence or absence of diagnoses classified as "major complication or comorbidities" (MCC), "complications or comorbidities" (CC), or "without MCC/CC" (non-CC).

What Does It Mean for the HCM?

This is probably the most significant change in reimbursement methodology since the introduction of the DRG payment system in 1983. The new reimbursement plan keeps the burden squarely on the hospital because physician reimbursement is not affected. Although Medicare claims that it will be revenue-neutral, analysts predict that hospitals' revenue stream will be either positively or negatively affected on the basis of case mix and levels of severity. In other words, payments would increase for hospitals serving more severely ill patients and decrease for serving patients who are less severely ill. To get the same or increased payment under the new MS-DRG system, clinical documentation and accurate coding will be key.

HCMs work closely with Clinical Documentation Improvement Program (CDIP) specialists. In hospitals where there is a real-time partnership between the case manager and the physician, query sheets about the medical documentation improvement opportunities are replaced with direct interactions. Regardless of vertical alignment of the CDIP specialists (are they working under the Health Information Management department, the Finance department, or the Case Management department?), there must be an avenue of regular communication between the CDIP specialists and the HCMs. In addition, HCMs should consider interpersonal communication tactics to motivate better medical documentation. A physician rarely responds to the plea for better documentation "so the hospital gets more reimbursement." Instead, the HCMs must ask themselves, "What incentive exists for the physician to spend more time in order to provide high quality documentation?"

Beyond the issue that good documentation is evidence of good quality care, the HCM must ask "what's in it for the physician?" Today and into tomorrow, the issues of pay for performance, provider selection, and public reporting are here to stay. The "boomer" generation patients, as active consumers of healthcare services, are predicted to expect and, in fact, demand ready access to comparative information to guide their healthcare choices. Good documentation leading to accurate coding will not only ensure appropriate hospital reimbursement but also aid in accurate data on physician performance. Although public reporting of physician-level performance data has been limited, it seems inevitable that it will increase. Just as hospital report cards are now available for public scrutiny, sooner, more than later, physician performance outcomes are sure to follow.

Buried in the new reimbursement rules, and lesser known, is a disclosure requirement. The rule requires written disclosure of physician ownership or investment interest in the hospital and the hospital must *provide the names of the physician owners upon request*. In addition, the rule requires a hospital to notify all patients in writing if a doctor of medicine or a doctor of osteopathy is not present in the hospital 24 hours a day, 7 days per week, and describe how the hospital will meet the medical needs of a patient who develops an emergency condition while no doctor is on site. The CMS has the authority to terminate a provider agreement for non-compliance with these disclosure requirements.

PRESENT ON ADMISSION

Every year, millions of Americans suffer needlessly from preventable hospital-acquired complications such as infections and medical errors. *Present on Admission* (*POA*) is a new policy adopted by the CMS that is effective October 2008. Essentially, it means that, unless there is documentation at the time of admission evidencing the presence of one of the listed hospital-acquired conditions (HACs), the CMS will no longer pay hospitals for the extra costs of treating these preventable errors, injuries, and infections. Put another way, if the condition arises as a result of the hospitalization itself, rather than any pre-existing or newly diagnosed condition, the hospital will not be reimbursed for the costs of treating the condition. The POA reimbursement rules are a good beginning for Medicare to use its clout to mobilize hospitals to improve care and keep patients safe. The CMS is targeting 11 preventable injuries:

1. Serious preventable event—objects left during surgery
2. Serious preventable event—air embolism
3. Serious preventable event—blood incompatibility
4. Catheter-associated urinary tract infections
5. Pressure ulcers (decubitus ulcers)
6. Vascular catheter-associated infection
7. Surgical site infection—mediastinitis after coronary artery bypass graft surgery
8. Hospital-acquired injuries—fractures, dislocations, intracranial injury, crushing injury, burn, and other unspecified effects of external causes

9. Surgical site infections following certain elective orthopedic procedures
10. Extreme blood glucose derangement in diabetics 11. Deep vein thrombosis/pulmonary embolism (formation/movement of a blood clot) following total knee & hip replacement

What Does It Mean for HCM?

Under the new rules, which went into full effect on April 1, 2008, severity of illness will be determined based only on what is documented at the time of admission, as opposed to the time of discharge, which is the current standard. Under POA rules, conditions that develop during an outpatient encounter, including emergency department, observation, or outpatient surgery are considered present on admission. Consistent and complete documentation is necessary to determine whether a condition is present on admission. In fact, many hospitals are performing screening surveillance and documentation improvement initiatives at the point of entry to capture all pre-existing conditions. This documentation must come from the provider, the physician, or the qualified healthcare practitioner who is legally responsible for establishing the patient's diagnosis. As with other diagnosis determinants based on medical documentation, POA information may not be gleaned from case manager documentation, although a query may be initiated in cases where documentation is inconsistent, missing, conflicting, or unclear.

Many HCMs are positioned to motivate better admission documentation, so it is evident that the diagnosis was present on admission. Emergency department notes, history and physician, or the admitting progress notes can be used. By making sure the information is documented at the time of admission, the physician will not be bothered by postdischarge queries. For example, a physician who includes a decubitus ulcer diagnosis in the history and physician would not need to be queried by a coding professional later. If the decubitus is not documented until the third day, the physician should note in the documentation that it was present at the time of admission.

It is the HCM's role as a patient advocate that has greater import to prevent nonreimbursable events. If HCMs are to serve as chief advocates and acute care navigators, they must also be quality ambassadors. It is their ethical obligation to question the rationale for certain medical practices. Under a

POA scenario, maintaining an indwelling catheter, for example, for convenience is not in the best interest of the patient. Neither is prolonged bed rest for the frail elderly, which significantly reduces functionality, making patients more prone to falls. This is another instance where making rounds with the physicians and nurses to help manage the patient benefits every stakeholder. For more information on POA log onto http://www.cms.hhs.gov/Hospital AcqCond/.

DURABLE MEDICAL EQUIPMENT, PROSTHETICS, ORTHOTICS, AND SUPPLIES

If you practice in 1 of the 10 communities selected as Phase 1 for the *Durable Medical Equipment, Prosthetics, Orthotics, and Supplies* (*DMEPOS*) project, then your discharge planning associate will be contacting 1 of the 325 suppliers who, through competitive bidding, have contracts with Medicare to provide supplies at lowest costs. The new program, which begins on July 2008 and will expand to 70 areas in the country in 2009, means that if Medicare beneficiaries need items such as hospital beds, glucose monitors, oxygen, and wheelchairs and the like, the new list of providers must be used. For a complete listing in your community, log onto http://www.medicare.gov/Supplier/Static/About/ DMEPOS.asp?dest=NAV|Home|AboutSupplier Directory|DME-POS#TabTop.

What Does It Mean for the HCM?

Post–acute care provider choice has been the hallmark of good post–acute care planning needs. Under the DMEPOS project, this choice will be honored as long as it is among those suppliers with current contracts with Medicare. Patients who choose to use suppliers outside of the contracted network may be both asked to sign an advanced beneficiary notice (ABN) and financially responsible for the expense, though there is a process where a current provider may apply to become a "grandfathered" supplier. HCMs should make sure they document the discussion with the patient/family concerning vendor selection. HCMs working in the demonstration communities should take the time to identify Medicare's contracted providers and instruct support staff accordingly. Educating patients, families, and physicians about patient choice and all its ramifications, continues to be an important component

of the HCM's role. This new rule does nothing to diminish that obligation.

HOSPITAL CONSUMER ASSESSMENT OF HEALTHCARE PROVIDERS AND SYSTEMS

Hospital Consumer Assessment of Healthcare Providers and Systems (*HCAHPS*) is a patient satisfaction survey supported by the CMS. In an age of new transparency, patients' perception of their experience with a hospital will now be reported with other quality metrics. The tool is a standardized, national patient survey, allowing public sharing of comparable data across acute care hospitals.

There are two stand-alone questions:

1. What number would you use to rate this hospital during your stay? (0 ! worst, 10 ! best)
2. Would you recommend this hospital to your friends and family?

The survey also asks two to three questions each from seven categories:

1. Communication with doctors
2. Communication with nurses
3. Communication about medicines
4. Cleanliness and quietness of physical environment
5. Discharge information
6. Pain control
7. Responsiveness of hospital staff

What Does It Mean for the HCM?

The CMS issued a rule stating that hospitals that are eligible for an annual payment update must submit their HCAHPS data or forfeit 2% of their annual reimbursement adjustment. The financial penalty varies from hospital to hospital on the basis of a number of factors, but it could be substantial. This approach to reimbursement may be the start of a more global payment process that ties reimbursement to quality outcomes. This new mandate is an opportunity to develop some scripting of conversations that address the seven categories that will be monitored, especially communication and discharge information. The "asking" must be linked with "actions" taken to address any dissatisfaction that may be uncovered. The HCM is in the perfect position to facilitate communication that will result in improved satisfaction and outcomes.

THE CARE INSTRUMENT

The Medicare Continuity Assessment Record and Evaluation (CARE) is a uniform patient assessment instrument designed to measure differences in patient severity, resource utilization, and outcomes for patients in acute care and post–acute care settings. The assessment is initiated at the acute level of care, and then the form accompanies the patient upon discharge to a post–acute care facility including nursing homes, home health agencies, and long-term care hospitals. The assessment form is an Internet-based tool developed by Northrup Grummon. Research Triangle International is managing the current demonstration project to test its effectiveness.

What Does It Mean for the HCM?

Although it is technically in the "demonstration" phase, this is one new regulation that actually makes sense! The CMS intends to eliminate all the legacy assessment forms (MDS, OASIS, etc) and use the single CARE format to measure change over the entire continuum beginning at the acute level of care. Because it is a Web-based tool, it is anticipated that the demographic information will be automatically populated, and, based on your hospital information system, clinical information may cross over as well. Case management leaders are urged to work with nursing, ancillary providers, and a hospital information system liaison to take full advantage of electronic capabilities to reduce manual data entries. This is also a great opportunity to review current patient assessment tools used in other provider areas that are often redundant and seek opportunities to condense, combine, and consolidated these tools to reduce redundancies and improve accuracy, compliance, and continuity.

MEDICAL NECESSITY FOR HOSPITAL ADMISSIONS

The CMS has revamped its set of *Hospital-Issued Notices of Noncoverage (HINNs)*, which inform patients of any potential financial liability if they receive services that are not medically necessary, are custodial in nature, or can be provided in another level of care such as at home with home healthcare or in a skilled nursing facility. Medicare does not cover these services, nor will it reimburse the hospital if the patient is no longer deemed eligible for acute care or if the hospital does not believe hospitalization is required. The HINN forms have undergone many iterations. The

following are the current forms for inpatients and observation/outpatients:

1. *Preadmission or Admission Hospital-Issued Notice of Noncoverage* replaces HINNs 1 and 9 and is used before a noncovered stay. The hospital should notify the patient that Medicare is not likely to pay for the admission because it is not considered to be medically necessary or it could be furnished safely in another setting. This form is especially helpful in social admission situations. Download form and sample notices at: www.cms.hhs.gov/BNI/downloads/PreadmissionadmissionHINN.pdf.

2. *Hospital-Requested Review (HRR)* notifies patients that the hospital has determined that the patient no longer meets Medicare criteria for a continued stay because the services are no longer medically necessary, *but the physician disagrees*. The HRR notifies the patient that the hospital is asking the quality improvement organization (QIO) to review the case and that the QIO will be contacting the patient to discuss the case. Download form and sample notices at: www.cms.hhs.gov/BNI/downloads/noticeofhos-pitalrequestedreview.pdf.

3. *HINN-11, Noncovered Services During a Covered Stay*, notifies Medicare beneficiaries that a diagnostic or therapeutic item or service may not be covered on the basis of medical necessity, but the patient still requires continued acute level of care. For example, if a patient comes in with an exacerbation of chronic obstructive pulmonary disease and the physician orders a mammogram for the patient's convenience. The item or the service must not be bundled into payment or treatment for the diagnosis that justified the inpatient stay. HINN-11 confirms the patient's acceptance of financial liability for the noncovered service, item, or procedure. Hospitals must give a copy to the patient, his or her physician, and to the QIO upon request. Download form and sample notices at: www.cms.hhs.gov/transmittals/downloads/R982CP.pdf.

4. The HINN-12, *Noncovered Continued Stay Notice*, is a new notice, which became effective July 2007 and notifies patients that the hospital believes Medicare may not continue to pay for their hospital stay beginning on a certain date. The notice states the reason in easy-to-understand language, and a statement from the business office estimating the cost of continued stay is included. The notice also encourages the patient to discuss

his or her pending discharge with the physician. Download form and sample notices at: www. cms.hhs.gov/BNI/downloads/HINN12non coveredcontinuedstay.pdf.

5. Medicare Advantage enrollees receive *Notice of Discharge and Medicare Appeal Rights (NOD-MAR)* once it is determined that inpatient hospital care is no longer necessary. If beneficiaries disagree with the hospital determination and remain in the hospital, they may immediately request that a QIO perform a review to determine if the issuance of the NODMAR was appropriate.

What Does It Mean for HCM?

Gatekeeping is quickly becoming a significant component of every hospital's case management program. Whether through the presence of an emergency department case manager or a formal patient access center, combining preadmission/admission medical necessity monitoring with bed management, gatekeeping systems to determine level of care and stem the loss of revenue is essential. The use of a preadmission/admission HINN is a significant tool in the effort to stop financial hemorrhaging, and, according to the Medicare manual, there is *no need* to obtain the admitting physician's concurrence, *nor do you have to notify the QIO* if the patient's SI/IS does not qualify for acute level of care. However, either the attending physician or the QIO must concur in order to issue an HRR, HINN 11, or HINN 12 for a service or continuing stay that the hospital believes will not be covered by Medicare.

HINN is not a popular strategy in many hospitals. Either administration is not aware of the practice or it is reluctant to implement it. The HCM leader should confirm administration's position on its use before initiating the practice. Even with the endorsement of the executive team and case management medical advisor, HCMs are often hesitant or reluctant to issue notices of noncoverage. Although no one wants to be the "bad guy," it is usually the HCM who must recognize and enforce Medicare requirements. Because the regulations have changed, it is good time to review the organizations utilization review plan to clarify processes and responsibilities and ensure compliance.

ADVANCED BENEFICIARY NOTICES

An *ABN* is a written notice from Medicare given to observation/outpatient patients before receiving services or items notifying them that Medicare may deny payment for a specific service, treatment, or procedure and that the beneficiary will be personally responsible for full payment if Medicare does deny payment. A single, revised ABN form went into effect on March 3, 2008, and replaces the previous ABN-G (Form CMS-R-131G), ABN-L (Form CMS-R-131L), and Notice of Exclusion from Medicare Benefits form (NEMB CMS-20007) (http://www.cms.hhs.gov/BNI/02_ABNGABNL.asp).

What Does It Mean for the Case Manager?

The ABN is used in situations where Part B provider and supplier services may not be covered by Medicare. This form is typically used for ambulatory outpatient services, but is also applicable among the growing observation population. Oftentimes, HCMs confront patients or families that insist on a full inpatient admission, although diagnosis remains vague or has not been identified as requiring acute level of care. The ABN form must be signed by the beneficiary, but if the patient refuses, the hospital may legitimately decide not to provide the items or services or a second person may witness the patient's refusal to sign the agreement and the service or treatment can be provided. The form is not required until September 1, 2008, but can be used immediately.

THE IMPORTANT MESSAGE FROM MEDICARE

Effective July 2, 2007, hospitals must deliver a revised version of the *Important Message from Medicare (IM)* to inform Medicare beneficiaries who are hospital inpatients about their hospital discharge appeal rights. Notice is required both for original Medicare beneficiaries and for those enrolled in Medicare Advantage health plans. In addition to a revised version of the IM, hospitals are now required to issue a duplicate of the notice to the patient no less than 2 days before discharge.

What Does It Mean for the HCM?

More than any other revised regulation, this probably had the greatest practical impact on HCMs. For years, hospital admission departments were responsible for issuing the IM—typically during the registration process. Even if the patient registration was delayed for whatever reason, admission personnel had to make sure that the patient/designee signed for the receipt of the notice that described the beneficiary rights to receive necessary care. The revised version, which grew out of a lawsuit filed against Medicare (*Weichardt v. Leavitt*, 2003)[1], includes wording to indicate that the patient has a right to appeal decisions about continued stay and includes language about how to appeal or request a review of the decision to be discharged. The new rules accompanying the revised IM requires that a duplicate of the notice must be given to the patient no more than 48 hr before discharge. It was this new requirement that caught hospital executives off-guard. What had been regarded as a perfunctory distribution requirement, took on new significance because the duplicate form was now tied to a discharge date. With so many disciplines potentially involved in discharge planning activities, and without any hard and fast rule about implementation, the question of distribution responsibility created widespread confusion among patients and hospital staff. Hospital admission departments claimed they would continue to be responsible for the initial notice, but could not do the follow-up notice because they had no idea of the patient's targeted discharge date. Also, nursing no longer saw themselves as keeper of the discharge plan, given the presence of case managers and nursing's irregular staffing schedules. With the deadline for implementation quickly advancing, many hospitals assigned distribution of the duplicate notice to the case management program, even in hospitals where not every patient required a case manager. Hospitals with greater resources either used volunteer staff or hired additional full-time equivalents to manage this unfunded mandate. To date, no one "best practice" has emerged and distribution of the duplicate notice remains problematic.

ACUTE CARE EPISODE

The CMS has proposed a new demonstration project that will bundle hospital reimbursement with physician reimbursement. The *Acute Care Episode* program with merge Part A and Part B payments to create a global payment for 28 cardiac and 9 orthopedic inpatient surgical services. These elective procedures were selected because profit margins and volume have historically been high, there is sufficient marketplace competition to ensure interested demonstration applicants, the services are easy to specify, and quality metrics are available for them. The demonstration project will take place in selected value-based care centers chosen from applicants in Oklahoma, Texas, New Mexico, and Colorado.

What Does It Mean for the HCM?

Currently, the CMS generally pays the hospital a single prospectively determined amount under the Inpatient Prospective Payment System for all the care it furnishes to the patient during an inpatient stay. The physicians who care for the patient during the stay are paid separately under the Medicare Physician Fee Schedule for each service they perform. The separate payment systems have always been a source of conflicting incentives that may affect decisions about what care will be ordered by the physician. Case managers working with physicians participating in this demonstration will be relying on their resource management skills more than ever to ensure that the patient is receiving services appropriate for an acute level of care.

RECOVERY AUDIT CONTRACTORS

Use of *recovery audit contractors* (*RACs*) is the latest strategy initiated by Medicare to reign in the excessive costs of healthcare. Authorized as a demonstration project by the Medicare Modernization Act of 2003,[2] RACs are private sector auditing firms contracted by the CMS to examine claims filed by hospitals and other medical providers. They were initially established in California, New York, and Florida, which account for more than 25% of Medicare spending. Under the Medicare Integrity Program, RACs must demonstrate success in (1) identifying underpayments and overpayments and (2) recouping overpayments under the Medicare program (for services for which payment is made under Part A or Part B of Title XVII of the Social Security Act). The CMS pays the RACs a contingency fee of approximately 22¢ for every recovered dollar. In fiscal year 2007, auditors identified $357 million in overpayments, $17.8 million or 7.1% of which were overturned on appeal, according to the CMS. Payments for contingency fees and other administrative expenses totaled $77.7 million. Auditors also found $14.3 million in Medicare underpayments. Up until recently, no incentive was present for the RACs to identify underpayments, but beginning with under-payments identified on or after March 1, 2006, the RACs will receive an equivalent percentage for all underpayment and overpayment identifications. The success of the RAC initiative resulted in expansion of the program nationwide (http://www.cms.hhs.gov/RAC/).

What Does It Mean for the HCM?

The RAC demonstration is the first time the Medicare program has ever paid a contractor on a contingency basis. It has been argued that this "bounty hunter" payment scheme creates perverse incentives to deny as many claims as possible and place the burden on providers to appeal these denials.

According to reports from hospitals in demonstration states New York, California, and Florida, the impact of the RAC audits is enormous. They have three main target areas: medical necessity for acute care and rehabilitation admissions; short-stay admissions level of care; and coding compliance. The process is arduous, and hospitals, depending upon its size, report that they have had to designate or hire personnel just to track the RAC review, repayment, and appeal processes. RAC teams as subgroups of the hospital's revenue cycle teams are not uncommon.

Although the RAC program is a financial program, depending upon your program structure, the HCM model, and scope of practice, the implications for case management may be broad. If your case management program includes gatekeeping systems to ensure that patients are qualified for inpatient stays or appropriately diverted to observation units, medical documentation improvement programs to promote accurate coding, capture of the correct disposition code, or applying evidence-based protocols for high-volume short stays (e.g., chest pain, congestive heart failure, back pain, gastroenteritis), then you can count on being involved in the RAC process as it expands to other states.

As of this writing, there is pending legislation to place a moratorium on the expansion of the RAC program. The Capps/Nunes bill-HR 4105 proposes to put a 1-year moratorium on further audits until expressed concerns about the process are resolved. Given the RAC's success in recovering money for the Medicare hospital-insurance trust fund, there is little expectation for the bill's passage.

NEW COVERAGE FOR DIALYSIS CENTERS

For the first time since 1976, Medicare has changed the *conditions of coverage for the 4,700 dialysis centers* currently certified by Medicare. The CMS reported that the new rules focus on patient rights, patient safety, and participation of patients with end-stage renal disease in developing a plan of care. Under the new rule, each facility is required to develop a quality assessment and performance improvement program, which will track a facility's performance in a patient's healthcare outcomes. The new rules promote broader use of computerized records to track patient care and encourage providers to follow nationally recognized standards.

What Does It Mean for the HCM?

Case managers often feel as though they are on the outside looking in when it comes to the care and services delivered by post–acute care providers. It often difficult to assess the quality of care being delivered beyond anecdotal accounts from patients and families. Part of the HCMs responsibility is to determine if post–acute care providers are indeed meeting the patients' needs and that they are satisfied with those services. Follow-up phone calls are a good way to assess whether or not the quality of these services meet expectations. Feedback about patient concerns should be given to the provider, and, if no action is taken to correct the issue, it may be necessary to report findings to the appropriate regulatory and licensing agencies. Involve your organization's risk and quality mangers whenever quality-of-care issues arise, regardless of the where the care is being delivered.

VALUE-BASED PURCHASING

The CMS is proposing a hospital *Value-Based Purchasing (VBP)* program that will link hospital reimbursement to performance outcomes. Also known as P4P (payment for performance), VBP projects have been underway since 2006 and have demonstrated success. It is the intent of the CMS to transform Medicare from a passive payer of claims to an active purchaser of high-quality, efficient care starting October 2008. Hospitals would be required to submit data on all quality measures applicable to their patient populations and service mix to qualify for the VBP program incentive payment. According to the American Hospital Association, the CMS would annually assess each hospital's performance and assign the hospital a performance rating for each measure. The incentive payment would be based on the rate of improvement for each measure.

What Does It Mean for the HCM?

In 2003, the CMS teamed with Premier to initiate a hospital quality incentive demonstration project to determine whether financial incentives are effective in raising the quality of hospital care. More than 260 hospitals participated and the results were published in various journals. Whether through case management involvement, use of protocol coordinators or documentation improvement specialists, patient management by hospitalists, new interest on evidence-based medicine, or any combination of these supporting variables, the CMS announced an overall quality increase of 11.8% on the basis of delivery of more that 25 quality measures.

Effective October 1, 2008, the CMS will begin a 3-year-plus phased VBP implementation plan under which incentives will be paid to top performers. These incentives will be based on quality measures performance, *not just reporting*. Organizations that do not meet specified performance standards will lose reimbursement. Physician-centric hospital case management models have the advantage of case managers working in partnership with physicians on a day-today basis. Whether assigned to specific physicians, service lines, or geographic areas, working alongside targeted physicians is probably the best strategy to promote *sustainable* change in physician practice behaviors and medical documentation improvement. A large portion of the hospital's revenue is going to be determined on outcomes, and as the CMS goes, so probably will commercial contracts follow. It is not enough to have a "good relationship" with members of the medical staff; it is now essential that partnerships are formed. Only in a trusting, respected partnership can one member influence the other, and in today's highly volatile hospital climate, influencing physician practice

decisions at the point of service is key to clinical and financial success.

Accessing the CMS Web site (http://www.cms.hhs.gov/home/tools.asp) can help the HCMs stay current. On the tools page, you can sign up for various mailing lists or access information related to your case management specialty. One of the resources we recommend is the federal *Quarterly Provider Update* that is published every month (http://www.cms.hhs.gov/quarterlyproviderupdates/emailupdates/ItemDetail.asp?ItemID!CMS1210830). The update reviews all the new regulations and rules proposed or issued and covers a wide variety of CMS services. By signing up, subscribers are immediately notified via e-mail of any regulations or program instructions released during the quarter that affect Medicare providers.

Another helpful resource is the Medicare Learning Network, a series of national articles designed to inform the physician, provider, and supplier community about the latest changes to the Medicare program. Articles are prepared in consultation with clinicians, billing experts, and CMS subject matter experts and are tailored in content and language to the specific provider type(s) who is affected by a particular Medicare change (http://www.cms.hhs.gov/MLNMattersArticles).

Several other CMS initiatives are in process or waiting in the wings. Many of them may not have direct or even indirect impact on hospital case management practice. Nevertheless, as the one group of hospital associates with interest in both clinical and financial excellence, it is important to stay current.

About the Authors

Stefani Daniels, MSNA, RN, ACM, CMAC, is the president and managing partner of Phoenix Medical Management, Inc and is the coauthor of the popular text *The Leader's Guide to Hospital Case Management*.

Marianne Ramey, RN, ACM, CPUR, is a partner at Phoenix Medical Management, Inc., specializing in case management program redesign and interim management and is the coauthor of the popular text *The Leader's Guide to Hospital Case Management*.

Notes

1. Weichardt v. Leavitt (C03-05490 VRW [N.D.Cal.]). CMS Manual System, Transmittal 1257, May 25, 2007. The Weichardt v. Leavitt class action lawsuit filed on December 5, 2003 contested the legitimacy of hospital notice procedures. A settlement agreement was signed on October 28, 2005 whereby CMS agreed to publication

of a proposed, and then a final rule setting forth revised discharge notice requirements for hospital inpatients who have Medicare. The Final Rule CMS-4105-F was published on November 27, 2006.
2. For more information on the Medicare Modernization Act (2003) go to http://www.cms.hhs.gov/mmaupdate/

Professional Case Management
Vol. 12, No. 2, 83–90

Designing a System of Case Management for a Rural Nursing Clinic for Elderly Patients With Depression

Marietta P. Stanton, PhD, RN, C, CNAA, BC, CMAC, CCM,
Jeri W. Dunkin, PhD, RN, CHCE, and L. Kathleen Williams Thomas, MS, FNP

ABSTRACT

This article provides an overview of the process and procedures used to develop and implement a system of case management for middle-aged and older depressed adults in a rural health nursing clinic. This system included on-site case management for elderly clients and telephonic follow-up by case managers on an ongoing basis.

This purpose of this article is to describe a pilot project for implementing a case management service for a cohort of rural elderly with depression at a rural nursing health center. The processes, tools, and procedures issued in the project are included for potential replication and modification. By re-creating similar services in other rural environments, case managers can continue to validate the cost-effectiveness and quality of care that is a product of these services. This will improve healthcare services for vulnerable rural populations, not just in the elderly, but also across the age continuum.

The management of chronic illness presents unique challenges within and among rural regions (Scott, 2000). These challenges have been addressed in several reports and initiatives. The reports provide direction and focus for improving healthcare for vulnerable populations especially in rural areas. In 2001, the Institute of Medicine (IOM) released the report *Crossing the Quality Chasm: A New Health System for the 21st Century*. Based on a large body of evidence documenting severe problems in the American healthcare system, the report identifies six aims for quality improvement. These are that healthcare should be:

1. Safe: prevents harm to patients (IOM, 2004).
2. Effective: refers to care that is evidence-based (IOM, 2001).
3. Patient-centered: addresses care that reflects the qualities of compassion, empathy, and responsiveness to the needs, values, and expressed preferences of the individual patient (IOM, 2001).
4. Timely: considers access to care as a critical factor influencing the quality of rural healthcare (IOM, 2001).
5. Efficient: refers to optimizing resources and minimizing waste to obtain the best value for investments in healthcare services and administration (IOM, 2001).
6. Equitable: ensures that the availability of care and quality services is based on an individual's healthcare needs and not on personal

characteristics such as gender, ethnicity, geographic location, and socioeconomic status (IOM, 2001).

The 2001 IOM report helped launch the Quality Chasm Initiative with a series of meetings where reports about healthcare were produced. In 2004, the report *Quality Through Collaboration: The Future of Rural Health* (2004) was published. In this report there was a series of key factors and recommendations. As to outcomes, the IOM committee developed a five-pronged strategy pertaining to health to address the related quality challenges in rural communities (IOM, 2004). The components of this strategy are that rural healthcare (IOM, 2004):

1. Adopt an integrated and prioritized approach to addressing both personal and population needs at the community level.
2. Establish a strong quality improvement support structure to improve quality.
3. Enhance the human resource capacity of rural communities including the education training and deployment of healthcare professionals.
4. Monitor rural health systems to ensure that they are financially stable.
5. Invest in building an information infrastructure.

The authors have no conflict of interest.

Address correspondence to Marietta P. Stanton, PhD, RN,C, CNAA,BC, CMAC, CCM, Capstone College of Nursing, University at Alabama, Box 870358, Tuscaloosa, AL 35487 (mstanton@bama.ua.edu).

This report has direct implications for rural health-care and underscores the important potential role of case management in rural healthcare.

LITERATURE REVIEW

Stanton and Packa (2001) proposed a model to provide case management for rural populations. This model incorporated the unique characteristics of rural populations; the quality, functional, clinical satisfaction, and financial outcome indicators that provide a gauge for the efficiency and effectiveness of rural case management processes; and the essential components of the case management process that would specifically address their healthcare needs. Stanton and Dunkin (2002) explored the unique characteristics of the rural case managers. Their research indicated that rural case management required a skill set more complex than those used in

urban settings and that case managers functioning as rural case managers needed at a minimum graduate-level preparation. Case management in rural settings has been shown to have a positive effect on healthcare outcomes (Barney, Rosenthal, & Speier, 2004), especially if the location and coordination of services are consistent with the needs of the rural population. Rural case management for chronic illness has the potential to impact outcomes if the program recognizes

a. characteristics of the population at risk;
b. characteristics of the health case delivery system in the rural setting;
c. current utilization of healthcare services by the population of rural persons with chronic illnesses;
d. perception of the healthcare system to rural persons with chronic illness; and
e. local and national health policy issues as they relate to the delivery of healthcare in rural settings (Scott, 2000).

Barney, Rosenthal, and Speier (2004) also found that there were important components when providing rural case management in their research. Case management was a success if the organization possessed positive attributes, such as good location, strong coordination of services, and support for professionals, that contributed to a positive case management experience for both staff and patients. In addition, the case manager required the knowledge, professional skills, and values, coupled with personal capabilities to practice in the rural setting. Silberman, Poley, James, and Slifkin (2002) found that case/disease management programs in a rural environment improved outcomes and compliance of Medicaid recipients with care regimens. Similarly, case management has proved to be an effective strategy to enhance outcomes with rural veterans (Ritchie, Wieland, Tully, Prachoda, et al., 2002).

In summary:

• case management has been found to be effective in enhancing outcomes in the rural environment,
• case management demands a different set of skills in the rural environment,
• case management needs to address the unique characteristics and requirements of rural residents and the rural healthcare environment, and
• the components of the case management process need tailoring to meet the needs of individuals in the rural environment.

DEVELOPMENT OF CASE MANAGEMENT IN THE RURAL CLINIC SETTING

Although there is much supportive research about what is needed in the rural setting for case management, there is little operational level information or guidance as to how to design, implement, and evaluate a case management program in the rural environment. Mullahy and Jensen (2004) and Swanson, Baker, Stanton, Godec, and Patton (2005) outline a process and goals for developing and implementing a case management program within a system. These goals include

1. establishing a case management information system (CMIS);
2. establishing standard outcomes and metrics;
3. establishing a model for case management services;
4. establishing senior case management leadership, mentoring, and operating procedures; and
5. achieving "buy-in" for the organizational innovation.

These components for developing a case management system have been used in the implementation of case management for a rural nurse-managed clinic. The initial group of patients was the elderly clients experiencing depression as their primary diagnosis. This article will demonstrate how this development process was adapted for a nurse-managed clinic. The group of patients selected to participate in a pilot program were selected because they have complex health problems and have a high rate of nonadherence with medications and plans of care.

A system of case management included one full-time on-site nurse practitioner dual hatted as an on-site case manager. The nurse practitioner was trained as a case manager. One part-time graduate student in the nursing case management program assisted with case management for patients on-site, on a limited basis, as part of her clinical experience. Two graduate-prepared case managers did telephonic case management. Patients receiving primary care and/or psychological counseling at the clinic were referred for telephonic case management by the on-site case managers. Telephonic case managers contacted patients between the clinic appointments. The case management process was similar to rural case management models described in the literature.

Goals of the Case Management Program

Prior to implementing the case management program, goals were established. These goals are described and then the progress that was made toward accomplishing the goals is discussed.

GOAL 1: ESTABLISH A CASE MANAGEMENT INFORMATION SYSTEM.

To establish a CMIS, several considerations are germane to the initial development. These are to

1. standardize terminology, documentation, and data management systems (Mullahy & Jensen, 2005; Powell, 2000; Swanson et al., 2005);
2. simplify data updates by tracking details required by the organization;
3. contain decision support systems that can turn data into actionable information;
4. provide outcome information;
5. provide the ability to run data in parallel with other systems, either real time or in batch mode;
6. act as a central repository for required patient information;
7. provide comprehensive patient data throughout the continuum of care;
8. provide patient census data;
9. store relevant clinical and administrative data for long-term population trends; and
10. eliminate double-data entry by same or multiple users.

A CMIS was developed for the Rural Healthcare Center. This included a standardized assessment tool, problem list, and progress notes. These documents helped define the content of the case management record. The assessment was completed on the initiation of services. At the completion of the assessment, the case manager completed a flag sheet. On this sheet were the major case management problems targeted for resolution. After each contact, the case manager documented observations and interventions on the case manager's progress note. The on-site case managers had oversight of the entire clinical record. The telephonic case managers were provided with access to the assessment and the case management flag list. Case information from the telephonic case management progress notes was provided to the on-site case managers during clinical conferences. This clinical documentation system is being piloted and will be automated at the completion of the pilot project.

GOAL 2: ESTABLISH STANDARD OUTCOMES AND METRICS. The population for the initial case management program was those patients diagnosed primarily with depression. The specific target population with that group were patients who were nonadherent with treatment and others who represented the highest risk for nonadherence. The patients were approved by the multidisciplinary team for inclusion in the case management program.

A template for clinical, financial, functional, and satisfaction outcomes was determined along with indicators related to each outcome. These outcomes are depicted in Table 1 and were derived from the rural case management model described by Stanton and Packa (2001). Protocols for clinical and case management intervention were drafted and approved by the multidisciplinary team. These protocols are based on evidence-based guidelines available at the National Guideline Clearinghouse Web site (www.ngc.gov). The Web site provides practice guidelines based on expert opinion and/or research. As part of the case management process, protocols were developed for case finding and screening.

The protocols used to determine the inclusion of patients in the case management process included the following.

1. Use of Global Depression Scale (Sheikh & Yesavage, 1986) to determine the presence of depression in patients older than 40 years: This instrument was administered to all middle-aged and elderly patients at the beginning and completion of the pilot project.

2. Referral of patients with a score greater than or equal to 4 on the Global Depression Scale to the geropsychology service.
3. Patient agreement to participate in case management services.
4. Assessment and monitoring of nonclinical functional outcomes during each clinic visit with documentation in the clinical record. The monitoring continues telephonically during followup.
5. Monitoring of patient satisfaction was measured before and after the pilot project.
6. Adherence to the treatment plan was monitored routinely by both on-site and telephonic case managers.
7. Patients were contacted telephonically at least once monthly.
8. Financial outcomes were monitored by case managers and clinic staff.

GOAL 3: ESTABLISH A MODEL FOR CASE MANAGEMENT SERVICES. The model used for case management service is based on the Cooperative Practice Team model developed by Stanton, Walizer, Graham, and Keppel (2000). This model utilizes a multidisciplinary team in which the case managers partner with the primary care physician/provider and other healthcare professionals as necessary to facilitate outcomes. The model was modified slightly for the purposes of this project. The on-site nurse case manager teamed with the psychological counselors who were also on site. The nurse practitioner and/or the collaborating physician worked with the on-site case manager to provide clinical care to patients selected for

TABLE 1 Capstone Rural Health Center Outcomes for Case Management

Clinical Outcomes	Functional Outcomes	Financial Outcomes	Satisfaction Outcomes	Quality Outcomes
Geriatric depression scale completed by patient with nurse practitioner	Pfizer vulnerable elders survey	Number of hours to after-hours clinic or emergency department (self-reported data)	Satisfaction questionnaire administered pre- and post case management	Clinical quality management checklist
	Age General health			
Target complaints—pre- and post completed by clinical psychologist	Activities (physical)	Unscheduled visits to clinic phone calls/ messages to clinics		
	Activities of daily living pre- and post treatment	Somatic complaints		

case management. The geropsychology counselor provided counseling and therapeutic intervention. The telephonic case managers worked with the on-site case manager and the counselors to provide follow-up and monitoring of outcomes between clinical visits. At different points in the case management process, responsibility for different aspects of care changes, or transitions from one provider to another occurred as it did in the original Cooperative Practice Team model.

GOAL 4: ESTABLISH CASE MANAGEMENT LEADERSHIP, MENTORING, AND OPERATIONAL PROCEDURES. The on-site case managers maintained leadership and operational oversight of the case management process for the duration of the project. A standard operating procedure and a case manager job description (see Appendices A and B) that were originally developed were used as a template for initiating services. All of the case managers were mentored by graduate faculty from the graduate program in rural nursing case management. Competencies were based on those used by Stanton, Swanson, and Baker (2005). A competency checklist is under development for use in integrating future MSN and geropsychology graduate students in the case management process at the rural health clinic. Standards for case management procedures were based on those developed by the Case Management Society of America (2002). Ongoing communication between all members of the multidisciplinary team, as well as the case managers, assisted in monitoring outcomes according to the standards.

GOAL 5: PROVIDE QUALITY OVERSIGHT FOR THE CASE MANAGEMENT PROCESS. The primary method of quality oversight in this process is, of course, the monitoring of patient outcomes on an individual basis and in the aggregate. However, the team wanted to monitor the documentation of client care and hence the monitoring of case managers and achievement of outcomes. A checklist for this review was developed and used for quality management. The criteria targeted quality standards and outcomes for the case management process for review by case managers (see Appendix C). This document will assist in determining achievement of quality outcomes.

GOAL 6: ACHIEVE "BUY-IN" BY STAFF FOR THE ORGANIZATIONAL INNOVATION. "Buy-in" was achieved prior to the implementation of this project. However, budgetary constraints inhibited the full implementation of case management services. Typically, agencies that provide funding or reimburse services for the rural health center do not cover case management services. Therefore, it is difficult to establish case management without reengineering existing staff and without the use of case manager volunteers. The nurse practitioner employed at the clinic obtained a post-master's degree in case management. She felt the distinct pull of both roles. Although students and faculty are available on a voluntary basis, it is difficult to build a case management service without some financial support. It is a goal to prove that the cost savings produced by case management would justify the addition of case management staff. This is a target goal for the project, but even with preliminary data proving the value of case management, there are no funds in the budget to fully underwrite costs. "Dual hatting" for the nurse practitioner to serve as an on-site case manager helped. However, the nurse practitioner perceived that she was attempting two full-time jobs at times. Volunteers and students extended the case management capability, but in the future, funding for a full-time case manager is necessary. Therefore, the "buy-in" that needs to occur is really from external payer agencies. Reimbursement for case management services by third party payers would provide needed support and motivation for agencies to deliver case management.

Lessons Learned

Implementing case management services at a rural nursing health center provided many challenges. The pilot project really identified major issues that need to be addressed when implementing a similar type program.

1. Expecting existing personnel to assume the case management function increases workload beyond the Full-Time Equivalent (FTE) for the existing position.
2. Agencies wishing to provide case management services need to provide some portion of an FTE to assume case management responsibilities. Volunteer faculty and staff may help, but are not as dependable as a dedicated position.
3. Communication is so important. Excellent communication between all members of the multidisciplinary term needs to be ongoing. Communication in the existing project was not as effective as it should have been to effect good patient and quality outcomes.

4. Organized, formal documentation systems, operating procedures, outcomes, metrics, and other standardized measures enhanced the effectiveness of the case management process in this project.

5. On-site, coupled with telephonic case management, enhances adherence and effective use of services. However, because residents are rural and poor for the most part, phone services or computer access can be limited. Funds to ensure that patients have access by phone or Internet is critical if this type of case management is going to be used on an ongoing basis. Consistent and frequent telephonic contact must be ensured to enhance case management effectiveness. Therefore, funds for phone service, cell phones, or Internet need to be budgeted where patients do not have good access.

6. Equally problematic for rural residents is access to transportation, especially for the rural elderly. At times, adherence to medication and attending appointments is not so much a choice for the rural elderly. They simply lack access to transportation. Transportation to and from appointments is of critical concern. Mechanisms for funding these for patients are being explored.

Recommendations

1. Case management targeting vulnerable groups must be a component of all rural healthcare services.

2. Processes and procedures for case management must be well delineated.

3. Studies to validate the cost savings of case management services in the rural healthcare environment need to be explored. Third party payers and other agencies that reimburse for healthcare

need to include an allocation for case management services.

CONCLUSION

It is abundantly obvious to the staff from an observational point of view that the case management with the telephonic follow-up worked well for clinic staff and patients. Adhering to the goals for case management and providing an organizational framework for implementing case management enhanced the effectiveness of the endeavor. Having staff, faculty, and students from different disciplines makes it necessary to have agreed-upon standards and forms. This helps facilitate communication and the accurate recording of information. The Standard Operating Procedure made it clear who was responsible for each aspect of the case management process. The job description for the case manager made it clear what their roles were in terms of both on-site and telephonic case management. The clinical quality checklist provided guidance as to the necessary documentation. The specification of outcomes for these patients assisted in communicating exactly what parameters would be measured. Case management intervention in the rural healthcare environment needs to be well organized to accommodate all the variables that can prevail with rural residents. There were approximately 20 individuals who were included in this initial pilot, and preliminary results seem to indicate that case management was a success from the patient's and the providers' perspective. There will be more conclusive evidence about case management's effectiveness in this situation when more definitive data can be collected and analyzed. Although there is no doubt after this pilot that case management provides a better standard of care and better follow-up, more precise measurement is required.

References

Barney, D., Rosenthal, C., & Speier, T. (2004). Components of successful HIV-AIDS case management in Alaska native villages. *AIDS Education and Prevention, 16*(3), 202. Retrieved March 30, 2006, from ProQuest database (660334061).

Case Management Society of America. (2002). *Standards of practice for case management.* Little Rock, AR: Author.

Institute of Medicine. (2001, March). *Crossing the quality chasm: A new health system for the 21st century.* Retrieved November 2, 2006, from http://www.iom.edu/cms/8089/5432.aspx

Institute of Medicine. (2004, November). *Quality through collaboration: The future of rural health.* Retrieved November 2, 2006, from http://www.iom.edu/cms/3809/13989/23359.aspx

Mullahy, C., & Jensen, D. (2004). *The case manager's handbook* (3rd ed.). Sudbury, MA: Jones & Bartlett.

Powell, S. (2000). *Case management: A practical guide to success in managed care.* Baltimore: Lippincott, Williams & Wilkins.

Ritchie, C., Wieland, D., Tully, C., Prachoda, K., Haddock, K., Boland, R., et al. (2002). Coordination and advocacy for rural elders (CARE): A model of rural case management with veterans. *The Gerontologist, 42*(3), 399–406. Retrieved March 30, 2006, from ProQuest database (125660831).

Scott, J. (2000). A nursing leadership challenge: Managing the chronically ill in rural settings. *Nursing Administration Quarterly, 24*(3), 21–33. Retrieved March 30, 2006, from ProQuest database (53861749).

Sheikh, J. I., & Yesavage, J. A. (1986). Geriatric Depression Scale (GDS): Recent evidence and development of a shorter version. In T. L. Brink (Ed.), *Clinical gerontology: A guide to assessment and intervention* (pp. 165–173). Binghamton, NY: Haworth Press.

Silberman, P., Poley, S., James, K., & Slifkin, R. (2002). Tracking Medicaid managed care in rural communi-

ties: A fifty-state follow-up. *Health Affairs, 21*(4), 255. Retrieved March 30, 2006, from ProQuest database (142204951).

Stanton, M., & Dunkin, J. (2002). Nursing case management: Nursing role variations. *Case Management, 2*(7), 48–55.

Stanton, M., & Packa, D. (2001). A model for rural case management. *Journal of Case Management, 2*(6), 96–103.

Stanton, M., Walizer, E., Graham, G., & Keppel, L. (2000). Case management: A case study. *Journal of Case Management, 5*(1), 37–45.

Swanson, C., Baker, R., Stanton, M., Godec, C., & Patton, L. (2005). The design and development of a case management system for RC Personnel. *U.S. Army Medical Departmental Journal, 8*(5), 60.

About the Authors

Marietta P. Stanton, PhD, RN, C, CNAA, BC, CMAC, CCM, is a Professor of Nursing and Director of the Graduate Program at The University of Alabama, Capstone College of Nursing (CCN). The focus of the CCN master's program is on case management for rural populations. She is also an Emeritus faculty from the University of New York at Buffalo School of Nursing. She has published a number of articles in case management, patient and provider education, and nursing education. Dr Stanton is also a Colonel in the U.S. Army Nurse Corps and a past Senior Case Manager of the Southeast Regional Medical Command.

Jeri W. Dunkin, PhD, RN, CHCE, is a Professor and Saxon Endowed Chair for Rural Nursing, Capstone College of Nursing, The University of Alabama. She is also the Director/CEO of Capstone Rural Health Center, a nurse-managed FQHC look-alike, in Parrish, AL.

L. Kathleen Williams Thomas, MS, FNP, provided primary healthcare to patients as a nurse practitioner at Capstone Rural Health Center for several years. She completed a post-master's program in nursing case management at the University of Alabama Capstone College of Nursing in 2006. She is currently employed at Northwest Alabama Mental Health Center in Jasper.

APPENDIX A

Case Manager

1. Act as a primary point of contact for patients regarding all clinical care.
2. Coordinate and communicate patients' clinical care when transferred between clinic and facilities.
3. Ensure timely and valid data entry into case management database.
4. Ensure that patient's flag list and progress reports are current and valid.
5. Ensure that functional assessment, satisfaction, and target behavior data instruments are initiated.
6. Coordinate and schedule all medical care and appointments for elderly depressed patients.
7. *Assessment.* Conduct a thorough and systematic assessment of patients' status within 24 hr of referral by the nurse practitioner for depression.
8. *Problem identification.* Coordinate with healthcare team to identify patients' clinical concerns/problems, including mental health concerns.
9. *Plan of care*
   a. Collaborate initially and at least weekly with telephonic case managers and other members of the medical team to identify immediate, short-term, and ongoing needs to develop, evaluate, and update plan of care.

b. Educate patients regarding clinical aspects of case management program, diagnosis, and plan of care, and assist the soldier to make informed decisions regarding plan of care.

c. Coordinate and communicate patients' appointments and referrals to patients and members of the team.

d. Coordinate with patients' family or significant other to ensure patients' compliance with scheduled appointments.

10. Monitor

a. Conduct ongoing assessment and document to monitor quality of care, achievement of outcomes, and whether healthcare goals are realistic or achievable.

b. Follow up with the telephonic case managers at least weekly and after each of the patient's clinic appointments, as appropriate and document interaction.

c. Maintain ongoing and regular communication with providers to coordinate adjustments or revisions to plan of care.

11. Evaluate

a. Engage the patient and the medical team to methodically and continuously evaluate the patient's response to healthcare and the case management process at least weekly.

b. Assist to evaluate when the patient meets optimal medical benefit.

APPENDIX B

Rural Health Center Standard Operating Procedure for Case Management of Rural Elderly Clients With Depression

1. *Purpose:* To provide case management (CM) services at the Capstone Rural Health Center for elderly patients with depression.

2. *Goals of the program:* The goals of the CM program for elderly patients with depression is to:

a. Implement case finding procedures to identify rural elderly aged 45 or more with depression.

b. Conduct CM intake to determine general medical/functional/mental health status, significant social and financial issues with or barriers to treatment, specific healthcare needs, adherence to medications profile, and CM plan.

c. Analyze financial, clinical, functional, and satisfaction outcomes for target population before and after CM services.

d. Develop a database for CM services.

e. Provide on-site and telephonic CM services for the target group.

f. Develop a long-term plan for CM services at the Capstone Rural Health Center.

3. *Procedure*

a. The nurse practitioner will administer the Geriatric Depression Scale (Short Form) to all patients 45 years or older as part of the history and physical. This form will be maintained in the patient record.

b. The nurse practitioner will refer all patients scoring 3 or more to on-site CM.

c. On-site CM will obtain permission or consent for patients to receive CM services and place consent in clinical record. On-site CM will initiate CM flag list and CM progress report. CM will coordinate appointments with clinical psychologist and check for adequacy of the transportation to and from appointments. CM will ensure that the patient is entered into CM database. These forms will be maintained in the patient record.

d. On-site CM will administer functional assessment tool and patient satisfaction instrument on intake visit. These forms will be maintained in the patient record.

e. Clinical psychologist will complete target complaint preassessment and psychology clinic SOAP note. A copy of these two documents will be added to the patient record.

f. The on-site CM will consult with the nurse practitioner and the clinical psychologist to complete CM plan and progress note. Plans for further medical and mental health follow-up will be documented in the patient record, and the CM plan will reflect actions that support the plan. The CM will update the patient CM database file.

g. On-site CM will notify telephonic case manager and provide plan of CM. Transmission of written patient data must be via secure fax and password protected if sent via e-mail.

h. Telephonic case manager will call the patient according to the following protocol. The number of calls per month by the telephonic CM will be based on the patient's score on the Geriatric Depression Scale. Patients who have severe depression will be called two times per week at a minimum and for moderate depression once a week. An electronic progress note will be forwarded to the on-site CM at least weekly.

APPENDIX C

Clinical Quality Checklist Case Management

Criteria	Comments	Y/N
1. *Assessment.* Conducted a thorough and systematic assessment of the patient's status within 24 hr of referral by the nurse practitioner for depression.		
2. *Problem identification.* Coordinated with the healthcare team to identify the patient's clinical concerns/problems, including mental health concerns.		
3. *Plan of care.* Collaborated initially and at least weekly with telephonic case managers and other members of the healthcare team to identify immediate, short-term, and ongoing needs to develop, evaluate, and update plan of care.		
a. Educated the patient regarding clinical aspects of case management program, diagnosis, plan of care, and assisted the patient to make informed decisions regarding plan of care.		
b. Coordinated and communicated the patient's appointments and referrals to the patient and members of the team.		
c. Coordinated with the patient's family or significant other to ensure the patient's compliance with scheduled appointments.		
4. Monitor		
a. Conducted ongoing assessment and documented to monitor quality of care, achievement of outcomes, and whether healthcare goals are realistic or achievable.		
b. Followed up with the telephonic case managers at least weekly and after each of the patient's clinic appointments, as appropriate and document interaction.		
c. Maintained ongoing and regular communication with providers to coordinate adjustments or revisions to plan of care.		
5. Evaluate		
a. Engaged the patient and the medical team to methodically and continuously evaluate the patient's response to healthcare and the case management process at least weekly.		
b. Assisted the healthcare team to evaluate when the patient met optimal medical/behavioral health benefit.		

CASE MANAGEMENT FOR PATIENTS WITH HEART FAILURE

A Quality Improvement Intervention

Louise C. Miller, Phd, Rn, and karen R. Cox, Phd, Rn

ABSTRACT

At-home case management is one strategy for improving quality of care for elderly patients with heart failure. Essential components of an effective heart failure case management intervention include frequent patient contact with the case manager and vigilant at-home monitoring of symptoms with responsive modifications to the treatment plan. It is just as important that the health care system (e.g., the acute care institution) is committed to assuring administrative support, financial backing, and dedicating clinical expert resources to achieve clinical quality improvements. In this article, the design, implementation, and outcomes of an at-home heart failure case management program are described, and challenges faced in implementing and sustaining the program are outlined.

In 1997, an Office of Clinical Effectiveness (OCE) was established within a 300-bed academic medical center in the Midwest to improve clinical outcomes in select patient populations. Since that time, all institutional clinical outcomes improvement projects have been guided by a 10-step continuous quality improvement model (Sidebar). The OCE adapted the 10-step model from a manual published by the University Health System Consortium (1997).

In 1999, the OCE was directed by the academic medical center's leadership to improve clinical outcomes among chronically ill patients with heart failure. As emphasized in this article, the selected improvement intervention (Step 7 of the 10-step model) was a case management model used when patients with heart failure were discharged from the hospital. The purpose of this article is to describe the authors' experiences using the 10-step improvement model and to explain why the authors believe the case management program intervention was unsuccessful.

The authors describe the 10-step improvement model with particular emphasis on the case management intervention (Step 7). The authors also indicate which aspects of this specific heart failure improvement processes proved particularly challenging. After 2 years, the case management program and its part-time OCE improvement coordinator were eliminated. The authors' hope is that practitioners will learn from these experiences and be better prepared to make decisions about improvement strategies targeted toward specific patient populations, particularly those patients with chronic diseases.

THE 10-STEP IMPROVEMENT MODEL

Steps 1, 2, and 3: Selection of the Problem, Champion, and Team

The academic medical center's leadership determined outcome for patients with heart failure was an area ripe for improvement because although the volume of hospitalizations for heart failure was ranked among the Top 10, financial losses were high (i.e., total reimbursements for hospitalizations and emergency department visits were insufficient to cover costs). An attending physician from the Cardiology Division specializing in heart failure agreed to champion the improvement team. When possible, team membership should include all stakeholders. In this case, physicians from each of the three services (i.e., Cardiology, Internal Medicine, Family Medicine) admitting patients with heart failure were asked to volunteer, along with nurses from representative care sites (inpatient and outpatient). Other team members should be invited to participate based on typical care needs of the selected patient population. For this program, the authors identified the need to involve a pharmacist, nutritionist, and social worker.

Steps 4, 5, and 6: Using Internal and External Data to Determine the Ideal Intervention(s)

Heart failure is a severe and progressive condition affecting nearly 5 million elderly individuals in the United States. Approximately 550,000 new cases are diagnosed annually. Nationally, hospital discharges for heart failure increased nearly threefold from 1979 to 2002, with 970,000 in 2002. Medicare beneficiaries were paid $3.6 billion in 1999 for heart failure reimbursement, averaging $5,456 per discharge. Total costs on heart failure are estimated at $27.9 billion in 2005, with $25.3 billion of that amount spent on direct care costs (American Heart Association, 2005).

Evidence suggests that when patients are taught self-management skills via a nurse-led case management program, clinical outcomes significantly improve, as do quality-of-life scores and patient satisfaction with factors under health care system control. Typical self-care skills that improve clinical outcomes include daily self-monitoring of blood pressure, weight, and dietary intake of salt and fluids (Rich et al., 1993; Rich et al., 1995; Riegel et al., 2002; Stewart, Pearson, & Horowitz, 1998). However, there are no common features for what should be included in case management interventions or how and when the intervention should be delivered. Studies varied by institutional commitment to services, availability and skill level of case managers, and numbers of patients available for enrollment in the program.

The literature reports variations in program design, suggesting clinical and financial results are "dose-related." Two studies reported increased readmission rates and longer lengths of hospital stay, along with lower quality-of-life scores in "case managed" heart failure patients (Oddone, Weinberger, Giobbie-Hurder, Landsman, & Henderson, 1999; Weinberger, Oddone, & Henderson, 1996). However, both of these studies used program designs involving only short-term (immediate post-discharge) interventions, such as phone calls and pre-discharge follow-up appointment scheduling.

Step 7: Case Management as the Targeted Intervention

Heart failure is one of many chronic conditions that lends itself to cooperative outpatient case management partnerships between patient and provider. Consistent with Orem's (2001) Self-Care Deficit Nursing Theory, the case manager identifies self-care actions that, when taken, will be successful in regulating heart failure from home. The case manager is expected to assess the patient's ability to take identified self-care actions and to develop an individualized plan for accomplishing these actions when the patient cannot make judgments about them or independently perform them. For example, patients with severe visual impairments may not be able to see the visual display from traditional equipment to monitor their

---

THE 10-STEP PROCESS TO ACHIEVE CLINICAL OUTCOMES IMPROVEMENTS

1. Choose a problem that is "ripe."
2. Identify a project champion.
3. Assemble the team.
4. Study the data.
5. Outline the current flow of care.

6. Research the literature and engage the experts.
7. Design targeted interventions.
8. Implement changes.
9. Monitor impact using data.
10. Use results to revise interventions.

Adapted from University Health System Consortium (1997).

daily weight and blood pressure. In this example, the case manager would need to arrange an alternate and reliable approach for these self-care activities.

Home-based self-care for heart failure requires attention to subjective and objective signs of deterioration, such as shortness of breath, changes in blood pressure and weight, as well as monitoring of medication effectiveness (e.g., diuretics). Over time, consistent patient contact and problem-solving by the case manager develops patients' capacity to care for themselves (self-care agency), thus empowering the patient to successfully regulate the condition at home.

In addition to the case manager's role, health care system factors also must be aligned for an effective at-home program. These health care system factors include:

- Prescribing appropriate medications.
- Allowing continuity of relationships to develop.
- Removing barriers to health care system access.
- Devoting time to developing the patient's capacity to care for self.

In designing this intervention, the authors considered the necessary elements to an effective heart failure case-manager-led program along with health care system factors.

The case management model for heart failure used in this article included successful interventions reported in the literature (Rich et al., 1993; Rich et al., 1995; Stewart et al., 1998). The multidisciplinary team (minimally including a physician, nurse, and pharmacist), established processes for developing self-management competencies while assuring both optimal prescriptions and ready access (e.g., "24/7" beeper coverage) to a familiar team member. Using a team model, treatment decisions were made in partnership to avert a crisis.

Developing self-management competency occurs over time through two primary methods. The first method is daily recording (diary) of symptoms and physiologic parameters (e.g., weight, blood pressure). The second is through frequent conversations between the nurse and patient. Nurses and patients can discuss the meaning of the patient's symptoms and any questions related to the patients' condition. Nurses and patients also use these conversations to discuss the variety of treatment decisions that could be made based on the information recorded in the patient's diary.

Health care system factors are optimized by establishing scheduled communication between health care providers and patients. Specifically, this includes appropriately-timed follow-up clinic appointments and free-flowing communication lines among providers, particularly when unexpected or preventable utilization (e.g., emergency department visits, hospitalizations) occur. Evidence shows that when case management models have "a healthy dose" of all four factors, patient quality of life scores improve—specifically patients' perception about personal health state—and case managed patients report a higher satisfaction with services (Rich et al., 1995; Riegel et al., 2002).

Steps 8, 9, and 10: Using Post-Implementation Results to Fine-Tune Intervention Success

Although clinicians and patients focus on improvement in disease symptomatology, evidence of heart failure program success is typically reported as utilization indicators. For example, when comparing patients who were case managed for heart failure with individuals who were not case managed, those who received case management had fewer unplanned

---

GUIDE TO INTERVIEW QUESTIONS

General Condition:

How has your health and your heart failure been in the past day/week/month?

Weight:

What is your weight today? How does it differ from yesterday/last week?

How are you weighing yourself? Same scale every day, same time every day, same clothes every day, scale on the same surface every day (hardwood vs. carpet)

Pedal Edema:

Do you have swelling in your ankles? If so, is it more or less than usual?

Is your swelling the same for both legs?

When you push with your finger, do you make a dent in the skin, and does it stay there?

If so, how long does it stay there?

Blood Pressure:

What is your blood pressure today?

What are your highest and lowest values in the past week?

How are you taking your blood pressure (e.g., sitting down, after activity, after resting?)

Who is taking your blood pressure?

What kind of equipment do you use?

What time of day are you taking your blood pressure? Is this a routine time?

Shortness of Breath:

Are you having shortness of breath today?

What is your pattern of shortness of breath?

Do you get short of breath with exercise?

Do you get short of breath if you lay down in bed?

If your shortness of breath is different today (or the past few days), what is different about it?

Energy Level:

How many steps can you climb without having to rest? Or, how many steps can you take across the floor without having to rest?

How is your energy level today? And the past several days?

Activities of Daily Living:

What kinds of activities do you/can you routinely do?

What are your normal daily activities? Can you do these activities?

Have you changed in your ability to do things that you normally do?

If so, are there reasons/events/issues that stop you from doing your normal activities?

Exercise:

What exercise do you do each day?

Can you do your prescribed routine from Cardiac Rehabilitation?

If you are not doing your exercises, what are the reasons?

Diet:

Have you eaten anything with extra salt (e.g., canned soup, convenience foods such as microwave or canned dinners, any commercially canned foods)?

Do you add salt at the table?

Have you had Chinese food?

Have you eaten any fast food? If so, what did you eat and where?

If you have a fluid restriction, have you stayed within that amount?

Smoking:

Are you smoking? If so, are you smoking more or less than before?

Medications

What medications are you taking now?

How much of each one (dose) are you taking?

When (time of day) are you taking your medications?

Have you made any adjustments in your medications, including medication you are taking or time/amount you are taking?

Has your physician, or other provider, made any adjustments in your medications?

Do you have any problems or concerns with your medications?

Medical Services:

Have you gone to another physician in your area other than your regular physician, or to an emergency department or hospital for care related to your heart failure or other conditions?

Have you gone to a pharmacy for care or questions related to your medical condition?

Are there any problems you know about now that would keep you from getting to your appointment?

If I hadn't called today, would you have needed to talk to someone about your heart failure or medical condition?

admissions. When read-missions did occur among patients who were case managed, length of hospital stay was decreased (Rich et al., 1995; Riegel et al., 2002; Stewart et al., 1998). Other comparisons between case managed and control group patients report heart failure readmissions decreased by one-fifth (Rauh, Schwabauer, Enger, & Mo-ran, 1999) to one-third (Rich et al., 1995; Riegel et al., 2002). Stewart et al. (1998) reported emergency department visits for heart failure exacerbations were reduced by nearly half. In contrast, the clinical outcomes the authors chose to compare (pre- and post-intervention) in this article included average length of stay, read-missions, quality of life, mortality, and internal financial indicators.

DISCUSSION

As previously mentioned, the leaders agreed to fund this heart failure case management intervention because both volume of geriatric patients and reimbursement losses associated with heart failure were high. Although the academic medical center is a tertiary referral center, geographic distribution of patients with heart failure was surprisingly regional with most visits confined to contiguous counties, and most patients cared for at the center by one of three medical specialty services (i.e., Cardiology, Internal Medicine, Family Practice). In this case, patient volume was not sufficient to support a dedicated provider, so the heart failure case management model was superimposed onto the mainstream of usual patient services. The OCE improvement specialist served a facilitative role, including such tasks as organizing agendas and meetings and providing day-to-day operational and evaluation expertise.

Successful improvement models involve a team (Step 3). The team identified best practices from the literature and agreed there should be a focus on frequent post-discharge patient contact to assure a continuity in relationship, enabling patients to successfully self-monitor and recognize meaningful symptoms to report. A case manager who develops continuity in relationships and is accessible to the patient can avert physiologic crises while continually teaching self-management skills. Unfortunately, these services are not directly reimbursed by Medicare or most other health plans.

Because heart failure is primarily seen in individuals older than 65, the most likely reim-

bursement source is Medicare. With Medicare, hospitalization payments are set by a contracted amount. Regardless of intensity of service or length of stay for hospitalization, the average national payment for heart failure (diagnosis-related group [DRG] No. 127) is $4,159.04 (Hart & Schmidt, 1999). In essence, the Medicare payment strategy allows increased profitability when patients are in crisis because emergency department and hospital care is reimbursed, but case management activities are not. Compounding economic challenges for these patients and the health care system is that effective medications might be too expensive for some patients, thus increasing the likelihood of emergency department visits and hospitalizations.

Although evidence shows that case management programs significantly reduce emergency department visits and hospitalizations related to heart failure exacerbations, arranging financial support from health care administrators for such programs can be difficult. If a health system administrator cannot be convinced to support a program because it is "the right thing to do" for community members, one should argue the benefits of shorter (less costly) hospital stay. In other words, program support is based on the assumption that when case managed patients are readmitted they are less sick, thus the length of stay is shorter, so costs for hospitalization will be less than the DRG payment, thus allowing profitability. Rauh et al. (1999), Rich et al. (1995), and Riegel et al. (2002) demonstrated that their case management programs resulted in decreased hospital readmissions, with savings of approximately $1,000 per admission for each program.

Costs associated with implementing a heart failure case management program have been calculated at less than $500 per patient. When this cost was combined with cost savings associated with fewer hospitalizations, one program realized a net savings of approximately $500 per patient (Riegel et al., 2002). An earlier study reported cost of care to be $460 less per patient who was case-managed compared to patients who were not case managed, with an average cost of $216 per patient to implement the case management intervention. In another model using a centralized outpatient heart failure clinic, the cost of the clinic was approximately $100,000. However, because of physician billing, revenues were calculated at more than $200,000 (Rauh et al., 1999).

PROGRAM DESIGN DECISIONS

After the program is approved, the first design decision is determining which patients would benefit from a case management program, and approaching these individuals. A total of 68 patients were enrolled in the case management program. Using the Specific Activity Scale (Goldman, Hasimo-to, Cook, & Loscalzo, 1981), New York Heart Association classification was determined and only Class II or III patients were prioritized for participation. New Class I and IV patients were not selected for enrollment because Class I patients are rarely hospitalized and require only sporadic clinic follow up and Class IV patients frequently use the hospital for regular complex medical and pharmacologic management.

During enrollment screening, the enrollment nurse evaluated patients for fluid retention and weight gain, shortness of breath, and cognitive function (especially information processing and memory), to assess acuteness of the condition and the patient's ability to effectively participate in a home self-management program. Baseline data including current medication regimen, evidence of frequent and recent medication changes, diet restrictions, and co-morbidities according to a modified Charlson Index measure were used to individualize the plan of care (Katz, Chang, Sangha, Fossel, & Bates, 1996). To participate, patients were required to have access to a telephone and the ability to hear and process information sufficiently to carry on a detailed telephone conversation about their heart failure symptoms and response to the treatment plan with the case manager.

After enrollment, patients were followed by a team of health care providers who were familiar with the patients' heart failure condition and were able to monitor the patients during inpatient admissions and outpatient clinic visits. Levels of expertise varied among the nursing personnel who case managed the patients, and included cardiology nurse practitioners and licensed practical nurses in general medicine clinics.

To standardize patient responses during telephone follow up, a script was developed to assure complete, consistent data collection in the case manager's log. This series of questions is summarized in the Sidebar. As a supplement to the scripted questions, patients were given a diary to record daily weight, blood pressure, medications taken, and symptom occurrence. Internal development monies from private contributions were used to provide appropriate at-home monitoring equipment (e.g., scales, blood pressure self-monitoring devices) for patients who did not have access to these resources.

Knowing that a case manager was going to call according to a defined schedule to discuss information from the patient's diary likely encouraged patient participation and reflection about daily heart failure self-assessments. Subtle changes in weight, shortness of breath, fatigue, blood pressure, exercise tolerance, medication, and diet adjustments were discussed during patient-case-manager conversations, often bringing about modifications to diet and medications, or earlier-than-expected referral to providers.

Standardized tools were used to assess patient response to medical and case management interventions (Step 9). The Minnesota Living with Heart Failure Questionnaire was used to collect patient data and quality of life scores at enrollment, 1 month, 3 months, and 6 months post-enrollment (Guyatt et al., 1989). This instrument provides a sum score of physical and emotional symptoms specific to heart failure. The tool was used outside of its standard application as an additional prompt for questions indicating symptoms of fluid retention, inability to perform daily activities, feelings of depression, and cost of care issues, among others. Particular attention was paid to questions scored as 4 or 5 on a 1 to 5 Likert-type scale by the patient, indicating significant limitations because of heart failure. Case managers followed these questions closely, monitoring for decreases in perceived severity score. Because data were collected on patients at multiple points in time, the tool served as a temporal indicator for improvement or deterioration in physical and emotional symptoms and could assist in making decisions or changes to the treatment plan.

Four process indicators were developed to monitor health care team members' use of the case management protocols (Step 9). These were:

- Case manager inbound and outbound phone calls.
- Pre-scheduled provider appointments that had been kept.
- Treatment plan updates faxed to provider prior to the scheduled appointment.
- Satisfaction with the program (both patients' and providers').

The protocol timeline describing the timing of key program components is outlined in the Table.

Heart Failure Case Management Activity Timeline

	Enrollment	1 to 4 Weeks	1 Month	3 Months	6 Months
Patient Visits	Assessment of: • Specific Activity Scale (SAS) for New York Heart Association classification • Ejection fraction • 6-minute walk • Living with heart failure (HF) quality-of-life (QOL) assessment • Presence or absence of symptoms including fluid retention, shortness of breath, fatigue • Medication plan • Diet restrictions • Comorbidities		SAS 6-minute walk QOL	SAS 6-minute walk QOL	SAS 6-minute walk QOL
Process	Case manager (CM) contact with patient Email/fax team members (TM)* Communication with patient's primary care provider (PCP) Scheduling of follow-up clinic appointments Patient education related to HF treatment plan, with complementary HF program video Provision of weight scales and blood pressure equipment, with instruction for daily use Instruction to patient on at-home data collection	CM call within 48 hours and at least weekly 2-week follow-up clinic visit and assessment by TM Communication with PCP and TM	CM biweekly calls Follow-up clinic visit and assessment by TM Communication with PCP and TM	CM biweekly/ monthly calls as indicated Follow-up clinic visit and assessment by TM as indicated Communication with PCP and TM	CM biweekly/ monthly calls as indicated Follow-up clinic visit and assessment by TM as indicated Communication with PCP and TM
Patient Data	Inpatient length of stay. Severity-of-illness scales	Readmissions Length of stay Emergency department (ED) visits Mortality Cost	Readmissions Length of stay ED visits Mortality Cost	Readmissions Length of stay ED visits Mortality Cost	Readmissions Length of stay ED visits Mortality Cost Event-free survival after 6 months

Team members are primary care provider, cardiologist case manager, pharmacist, dietitian, social worker, cardiac rehabilitation.

PROGRAM OUTCOMES

After 1 year, utilization-based outcome measures were less than anticipated (Step 10). The rate of 90-day re-admission was essentially unchanged at 1.3 visits per patient, and similar to the baseline rate of 1.4 visits. The rate of re-admissions at 1 year im-proved from 2 per patient at baseline to 1.3 in the case managed group. The rate of event-free survival (i.e., no readmission or death within 12 months) was 86%—again close to the baseline rate of 82%.

In keeping with optimal heart failure pharma-cotherapy standards (Gomberg-Maitland, Baran, &

Fuster, 2001), almost all patients without contraindications were managed with angiotensin-converting enzyme inhibitors, beta-blockers, and spironoloactone subsequent to enrollment in the program. In the 24 patients who completed the case management program, quality-of-life change scores on the Minnesota Living with Heart Failure tool improved in 19 patients, with patient scores of 4 and 5 improving to scores of 3 or less. Patients who participated in the program for 6 months reported satisfaction, particularly with the working and responsive relationship with the individual case managers.

Even though improvement in utilization outcomes were modest, the quality-of-life improvements were exciting. However, only one-fourth of eligible patients were ever approached for case management enrollment. The effort to overlay the heart failure case management process on a large number of otherwise busy clinicians resulted in a fragmented and inconsistently implemented program. The program was delivered across diverse inpatient and outpatient settings, using multiple nurse providers with different levels of expertise and skills. It was the expectation that case management services would be incorporated into already heavy workloads.

Although communication among team members was possible using electronic mail, implementation of the program by multiple individuals with various heart failure proficiency as opposed to by a dedicated coordinator with heart failure expertise, often led to poor coordination of services. The lack of commitment to creating a small, core clinician team dedicated to providing this service led to poor accountability by case managers. However, some case managers were able to function effectively despite a weak system. Successful case managers were able to document positive clinical and financial outcomes, measured by early medical management intervention (e.g., medication changes, dietary modifications), appropriate hospital admissions, timely referrals, and increased patient disease-management skills.

Funding for a dedicated heart failure case manager was not approved for the heart failure improvement project because the case manager salary could not be offset by billable revenue. Physician commitment to the program was varied. Specialty physicians and the institution receive greater financial return on patient visits and procedures compared to savings from an at-home case management strategy. This lack of financial benefit to the institution and physicians likely led to overall disinterest in investing in the program. Lack of institutional attention allowed an opportunity for some case managers to be lax in providing services as outlined in the program protocol. Successful programs reported in the literature demonstrate institutional and physician commitment and advocacy for program components.

Poor outcomes in terms of cost reduction, lack of revenue generated, and mediocre clinical successes led to the program's demise. The authors' caution to readers is to understand the clinical and financial incentives that can affect a well-intended,

---

KEYPOINTS
Heart Failure Intervention

Miller, L.C., & Cox, K.R. Case Management for Patients with Heart Failure: A Quality Improvement Intervention. *Journal of Gerontological Nursing*, 2005, *31*(5): 20–28.

1. A 10-step systematic improvement model was used by a multidisciplinary team whose goal was to improve patient outcomes following hospitalization for heart failure.
2. The team identified best practices from the literature, and the nurse case managers followed up with patients post-discharge to help them to self-monitor their condition and recognize symptoms to report.
3. Patients who received the case management intervention reported satisfaction with care, had improved quality-of-life scores, and experienced fewer exacerbations requiring emergency department or hospital treatment.
4. Although aspects of the program were unsuccessful, the authors' experience may help nurses to make decisions about improvement strategies targeted toward specific patient populations, particularly those patients with chronic disease.

valuable program. Further, careful consideration and planning related to delivery of, and accountability for, program components are equally essential.

CONCLUSION

The case management intervention implemented in this program and those reviewed in the literature can accomplish the goals of individualized, holistic services, and enhanced patient ability for self-care through the continuum of care (Llewellyn & Moreo, 2001). Patients who received the case management intervention as designed expressed satisfaction with care, had improved quality-of-life scores, and experienced fewer exacerbations requiring emer-

gency department or hospital treatment. Consistent with the goals of the case management program, these patients were able to maintain their independence and self-sufficiency at home, and functioned at a higher level of symptom control. Unfortunately, the current Medicare reimbursement structure does not necessarily support activities that develop self-care agencies. For now, the implementation of a sustainable case management program should only be designed to fit within the context of an institution's priorities—specifically so a balance can be created between evidence-based care and an investment of dedicated resources to improve that care.

References

American Heart Association. (2005). Congestive heart failure. In *Heart and stroke statistical update* (chap. 9). Retrieved April 11, 2005, from www.americanheart.org/downloadable/heart/1105390918119HDSStats2005Update.pdf

Goldman, L., Hasimoto, B., Cook, E.J., & Loscalzo, A. (1981). Comparative reproducibility and validity of systems for assessing cardiovascular functional class: Advantages of a new specific activity scale. *Circulation, 64,* 1227–1234.

Gomberg-Maitland M., Baran D.A., & Fuster V. (2001). Treatment of congestive heart failure: Guidelines for the primary care physician and the heart failure specialist. *Archives of Internal Medicine, 161,* 342–352.

Guyatt, G.H., Nogradi, S., Halcrow, S., Singer, J., Sullivan, M.J.J., & Fallen, E.L. (1989). Development and testing of a new measure of health status for clinical trials in heart failure. *Journal of General Internal Medicine,* 101–107.

Hart, A.C., & Schmidt, K. (Eds.). (1999). *St. Anthony's DRG guidebook.* Reston, VA: St. Anthony's Publishing.

Katz, J.N., Chang, L.C., Sangha, O., Fossel, A.H., & Bates, D.W. (1996). Can comorbidity be measured by questionnaire rather than medical record review? *Medical Care, 34,* 73–84.

Llewellyn A., & Moreo, K. (2001). *Case management review & resource manual: The essence of case management.* Washington, DC: Institute for Research, Education, and Consultation at ANCC.

Oddone, E.Z., Weinberger, M., Giobbie-Hur-der, A.N., Landsman, P., & Henderson, W. (1999). Enhanced access to primary care for patients with congestive heart failure. *Effective Clinical Practice, 2,* 201–209.

Orem, D.E. (2001). *Nursing: Concepts of practice* (6th ed.). St. Louis, MO: Mosby.

Rauh, R.A., Schwabauer, N.J., Enger, E.L., & Moran, J.F. (1999). A community hospital-based congestive heart failure program: Impact on length of stay, admission and re-admission rates, and cost. *American Journal of Managed Care, 5*(1), 37–43.

Rich, M.W., Beckham, V., Wittenberg, C, Lev-en, C.L., Freedland, K.E., & Carney, R.M. (1995). A multidisciplinary intervention to prevent the readmission of elderly patients with congestive heart failure. *New England Journal of Medicine, 333,* 1190–1195.

Rich, M.W, Vinson, J.M., Sperry, J.C, Shah, A.S., Spinner, L.R., Chung, M.K., Davila-Roman, V. (1993). Prevention of readmission in elderly patients with congestive heart failure. *Journal of General Internal Medicine, S,* 585–590.

Riegel, B., Carlson, B., Kopp, Z., LePetri, B., Glaser, D., & Unger, A. (2002). Effect of a standardized nurse case-management telephone intervention on resource use in patients with chronic heart failure. *Archives of Internal Medicine, 162,* 705–712.

Stewart, S., Pearson, S., & Horowitz, J.D. (1998). Effects of a home-based intervention among patients with congestive heart failure discharged from acute hospital care. *Archives of Internal Medicine, 158,* 1067–1072.

University Health System Consortium. (1997). *Clinical Process Improvement Manual.* Chicago: Author.

Weinberger, M., Oddone, E.Z., & Henderson, WG (1996). Does increased access to primary care reduce hospital readmissions? *New England Journal of Medicine, 334,* 1441–1447.

About the Authors

Dr. Miller, is former Office of Clinical Effectiveness Improvement Specialist, is Assistant Professor of Clinical Nursing, Sinclair School of Nursing, University of Missouri- Columbia, Columbia, Missouri. Dr. Cox is Coordinator, Quality Improvement, Office of Clinical Effectiveness, University of Missouri- Columbia Health Care, Columbia, Missouri.

Address correspondence to Louise C Miller, PhD, RN, S303 School of Nursing Building, University of Missouri-Columbia, Columbia, MO 65211.

A Taxonomy for Disease Management: A Scientific Statement From the American Heart Association Disease Management Taxonomy Writing Group

Harlan M. Krumholz, Peter M. Currie, Barbara Riegel, Christopher O. Phillips,
Eric D. Peterson, Renee Smith, Clyde W. Yancy and David P. Faxon *Circulation*
2006;114;1432–1445; originally published online Sep 4, 2006; DOI:
10.1161/CIRCULATIONAHA.106.177322

Circulation is published by the American Heart Association. 7272 Greenville Avenue,
Dallas, TX 72514

Copyright © 2006 American Heart Association. All rights reserved. Print ISSN:
0009-7322. Online ISSN: 1524-4539

The online version of this article, along with updated information and services, is located
on the World Wide Web at: http://circ.ahajournals.org/cgi/content/full/114/13/1432
Data Supplement (unedited) at: http://circ.ahajournals.org/cgi/content/full/
CIRCULATIONAHA.106.177322/DC1

Subscriptions: Information about subscribing to Circulation is online at
http://circ.ahajournals.org/subscriptions/

Permissions: Permissions & Rights Desk, Lippincott Williams & Wilkins, a
division of Wolters Kluwer Health, 351 West Camden Street, Baltimore, MD
21202-2436. Phone: 410-528-4050. Fax: 410-528-8550. E-mail:
journalpermissions@lww.com

Reprints: Information about reprints can be found online at
http://www.lww.com/reprints

Downloaded from circ.ahajournals.org at UNIV OF CINCINNATI on
January 13, 2009

AHA SCIENTIFIC STATEMENT

A Taxonomy for Disease Management: A Scientific Statement From the American Heart Association Disease Management Taxonomy Writing Group

Harlan M. Krumholz, MD, FAHA; Peter M. Currie, MHS; Barbara Riegel, DNSc, RN, CS, FAHA; Christopher O. Phillips, MD, MPH; Eric D. Peterson, MD, MPH; Renee Smith, MPA; Clyde W. Yancy, MD, FAHA; David P. Faxon, MD, FAHA

Background: Disease management has shown great promise as a means of reorganizing chronic care and optimizing patient outcomes. Nevertheless, disease management programs are widely heterogeneous and lack a shared definition of disease management, which limits our ability to compare and evaluate different programs. To address this problem, the American Heart Association's Disease Management Taxonomy Writing Group developed a system of classification that can be used both to categorize and compare disease management programs and to inform efforts to identify specific factors associated with effectiveness.

Methods: The AHA Writing Group began with a conceptual model of disease management and its components and subsequently validated this model over a wide range of disease management programs. A systematic MEDLINE search was performed on the terms *heart failure, diabetes,* and *depression,* together with *disease management, case management*, and *care management*. The search encompassed articles published in English between 1987 and 2005. We then selected studies that incorporated (1) interventions designed to improve outcomes and/or reduce medical resource utilization in patients with heart failure, diabetes, or depression and (2) clearly defined protocols with at least 2 prespecified components traditionally associated with disease management. We analyzed the study protocols and used qualitative research methods to develop a disease management taxonomy with our conceptual model as the organizing framework.

Results: The final taxonomy includes the following 8 domains: (1) *Patient population* is characterized by risk status, demographic profile, and level of comorbidity. (2) *Intervention recipient* describes the primary targets of disease management intervention and includes patients and caregivers, physicians and allied healthcare providers, and healthcare delivery systems. (3) *Intervention content* delineates individual components, such as patient education, medication management, peer support, or some form of postacute care, that are included in disease management. (4) *Delivery personnel* describes the network of healthcare providers involved in the delivery of disease management interventions, including nurses, case managers, physicians, pharmacists, case workers, dietitians, physical therapists, psychologists, and information systems specialists. (5) *Method of communication* identifies a broad range of disease management delivery systems that may include in-person visitation, audiovisual information packets, and some form of electronic or telecommunication technology. (6) *Intensity and complexity* distinguish between the frequency and duration of exposure, as well as the mix of program components, with respect to the target for disease management. (7) *Environment* defines the context in which disease management interventions are typically delivered and includes inpatient or hospital-affiliated outpatient programs, community or home-based programs, or some combination of these factors. (8) *Clinical outcomes* include traditional, frequently assessed primary and secondary outcomes, as well as patient-centered measures, such as adherence to medication, self-management, and caregiver burden.

Conclusions: This statement presents a taxonomy for disease management that describes critical program attributes and allows for comparisons across interventions. Routine application of the taxonomy may facilitate better comparisons of structure, process, and outcome measures across a range of disease management programs and should promote uniformity in the design and conduct of studies that seek to validate disease management strategies. (*Circulation.* 2006; 114:1432-1445.)

Key Words: AHA Scientific Statements ■ disease management ■ chronic disease delivery of health care ■ classification ■ heart failure

The American Heart Association makes every effort to avoid any actual or potential conflicts of interest that may arise as a result of an outside relationship or a personal, professional, or business interest of a member of the writing panel. Specifically, all members of the writing group are required to complete and submit a Disclosure Questionnaire showing all such relationships that might be perceived as real or potential conflicts of interest.

This statement was approved by the American Heart Association Science Advisory and Coordinating Committee on June 16, 2006. A single reprint is available by calling 800-242-8721 (US only) or writing the American Heart Association, Public Information, 7272 Greenville Ave, Dallas, TX 75231-4596. Ask for reprint No. 71-0371. To purchase additional reprints: Up to 999 copies, call 800-611-6083 (US only) or fax 413-665-2671; 1000 or more copies, call 410-528-4121, fax 410-528-4264, or e-mail kelle.ramsay@wolterskluwer.com. To make photocopies for personal or educational use, call the Copyright Clearance Center, 978-750-8400.

Expert peer review of AHA Scientific Statements is conducted at the AHA National Center. For more on AHA statements and guidelines development, visit http://www.americanheart.org/presenter.jhtml?identifier=3023366.

The past decade has witnessed increasing prevalence of chronic disease in the United states. This trend has contributed to skyrocketing healthcare costs and highlighted the fragmented nature of care available to chronically ill patients.[1] Consequently, many public policy makers and organizations have embraced disease management as a means of reorganizing medical treatment for chronic illness, shifting the emphasis toward an integrated, patient-centered approach to care. The purported benefits of disease management include improved health outcomes, greater patient satisfaction, better quality of life, and reduced healthcare costs.[2]

Despite the promise offered by disease management programs, questions remain about their potential for widespread application. Randomized trials of disease management have demonstrated improved outcomes for conditions such as heart failure, diabetes mellitus, and chronic kidney disease, but these studies generally have been conducted at single sites, and it is not known how successfully their results can be generalized to larger patient populations. In addition, many disease management programs are multidimensional, and the essential program elements that are associated with efficacy have yet to be established. These challenges are further complicated by a lack of standardization: The term *disease management* has entered into common usage without a shared, specific understanding of its meaning. Instead, multiple definitions of disease management and a variety of related models exist. Although disease management programs generally share core elements such as risk management and coordination of care, individual program components are highly variable. This variability presents difficulties in comparing and contrasting models, programs, outcomes, and effectiveness. The heterogeneity also impedes the development of policies that will provide incentives for the provision of disease management.

In response to these challenges, the American Heart Association (AHA) formed an interdisciplinary Disease Management Taxonomy Writing Group to develop a classification system for disease management. The work of the AHA Writing Group builds on the previous efforts of the AHA's Expert Panel on Disease Management to establish core principles for the application of disease management to cardiovascular disease and stroke (Table 1).[3] The taxonomy outlined in the present statement provides a conceptual framework that can be used both to compare the diverse range of disease management programs and to inform efforts to identify specific factors associated with effectiveness.

BACKGROUND

The challenge in identifying a precise definition for disease management lies partially in its complex origins and historical evolution. Although the term *disease management* was first coined in the early 1990s, many of its components were used informally throughout much of the history of medical practice.[4] Common attributes of disease management, such as formal and informal best practices and multidisciplinary care teams, had long been used to identify and treat patients. However, these techniques were inconsistently applied. In addition, throughout most of the 20th century in the United States, disease management components were implemented in a healthcare system characterized by fragmentation and poorly aligned reimbursement priorities.[5] The shift toward a model of care organized around the principles of disease management, with an emphasis on coordinated care, evidence-based practice, and outcomes evaluation, has been a relatively recent phenomenon.

Managed care organizations were among the first to adopt disease management concepts, in part because of their structure for sharing economic risk.[6] Because hospital costs represent a significant portion of patients' overall healthcare resource utilization, disease management strategies to reduce hospitalization rates and length of stay offered attractive financial incentives to these organizations.

TABLE 1   Principles and Recommendations from the AHA's Expert Panel on Disease Management[3]

1. The main goal of disease management should be to improve the quality of care and patient outcomes.
2. Scientifically derived, peer-reviewed guidelines should be the basis of all disease management programs. These guidelines should be evidence based and consensus driven.
3. Disease management programs should help increase adherence to treatment plans based on the best available evidence.
4. Disease management programs should include consensus-driven performance measures.
5. All disease management efforts must include ongoing and scientifically based evaluations, including clinical outcomes.
6. Disease management programs should exist within an integrated and comprehensive system of care in which the patient–provider relationship is central.
7. To ensure optimal patient outcomes, disease management programs should address the complexities of medical comorbidities.
8. Disease management programs should be developed for all populations and should particularly address members of underserved or vulnerable populations.
9. Organizations involved in disease management should scrupulously address potential conflicts of interest.

Other early disease management initiatives included pharmaceutical company programs developed in response to concerns that health maintenance organizations (HMOs) might decrease payments for drugs.[7] Pharmaceutical companies began identifying patients with chronic illnesses, determining their level of risk, and offering educational services to promote medication adherence and behavior change. By bundling prescription drugs with these ancillary services, companies sought to add value to their products and to increase the likelihood that they would be included on HMO formularies.[8]

It was not until the mid-1990s that disease management strategies were adopted by the healthcare industry on a wider scale, though still principally as a means of controlling costs. This widespread adoption coincided with a period of significant transition within the US healthcare delivery system: The promise of long-term cost savings offered by HMOs had begun to wane, and consumer dissatisfaction with managed care was high.[9] At the same time, the chronic disease burden continued to drive healthcare spending and utilization rates.[10] In response to these conditions, disease management emerged in the healthcare marketplace as an attractive new model for controlling costs.[5]

A body of medical literature evaluating disease management also began to emerge in the mid-1990s. In 1995, Rich et al[11] published a landmark article that reported results of a prospective, randomized trial of a nurse-directed, multidisciplinary intervention on the rates of readmission within 90 days of hospital discharge, quality of life, and costs of care for high-risk patients >70 years of age who were hospitalized with heart failure. Readmissions for heart failure were reduced by 56%, and the program saved almost $500 for each person enrolled. The study provided strong validation for the concept of disease management and was soon followed by many other trials of disease management interventions. Phillips and colleagues,[12] in a review of this literature, studied 18 trials and found that during a pooled mean observation period of 8 months, the risk of readmission was reduced by 25%.

Once the disease management trend took hold, it spread rapidly.[13] Numerous healthcare companies—including HMOs, pharmaceutical manufacturers, pharmaceutical benefits managers, medical groups and hospitals—organized quickly to meet the demand for comprehensive initiatives that would improve chronic disease care while reducing expenditures. By 1999, some 200 disease management programs were in place for conditions such as congestive heart failure, diabetes, and asthma.[13] These disease-specific programs shared certain common features, including an integrated approach to care, patient education, and the collection of outcomes data. Ultimately, though, the proliferation of disease management programs was characterized by variety rather than uniformity. Market forces encouraged companies to develop proprietary treatment algorithms and unique component packages in an effort to gain a competitive advantage. As a result, private sector disease management developed as a diverse field exhibiting a wide range of programmatic features.

Government interest in disease management also evolved during this period. Motivated in part by private sector developments, in the late 1990s Congress authorized several demonstration projects to evaluate disease management strategies under fee-for-service Medicare (see Table 2). President Clinton's 1999 Medicare Modernization proposal named disease management as an important new

---

TABLE 2 Medicare Disease Management Initiatives

1. Medicare Coordinated Care Demonstration[15]
2. Disease Management Demonstration for Severely Chronically Ill Medicare Beneficiaries With Congestive Heart Failure, Diabetes, and Coronary Heart Disease[16]
3. Physician Group Practice Demonstration[17]
4. Capitated Disease Management Demonstration for Beneficiaries with Chronic Illnesses[18]
5. End-Stage Renal Disease—Disease Management Demonstration[19]
6. Care Management for High-Cost Beneficiaries Demonstration[20]
7. Disease management initiatives authorized by the Medicare Modernization Act:
   - Pilot Project for Consumer-Directed Chronic Outpatient Services[21]
   - Medicare Care Management Performance Demonstration[22]
   - Voluntary Chronic Care Improvement Programs[23]

tool for modernizing the Medicare program.[14] As part of the 2003 Medicare Modernization Act, Congress authorized Medicare Health Support, which constitutes the largest randomized evaluation of disease management to date.[23] Under this pilot program, approximately 160 000 Medicare beneficiaries with congestive heart failure and complex diabetes among their chronic conditions will be randomized to either an intervention or a control group; those assigned to the intervention group will be able to accept or decline participation. Eligible beneficiaries will be identified through a population-based approach that uses Medicare claims data. Patients in the intervention group will receive guidance to promote medication adherence, self-management, and access to covered healthcare services. Disease management interventions will be delivered by private healthcare organizations, which must guarantee effective management of comorbidities, reduced healthcare costs, improved quality of care, and improved provider and patient satisfaction. After 2 years, pending successful interim results, this pilot may be expanded nationally.

These initiatives represent a landmark effort to determine whether disease management programs can be effective in improving health and cost outcomes for selected subgroups of chronically ill Medicare beneficiaries. Collectively, the demonstration and pilot projects comprise the largest evaluation of disease management to date, and their outcomes will undoubtedly influence future public and private sector approaches to disease management.

States also have been permitted to develop disease management programs for their primary care case management and fee-for-service Medicaid populations; to date, 28 states have done so.[24] These programs may be designed and operated by health plans or state Medicaid agencies, or they may be contracted out to disease management organizations.[25] Because of this flexibility, state disease management programs vary widely in their scope and impact. Many are still at an early stage of development, so effectiveness cannot be evaluated.[26]

DISEASE MANAGEMENT DEFINITIONS AND RELATED MODELS

Numerous definitions of disease management exist. They have evolved over time in response to the changing conditions outlined above, and they feature varying levels of specificity, ranging from the highly conceptual to the highly detailed. A sample of published definitions is provided in Tables 3 and 4 to illustrate the diversity of opinion that exists in the field. Each of these definitions shares a common theme—the transition from a traditional system of care, characterized by fragmentation and resource-intensive acute care, to a more integrated model—but their specific points of emphasis differ significantly. Epstein and Sherwood[4] reference risk-based patient identification and outcomes measurement, whereas Zitter[5] discusses organization of care and reimbursement practices. Faxon et al[3] draw attention to quality of care, the use of science-based guidelines, the management of comorbid conditions, and the role of the physician. Given this degree of divergence, it is challenging to identify specific components that truly define a disease management program.

The Disease Management Association of America (DMAA), a nonprofit trade association representing stakeholders in the disease management industry, responded to this problem by publishing a comprehensive definition that has gained widespread acceptance in recent years (Table 4). However, the DMAA definition is not used universally, and many programs that fail to meet its standards are nonetheless described as disease management programs in the medical literature.[28] It is also not clear

---

TABLE 3   Selected Disease Management Definitions

1. "[disease management] refers to the use of an explicit systematic population-based approach to identify persons at risk, intervene with specific programs of care, and measure clinical and other outcomes."[4]

2. ". . . . *disease management* is generally defined as a comprehensive, integrated approach to care and reimbursement based on a disease's natural course.

   The goal of disease management is to address the illness or condition with maximum effectiveness and efficiency regardless of treatment setting(s) or typical reimbursement patterns."[5]

3. ". . . . disease management typically refers to multidisciplinary efforts to improve the quality and cost-effectiveness of care for selected patients suffering from chronic conditions. These programs involve interventions designed to improve adherence to scientific guidelines and treatment plans."[3]

TABLE 4 DMAA Definition of Disease Management[27]

Disease management is a system of coordinated healthcare interventions and communications for populations with conditions in which patient self-care efforts are significant. Disease management:

supports the physician or practitioner/patient relationship and plan of care;

emphasizes prevention of exacerbations and complications through the use of evidence-based practice guidelines and patient empowerment strategies; and

evaluates clinical, humanistic, and economic outcomes on an ongoing basis with the goal of improving overall health.

Disease management components include:

population identification processes;

evidence-based practice guidelines;

collaborative practice models to include physician and support-service providers;

patient self-management education (may include primary prevention, behavior modification programs, and compliance/surveillance);

process and outcomes measurement, evaluation, and management; and

routine reporting/feedback loop (may include communication with patient, physician, health plan, and ancillary providers, and practice profiling).

Full-service disease management programs must include all 6 components. Programs consisting of fewer components are disease management support services.

---

that this definition can be supported empirically, as the optimal mix of ingredients for a successful disease management program is not yet known.[6] For these reasons, the AHA Writing Group believes that a broad definition is necessary as research continues to define the key components associated with positive outcomes.

The development of alternative care management models, many of which are considered under the overarching heading of disease management, has further complicated the search for a standard definition. Terms such as *case management, coordinated care,* and *multidisciplinary care* have been used interchangeably with disease management, but their unique characteristics are rarely enumerated. Because disease management programs have historically provided narrowly tailored medical solutions focused on one dominant health problem, several of these alternative models have arisen in an attempt to provide a more integrated approach to care, directing attention to the wide range of patient comorbidities.[29] Boundaries between models have increasingly blurred, however, as disease management programs have started to evolve to encompass both comorbid conditions and a greater constellation of outpatient services. Below is a discussion of the most commonly referenced disease management–related models.

Case management is characterized by intensive postdischarge monitoring by a case manager (usually a nurse) who connects patients to community-based, nonmedical support services.[30] (It is important to distinguish between case management services provided by nurses or physicians and those provided by nonlicensed personnel. Described both as case managers and care managers, this latter group typically provides functional assistance to patients who are incapacitated and facilitates communication among patients, caregivers, and providers. However, these individuals may not possess the training and expertise necessary to address the complex physiological issues associated with conditions such as heart failure or diabetes.) Case management programs provide individually tailored care plans for patients who are at high risk socially, financially, and medically. These plans frequently include education designed to reduce harmful behaviors and promote beneficial ones. Because many high-risk patients' problems are social or functional in nature, coordinating access to community resources and social support services—such as respite care, home-delivered meals, and transportation assistance—is integral to the case management approach. Family and caregivers are often engaged to provide social support, and the majority of patients' interaction with the healthcare system is through case managers.[30] Some case management programs—particularly those deployed in the Medicaid environment— create a more prominent "gatekeeping" role for the primary care provider.[31] Traditionally a physician, this individual is responsible for approving referrals and other non–primary-care service utilization in an effort to contain costs.[32] Primary care case management usually operates as a blended fee-for-service/capitation model: All medical services are paid on a fee-for-service basis, but the primary care provider also receives an additional per capita management payment to cover administrative expenses. Physician case management may also involve nurse care coordinators who assume many of the standard case management duties described above.[31]

Coordinated care involves the development and implementation of a therapeutic plan designed to integrate the efforts of medical and social service providers.[33] Care coordination programs may designate a specific individual to manage provider collaboration, similar to the gatekeeping case management role discussed above.[34] Traditionally, coordinated care initiatives have targeted the healthcare system in an attempt to reduce inappropriate utilization of resources, rather than explicitly aiming to improve health outcomes.

Multidisciplinary care mirrors the holistic approach of case management by adapting treatment plans to the medical, psychosocial, and financial needs of each patient. It differs, however, by involving a greater range of medical and social support personnel. Multidisciplinary disease management typically draws on the expertise of physicians (including the primary care provider), nurses, pharmacists, dietitians, social workers, and others to facilitate the transition from inpatient acute care to long-term, outpatient management of chronic illness.[6] Some multidisciplinary disease management programs have incorporated a "health coaching" approach, in which health professionals promote patient empowerment to achieve behavior modification and treatment compliance.[35] Other multidisciplinary programs have also sought to improve patient access to home health care, hospice care, and palliative care.[36]

The **chronic care model** (CCM) is the most comprehensive of the disease management–related models included here.[37] Originally developed by Wagner et al,[38] the CCM is founded on an understanding and appreciation of the overlapping domains in which health care occurs. These domains include (1) the entire community, (2) the healthcare system, and (3) the provider organization. The CCM further identifies 6 essential elements within these domains that are necessary to ensure optimal chronic care: (1) community resources and policies, (2) healthcare organization, (3) self-management support, (4) delivery system design, (5) decision support, and (6) clinical information systems.[39] These elements are intended to provide a practical guide for restructuring the management of chronic care, incorporating sufficient flexibility to allow customization for different treatment settings. In contrast to models such as case management or multidisciplinary care, the CCM does not focus on the roles of specific personnel. Instead, it aims to coordinate activities within primary care systems to improve organizational and health outcomes.[40]

A TAXONOMY FOR DISEASE MANAGEMENT

The AHA's Disease Management Taxonomy Writing Group supports the effort to establish a comprehensive, theory-based definition of disease management. However, the group also recognizes that many, if not the majority, of existing disease management interventions fail to meet the full range of criteria required under the comprehensive approach advocated by DMAA. By adopting an empirical approach based on published reports of disease management, we aimed to develop a taxonomy that could account for this diversity. Consequently, although aspects of the DMAA definition and the AHA taxonomy are in agreement, our different methodologies also produced divergent results. For example, the DMAA requires full-service disease management programs to incorporate routine reporting and feedback, which roughly corresponds with our "Method of Communication" domain. However, the AHA taxonomy expands this category to describe different options for communication format (one on one, in a group setting, or electronically mediated), medium (face to face, by telephone, or through the Internet), and function (symptom monitoring, patient education, or pharmacological management). Moreover, no evidence suggests that all features of any one definition need be satisfied for the intervention to be effective. Among the studies reviewed for the present statement, positive outcomes were associated with simple, single-intervention designs[41] as well as with highly complex programs.[42] Thus, the need remains for a broad-based taxonomy that can adequately classify all types of disease management programs, from the most comprehensive to those that are more selective in what they offer. Such a taxonomy would facilitate the description and comparison of different programs.

The taxonomy that follows is designed to meet this need through both descriptive and prescriptive analysis. It is based on a conceptual model developed by the AHA Writing Group that was refined through a review of published reports of disease management strategies for heart failure, depression, and diabetes. A complete listing of these published reports is available as an online Data Supplement. The conditions of heart failure, depression, and diabetes were chosen because of their lengthy history as targets for disease management intervention and because of the relative abundance of published studies evaluating those interventions. Beyond this focus, however, the taxonomy is intended to be applicable to disease management programs across myriad chronic disease states and to both current and future models. The AHA Writing Group strongly encourages researchers and publishers to report the results of disease management trials according to the taxonomic framework described here. Although detailed reporting requirements may vary by study design or disease state, at a minimum, every article on disease management should include information addressing the 8 domains (and respective subdomains) of the taxonomy.

METHODS

The AHA Writing Group began by establishing a conceptual model that categorized common disease management components into categories of increasing specificity. The initial model consisted of 4 domains, selected because of their broad relevance to disease management programs: target population, intervention design, method of communication, and intensity. This model was then refined through an iterative process of comparison with a wide range of disease management protocols drawn from the academic literature. Published reports of disease management programs were deconstructed, and an inductive analytical approach was used to identify additional categories of program components. After further discussion, we conceptualized these categories into an expanded disease management taxonomy, with our original model of disease management components used as the organizing framework.

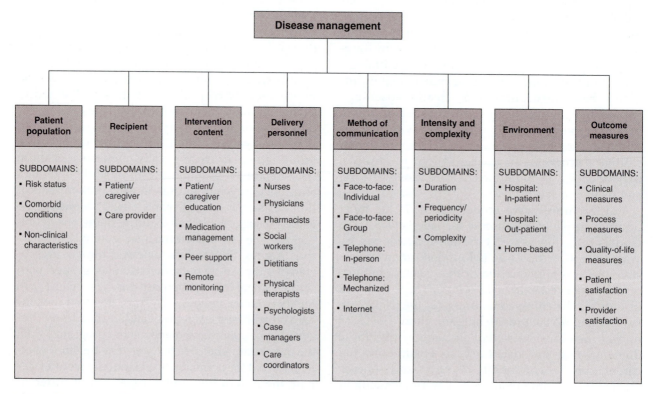

Disease Management Taxonomy

SEARCH STRATEGY

To identify study protocols for evaluation, a MED-LINE literature search was performed on the terms *heart failure, diabetes,* and *depression* in tandem with *disease management, case management,* and *care management.* The initial search was limited to articles published in English between January 1995 and January 2005. However, further screening of the reference list of each article yielded several additional relevant publications, some of which fell outside of the original date range. The reference screening process was continued until no new articles were identified, resulting in a final date range of December 1987 to April 2005.

Articles were selected according to the following criteria: (1) They described interventions designed to improve outcomes and/or reduce medical resource utilization in patients with heart failure, diabetes, or depression; and (2) they used clearly defined protocols incorporating at least 2 prespecified components traditionally associated with disease management (such as patient education, involvement of nonphysician personnel, or intensive follow-up). Because study outcomes were not formally evaluated or statistically compared, the review was able to accommodate a heterogeneous mix of interventions and study designs. Indeed, these broad inclusion criteria were deliberately established to encourage the assessment of a wide range of interventions to best capture the full spectrum of disease management–related activities.

TAXONOMY

On the basis of our conceptual model and subsequent refinement, the Writing Group developed a taxonomy that includes the following 8 domains: (1) patient population, (2) intervention recipient, (3) intervention content, (4) delivery personnel, (5) method of communication, (6) intensity and complexity, (7) environment, and (8) clinical outcomes. Within each of these domains, additional levels of detail, or subdomains, were identified. For example, intervention design can be more precisely specified according to subdomains such as patient education, medication management, and peer support care. A graphic representation of the taxonomic structure is found in the Figure, and the taxonomy is used to compare 2 heart failure disease management programs in Table 5.

Because the taxonomy was refined through comparison with reports from the academic literature, its content and structure reflect the attributes of programs described in those reports. However, the taxonomy was constructed to accommodate future developments in the field. The domains and subdomains outlined below represent a framework for the content that reports of disease management should include, as well as the level of detail with which that content should be described. This framework incorporates sufficient flexibility to accommodate the evolving nature of disease management and novel approaches that may be developed in the future.

1. Patient Population

To classify disease management interventions, or to compare disease management programs, it is critical that their target patient populations be clearly defined. Although narrowly tailored selection criteria may facilitate the conduct of research, this approach fundamentally limits our ability to understand the impact of disease management in the broader population of chronically ill patients. The following subdomains should be addressed in a patient population definition.

RISK STATUS The patient populations included in the review differed widely in their levels of risk. In disease management interventions for heart failure, this included variability in such important factors as age, degree of left ventricular dysfunction, and NYHA class. Among diabetes programs, patients differed in their diabetes type, degree of glycemic control, and the presence of complications. The impact of disease management can vary widely depending on the fit between the intervention and the risk status of the patient population. High-risk groups—such as older patients, patients with a history of prior hospitalizations, and patients with significant comorbidities—may experience fewer hospitalizations in response to disease management. Failure to account for the risk status of the target population can therefore lead to inappropriate comparisons between interventions. For example, we could draw few meaningful conclusions about the relative efficacy of 2 programs by comparing the outcomes of the 52-year-old heart transplantation candidates studied by Fonarow et al[42] with those of the 80-year-old patients with chronic heart failure examined by Ekman and colleagues.[43]

TABLE 5 Comparison of Two Disease Management Programs

Taxonomic Domain	Disease Management Program A[43]	Disease Management Program B[42]
Intervention recipient	Patients	Patients
Patient population	Diagnosis of heart failure or cardiomyopathy	Diagnosis of severe heart failure; eligible for elective heart transplantation
	Mean age: 80.3 years	Mean age: 52 years
	NYHA class III or IV	NYHA class III or IV
	Patients were excluded if any of the following applied: • need for permanent nursing home care, • serious or life-threatening illness, or • communication problem. Unspecified demographic and psychosocial information was collected.	Mean left ventricular ejection fraction: 0.21 Mean VO_{2max}: 11.0
Intervention content	Patient meeting with study nurses	Detailed baseline evaluation
	Development of individual patient care plans	Medication therapy optimized for each patient
	Treatment based on established guidelines	Treatment based on established guidelines
	Patient education on weight monitoring, medication adherence, symptom recognition, and diet	Patient/caregiver education on diet, exercise, self-monitoring, and symptom recognition
	Regular updates to patients' primary care providers or home health staff	
Delivery personnel	Specialty-trained research nurses	Heart failure clinical nurse specialist
	Home health nurses (for select patients)	Study cardiologists
	Physicians	Referring physician
Method of communication	Face to face: individual	Face to face: individual
	Telephone: in person	Face to face: group
		Telephone: in person
Intensity and complexity	Patients were followed up for 6 months.	Patients were followed up for 6 months.
	Frequency of contact was variable because patients were responsible for initiating contact with study nurses. At a minimum, all patients were contacted at baseline, week 1, and monthly thereafter. Program featured a high level of complexity.	Patient contact occurred: • within 3 days of hospital discharge, • weekly until criteria for clinical stability were met, • 2 to 3 days after any major medication change, and • at routine intervals between weeks 2 and 8. Program featured a high level of complexity.
Environment	Hospital based, outpatient	Hospital based, outpatient
Clinical outcomes	Percentage of patients who did not visit the study nurse	Patient functional status
	Change in NYHA class	
	No. of hospital readmissions	No. of hospital readmissions
	If readmitted, length of hospital stay	Estimated hospital costs

VO_{2max} indicates peak exercise oxygen consumption.

MEDICAL COMORBIDITIES All studies included in the review identified a primary condition targeted by the disease management intervention. However, few of the reports explicitly discussed the management of comorbid conditions in addition to the primary diagnosis.[44–48] The remainder either excluded patients with comorbidities from participation or noted their presence without taking steps to manage those conditions. A large proportion of patients with chronic illness suffer from medical comorbidities, and some of the greatest challenges in caring for these patients involve the complex interactions of different disease states. As disease management evolves to meet the full range of medical needs experienced by chronically ill patients, programs and interventions may similarly evolve to address comorbidities more comprehensively.

NONCLINICAL CHARACTERISTICS In addition to defining the clinical parameters of the target population, researchers must consider other nonclinical characteristics when describing a disease management intervention. A number of studies in the review identified potentially significant patient characteristics such as education level, annual income, literacy, and marriage status. Riegel and LePetri[6] have noted that the specific role played by these factors is unclear; it may vary with the nature of the disease management intervention. Patients with higher levels of education and greater self-efficacy may be more responsive to self-management strategies while exhibiting no difference in their response to medication management. A more systematic attempt to document and report nonclinical characteristics of the target population will improve the comparability of study results and may facilitate elucidation of the specific mechanisms underlying improved outcomes.

2. Intervention Recipient

The patient population that is expected to benefit from disease management (see *Patient Population* above) should be differentiated from the individuals who are targeted by the intervention. In most studies these 2 groups overlapped: Heart failure patients who received education about diet, exercise, and weight monitoring were also intended to receive direct benefit as a result. However, the literature also describes disease management interventions designed to benefit patients indirectly by influencing provider behavior. Under this alternative strategy,

healthcare providers receive instruction (often developed from evidence-based guidelines) about optimal care for the target population, are given feedback on the results of care received by their patients, or alter the organization of care processes. In our review, the provider education approach was used less frequently in the heart failure studies reviewed[49–51] but was common in disease management programs for depression[52] and diabetes.[53–58]

3. Intervention Content

Intervention content is another key domain in describing any disease management program. Disease management interventions range widely from a single educational session to remote electronic monitoring to comprehensive programs involving multidisciplinary care teams. This variety reflects the perspective of those providing the intervention (e.g., physician, nurse, or pharmacist), issues specific to the patient population, and the goals of the funding organization. Specifically, the content of a disease management program led by a clinical pharmacist will probably address pharmacological therapy, whereas that led by a nurse may emphasize patient education to improve self-care. A disease management program for heart failure would likely aim to reduce hospitalization costs, whereas the program for a patient with diabetes might emphasize glucose control. The content of a program funded by a hospital may address ways to shorten hospital stays, but an intervention paid for by an HMO would want to limit readmissions. These different perspectives contribute significantly to the variety found among disease management programs.

Patient education is the cornerstone of all disease management programs, and the majority of those reviewed incorporated patient education on topics such as the consequences of illness in daily life. For heart failure patients, this included recognition of warning signs of deterioration; advice on diet, fluid, and sodium management; and the importance of daily weighing. Diabetic patients received education about weight and caloric intake control, blood glucose self-monitoring, and foot measurement and care. Educational interventions also addressed behavioral strategies to improve patient compliance with prescribed diet, exercise, and medication regimens. A smaller number reinforced educational messages with ancillary materials, such as brochures or videos.

Peer support was one component that was regularly present in disease management programs for depression but has been used less frequently as part of cardiac disease management.[59] In disease management for depression, peer support was provided by trained individuals, linked with study subjects of similar age and sex, who had experienced an episode of major depression. These individuals were expected to make telephone or in-person contact with the patient for at least 6 months; during these encounters, peer supporters were supposed to model and share their successful coping skills, provide emotional support, and encourage self-monitoring and continued medical treatment.

Though less structured than the peer support intervention described above, disease management programs for diabetic patients routinely educated participants in a group setting.[46,48,60–63] Groups ranged in size from 4 to 28 patients, and their educational content was similar to that offered in studies that used one-on-one sessions. Group education sessions were reinforced by encouraging patients to interact between sessions and by follow-up nurse contact.

4. Delivery Personnel

The type of delivery personnel is another key domain. Programs with similar patient populations and intervention content may vary substantially in the qualifications of the individuals who deliver the content, which may in turn influence program effectiveness.

The programs reviewed generally emphasized a multidisciplinary approach to care; however, the specific disciplines represented, as well as the number of personnel involved, varied significantly across programs. It has been noted elsewhere[64] that the optimal mix of program delivery personnel is not yet known: Small teams may be as likely to improve outcomes as large ones, and alternative models (involving personnel such as health educators) have yet to be thoroughly explored. The following list therefore includes a range of delivery personnel commonly represented in disease management programs, but we do not claim the list to be exhaustive.

NURSES Nursing staff were integral to nearly all of the disease management strategies included in the review. Their duties were broad in scope, consisting of patient education, inpatient and outpatient evaluations, and making treatment or patient support recommendations to physicians. Among these, the most common theme was reliance on nurse expertise to provide patient education and frequent follow-up to relay clinically relevant findings to the patient's physician, thereby effecting more intensive management of the disease. In some studies, nurses also made home visits to optimize medication management, identify early signs of deterioration, and intensify medical follow-up as needed.[65–67]

CASE MANAGERS A subset of studies also cast nurses in the role of case manager. The precise duties associated with this title were not always clearly articulated, though it generally connoted a more supervisory role in patient care. Case managers assessed patients in person and via telephone; monitored and participated in education sessions for patients and caregivers; relayed information to patients about symptoms and medication side effects; collected information about medication use, symptoms, and vital signs; discussed patients' status with treating physicians; and coordinated care with ancillary patient services, such as physical therapy or social work consultations. Some qualified case managers independently managed patients' medication.

PHYSICIANS Physician involvement tended to be greatest during the early stages of disease management intervention. Specialist physicians (cardiologists, psychiatrists, or endocrinologists) routinely conducted an initial consultation with each patient, involving a comprehensive assessment of the patient's status, with follow-up review as required. This was followed by the establishment of individualized treatment plans, with particular attention to the optimization of medication. Ongoing evaluation of patients' progress was performed by a combination of different personnel, including specialist physicians, nurses, and primary care physicians. Despite their inclusion in many of the interventions, however, the role of the primary care physician was variable and often ill defined. In some cases, they were encouraged to conduct regular patient monitoring and to modify the treatment plan as needed; in others, they were merely kept apprised of their patients' status.

PHARMACISTS A small number of studies[48,66,68–71] evaluated the addition of a pharmacist to the care team. In these studies, the pharmacist reviewed patient histories and medication regimens and provided recommendations to physicians to optimize drug therapy. The pharmacist also communicated directly with patients, discussing medication changes, emphasizing the importance of adherence, and conducting telephone follow-up.

SOCIAL WORKERS Social workers participated in both heart failure and depression interventions to help coordinate social services. This included assessment of patients' living arrangements, economic status, cognitive abilities, and existing sources of social support. Social workers also helped connect patients to legal resources, meal delivery services, therapy, and live-in caregivers.[72] In one study of depression, a psychiatric social worker screened volunteers who had expressed interest in providing structured peer support for subjects.[73]

DIETITIANS Multidisciplinary heart failure disease management programs routinely included dietitians who provided individualized dietary assessment and instruction. Dietitians were also a regular feature in diabetes disease management because of the importance of weight and blood glucose control for diabetic patients.

PHYSICAL THERAPISTS Patients were offered a physical therapy assessment in both heart failure and diabetes studies, and physical therapists designed personalized exercise programs to improve patients' strength and endurance.

PSYCHOLOGISTS Although many depression disease management studies augmented physician services with nursing support, a smaller number also included psychologists among the members of the care team.[74,75] Psychologists were not specifically identified in any of the heart failure or diabetes studies reviewed.

INFORMATION SYSTEMS SPECIALISTS A subset of disease management programs used electronic devices or automated telephone messages to deliver content to patients.[41,76,77,79–81] In addition to monitoring clinical information such as blood pressure, weight, and blood glucose, these programs offered programmed education in areas such as medication adherence and behavior change.

5. Method of Communication

The methods used to deliver disease management interventions are increasingly important to consider, particularly as information technology has become a more prominent feature in many disease management programs. In most studies, care providers communicated directly with patients through face-to-face interaction. However, a significant number either replaced or augmented face-to-face contact with a mediated form of communication. Remote electronic monitoring systems were used in a subset of heart failure studies[41,76,77,79,80] to record measurements of patients' weight, blood pressure, heart rate, and oxygen saturation. These systems required the installation of electronic equipment in patients' homes to transmit data to a central location via telephone or the Internet. Telephone monitoring was more common than remote electronic monitoring in heart failure, diabetes, and depression interventions. Disease management interventions that closely monitored symptoms and vital signs also tended to emphasize intensive management of patients' pharmacological therapy.

Telephone contact also provided an opportunity for care providers to reinforce educational content, offer encouragement, and respond to patient questions. In one study of diabetes, an automated telephone care program was used as the primary method of patient education, with additional telephone reinforcement by a nurse educator.[81]

Only one study[82] specified the use of the Internet as a means of transmitting educational information to patients; however, the use of advanced technology is expected to increase.

6. Intensity and Complexity

Disease management programs differ both in the intensity with which interventions are delivered and in their structural complexity.

A recent systematic review of disease management interventions for depression found that patient outcomes were improved by complex strategies incorporating clinician education, nurse case management, and greater interaction between primary and secondary care. However, the same review also identified improved outcomes associated with simpler, less expensive interventions such as telephone medication counseling.[83] If a basic program is able to deliver the same benefits as a more costly one, it is more likely to be implemented on a wider scale. It is therefore critical that disease management interventions are reported and analyzed not only in terms of their individual components, but also in terms of the relationship between these components and the intensity with which they are delivered.

DURATION   The duration of patient participation in the disease management interventions reviewed varied significantly. Most programs typically involved structured intervention (some combination of education, medication management, and counseling) for no more than a 6-month period. A few provided less intensive telephone follow-up ranging from 3 months to 2 years.

FREQUENCY/PERIODICITY   For hospital-based programs, patient–provider interaction occurred most frequently during the inpatient phase. However, outpatient interventions could also be intensive and time consuming: Ledwidge et al[84] required heart failure patients to complete 3 scheduled clinic visits and 10 separate clinic-led consultations during the 3 months immediately after discharge. Home-based interventions and telephone support programs involved significantly less face-to-face contact. Stewart and Horowitz[85] found evidence of reduced hospital readmissions for heart failure patients after only 1 home visit by a cardiac nurse with reinforcement by a community pharmacist, and Krumholz et al[86] required only 1 in-person education session. Structured telephone contact tended to take place weekly during the immediate postdischarge period, with the frequency decreasing over time.

COMPLEXITY   The individual components of disease management contribute to overall program structure, such that disease management programs can also be characterized by their complexity. On the basis of their mix of individual components, programs were quite heterogeneous in this respect. Highly complex programs maximized the application of many different disease management components, involved a wide variety of delivery personnel, and were more likely to tailor the application to the individual needs of each patient. For example, Naylor et al[87] evaluated a highly complex hospital discharge protocol administered by advanced practice nurses in conjunction with patients' physicians, caregivers, and other home-based service providers. Program components included individualized discharge planning; assessment of functional, cognitive, and emotional health; extensive self-management education; and regularly scheduled home visits and telephone contact. By contrast, the least complex programs were characterized by far fewer disease management components, with fewer disciplines represented among delivery personnel and a more uniform approach to patients. A simple home-based telemonitoring intervention studied by Cordisco and colleagues[41] involved only electronic transmission of patients' weight and symptoms, with daily review by a nurse. Finally, programs of intermediate complexity could be recognized by the incorporation of some, but not all, of the intervention components and delivery personnel described in the preceding sections of the taxonomy. Krumholz and colleagues[86] investigated a program of intermediate complexity in which heart failure patients received a nurse-led hour-long education session shortly after discharge, followed by telephone-based reinforcement for 1 year. Although the program did not provide individualized care plans, nurses could encourage physician contact during the telemonitoring phase if patients' status deteriorated.

Finding a reliable coding system for complexity may be challenging, but any adequate description of a disease management program should provide a description of the operational aspects of the program. Program complexity may significantly affect clinical outcomes, intervention costs, and overall costs of care; however, few analyses have examined the association between program complexity and these factors. This is an area for further exploration, as it is important to identify the types of disease management program structure that optimize chronic care at the level of individual patients or targeted patient communities.

7. Environment

The environment in which disease management interventions are delivered also has the potential to affect both patient and financial outcomes, though it is not yet clear which environmental factors are associated with success. The majority of studies included in the review implemented disease management interventions in the outpatient setting, incorporating a mix of hospital-based clinic visits and telephone contact. In some cases (particularly those involving patients with more advanced progression of disease or limited mobility), disease management interventions were delivered in patients' homes, either electronically or by program staff (see *Method of Communication* above). Other programs specifically targeted the hospital-to-home transition, reinforcing inpatient education and medication management with subsequent outpatient contact and monitoring.

Program environment also varied with the disease being targeted. Heart failure programs were significantly more likely to incorporate an inpatient component because of the high hospitalization rate for patients with heart failure. Alternatively, disease management interventions for depression and diabetes were more often administered from primary care clinics.

In addition to the physical location of a disease management program, organizational factors may have a significant environmental impact. Organizations responsible for funding and executing disease management programs range widely, including government agencies, health insurers, physician groups, hospitals, and private disease management companies. It is not yet known whether these different organizational environments, and the different financial motivations that accompany them, impact the cost or efficacy of disease management programs.

8. Clinical Outcomes

A description of a disease management program should also include a clear description of its goals—that is, the outcomes it is designed to influence. Although interventions to improve patient and/or caregiver knowledge, self-care behavior, medication adherence, and overall quality of life were common components of disease management programs, outcomes specific to these interventions were not assessed or reported with consistency in the heart failure literature reviewed. Instead, patient mortality and hospital readmission rates were often the primary outcomes assessed and reported with consistency. This trend reflects a design bias in favor of programs targeting costs Reductions in readmission rates tended to reduce their costs while producing economic loss for hospitals charged with implementing disease management programs. For payers, there may be little enthusiasm for implementing disease management if it results in economic loss to the system. Few other interventions in medicine are required to be cost saving. However, a shift in the domains of program evaluation toward patient-centered outcomes such as quality of life, changes in caregiver burden, and overall societal costs may facilitate a change in perspective by hospital systems through increased demands by patients for these beneficial programs and a change in reimbursement priorities by private and public payers.

Non–hospital-based programs for depression and diabetes tended to report on a wider range of outcomes. For depression, these included medication adherence, frequency of mental health visits, satisfaction with treatment, symptoms of depression, and general mental and physical functioning. Diabetes disease management programs generally reported change in glycosylated hemoglobin value as the primary outcome measure, though secondary outcome variables, including weight, blood pressure, lipid profile, eye and foot examinations, diabetes knowledge, and health-related quality of life were also reported with regularity.

CONCLUSION

Conceptually, disease management should include key elements such as a coordinated system of care, delivery system support, support for patient self-care, identification of at-risk populations, a continual feedback loop between patients and care providers, measures of clinical and other outcomes, and the goal of improving overall health. In practice, however, disease management programs contain myriad different elements and vary significantly in their comprehensiveness. The taxonomy outlined in this statement is intended to advance the field by providing a system to classify these diverse elements and programs. It does not attempt to certify which particular programs or components qualify as disease management, but rather establishes a framework for understanding the programs that exist. The taxonomy represents a first step toward establishing a common language for evaluation of disease management and should ultimately facilitate more rapid identification of effective program components.

Disclosures

Writing Group Disclosures

Writing Group Member	Employment	Research Grant	Other Research Support	Speakers' Bureau/ Honoraria	Ownership Interest	Consultant/ Advisory Board Member	Other
Harlan M. Krumholz	Yale University	None	None	None	None	None	None
Peter M. Currie	Georgetown University Law Center*	None	None	None	None	None	None
David P. Faxon	University of Chicago	None	None	None	None	None	None
Eric D. Peterson	Duke University	Millennium Pharmaceuticals,[†] Schering Plough[†]	Bristol Myers Squibb/ Sanofi[†]	None	None	Millennium Pharmaceuticals[‡]	None
Christopher O. Phillips	Cleveland Clinic	None	None	None	None	None	None
Barbara Riegel	University of Pennsylvania	American Heart Association, Pfizer[‡]	None	None	None	Pfizer[‡]	None
Renee Smith	None*	None	None	None	None	None	None
Clyde W. Yancy	University of Texas Southwestern Medical Center	GlaxoSmithKline,[‡] Medtronic, Inc.,[‡] Nitromed,[‡] Scios, Inc.[‡]	Scios, Inc.[‡]	GlaxoSmith Kline,[‡] Medtronic,[‡] Medtronic,[‡] Novartis, [‡] Scios, Inc.[‡]	None	AstraZeneca,[‡] CHF Solutions,[‡] GlaxoSmithKline,[†] Medtronic,[‡] Novartis,[‡] Scios, Inc.[‡]	None

This table represents the relationships of writing group members that may be perceived as actual or reasonably perceived conflicts of interest as reported on the Disclosure Questionnaire, which all members of the writing group are required to complete and submit. A relationship is considered to be "significant" if (a) the person receives $10 000 or more during any 12-month period, or 5% or more of the person's gross income; or (b) the person owns 5% or more of the voting stock or share of the entity, or owns $10 000 or more of the fair market value of the entity. A relationship is considered to be "modest" if it is less than "significant" under the preceding definition.

*Dr. Currie and Ms. Smith were employed at the American Heart Association during the writing of this statement.
[†]Significant.
[‡]Modest.

(Continued)

Reviewer Disclosures

Reviewer	Employment	Research Grant	Other Research Support	Speakers' Bureau/ Honoraria	Ownership Interest	Consultant/ Advisory Board Member	Other
Debra K. Moser	University of Kentucky	R01 from NIH, National Institute of Nursing Research, Biobehavioral Intervention in Heart Failure	None	None	None	None	none
Michael Rich	Washington University School of Medicine	None	None	None	None	None	None
W.H. Wilson Tang	Cleveland Clinic Foundation	None	None	Takeda Pharmaceuticals, Medtronic Inc	None	Medtronic Inc, Neurocrine Biosciences, MedImmune, F-Hoffman La Roche	None
Randall Williams	Pharos Innovations, LLC; Midwest Heart Specialists	None	None	None	Pharos Innovations	ResMed Sleep Foundation	Williams Foundation— Director

This table represents the relationships of reviewers that may be perceived as actual or reasonably perceived conflicts of interest as reported on the Disclosure Questionnaire, which all reviewers are required to complete and submit.

References

1. Centers for Disease Control and Prevention. *The Burden of Chronic Diseases and Their Risk Factors: National and State Perspectives 2004*. Available at: http://www.cdc.gov/nccdphp/budenhook2004. Accessed August 1, 2005.

2. Congressional Budget Office. *An Analysis of the Literature on Disease Management Programs*. October 13, 2004. Available at: http://www.cbo.gov/showdoc.cfm?index35909&sequence30. Accessed August 1, 2005.

3. Faxon DP, Schwamm LH, Pasternak RC, Peterson ED, McNeil BJ, Bufalino V, Yancy CW, Brass LM, Baker DW, Bonow RO, Smaha LA, Jones DW, Smith SC, Ellrodt G, Allen J, Schwartz SJ, Fonarow G, Duncan P, Horton K, Smith R, Stranne S, Shine K. Improving quality of care through disease management: principles and recommendations from the American Heart Association's Expert Panel on Disease Management. *Circulation*. 2004;109:2651–2654.

4. Epstein RS, Sherwood LM. From outcomes research to disease management: a guide for the perplexed. *Ann Intern Med*. 1996;124:832–837.

5. Zitter M. A new paradigm in health care delivery: disease management. In: Todd WE, Nash D, eds. *Disease Management: A Systems Approach to Improving Patient Outcomes*. Chicago, Ill: American Hospital Publishing, Inc; 1997:1–26.

6. Riegel B, LePetri B. Heart failure disease management models. In: Moser DK, Riegel B, eds. *Improving Outcomes in Heart Failure: An Interdisciplinary Approach*. Gaithersburg, Md: Aspen Publishers, Inc; 2001: 267–281.

7. Bodenheimer T. Disease management—promises and pitfalls. *N Engl J Med*. 1999;340:1202–1205.

8. Homer CJ. Asthma disease management. *N Engl J Med*. 1997;337: 1461–1463.

9. Blendon RJ, Brodie M, Benson JM, Altman DE, Levitt L, Hoff T, Hugick L. Understanding the managed care backlash. *Health Aff (Millwood).* 1998;17:80–94.

10. Hoffman C, Rice D, Sung HY. Persons with chronic conditions: their prevalence and costs. *JAMA.* 1996; 276:1473–1479.

11. Rich MW, Beckham V, Wittenberg C, Leven CL, Freedland KE, Carney RM. A multidisciplinary intervention to prevent the readmission of elderly patients with congestive heart failure. *N Engl J Med.* 1995;333: 1190–1195.

12. Phillips CO, Wright SM, Kern DE, Singa RM, Shepperd S, Rubin HR. Comprehensive discharge planning with postdischarge support for older patients with congestive heart failure: a meta-analysis [published correction in *JAMA.* 2004;292:1022]. *JAMA.* 2004;291:1358–1367.

13. Bodenheimer T. Disease management in the American market. *BMJ.* 2000;320:563–566.

14. Clinton Administration, National Economic Council, Domestic Policy Council. *The President's Plan to Modernize and Strengthen Medicare for the 21st Century.* July 2, 1999.

15. 65 *Federal Register* 46,466 (July 28, 2000).

16. 67 *Federal Register* 8,267 (February 22, 2002).

17. 67 *Federal Register* 188 (September 27, 2002).

18. 68 *Federal Register* 9,673 (February 28, 2003).

19. 68 *Federal Register* 33,495 (June 4, 2003).

20. 69 *Federal Register* 193 (October 6, 2004).

21. Medicare Prescription Drug, Improvement, and Modernization Act. USC §648 (2003).

22. Medicare Prescription Drug, Improvement, and Modernization Act. USC §649 (2003).

23. Medicare Prescription Drug, Improvement, and Modernization Act. USC §721 (2003).

24. Kaiser Family Foundation. Medicaid cost containment actions taken by states, FY2005. Available at: http://www.statehealthfacts.kff.org/cgi-in/ health-facts.cgi?action3compare&category3Medicaid3%263 SCHIP&subcategory3Medicaid3Cost3Containment &topic3Medicaid3Cost3Containment3Actions. Accessed May 23, 2005.

25. Wheatley B. Medicaid disease management: seeking to reduce spending by promoting health. State Coverage Initiatives Issue Brief, Academy-Health, August 2001. Available at: http://www.statecoverage. net/pdf/issuebrief0801.pdf. Accessed May 25, 2005.

26. Gillespie JL, Rossiter LF. Medicaid disease management programs: findings from three leading US state programs. *Dis Manage Health Outcomes.* 2003; 11:345–361.

27. Disease Management Association of America. Definition of disease management. Available at: http://www.dmaa.org/definition.html. Accessed May 25, 2005.

28. Gonseth J, Guallar-Castillón P, Banegas JR, Rodríguez-Artalejo F. The effectiveness of disease management programmes in reducing hospital re-admission in older patients with heart failure: a systematic review and meta-analysis of published reports. *Eur Heart J.* 2004;25:1570–1595.

29. Brass-Mynderse NJ. Disease management for chronic congestive heart failure. *J Cardiovasc Nurs.* 1996; 11:54–62.

30. Chen A, Brown R, Archibald N, Aliotta S, Fox PD. *Best Practices in Coordinated Care.* Centers for Medicare and Medicaid Services, US Department of Health and Human Services. March 22, 2000. MPR Reference No. 8534-004.

31. Silberman P, Poley S, Slifkin R. Innovative primary care case management programs operating in rural communities: case studies of three states. Working Paper No. 76, North Carolina Rural Health Research and Policy Analysis Program. January 3, 2003.

32. Berenson RA, Horvath J. Confronting the barriers to chronic care management in Medicare. *Health Aff (Millwood).* 2003;(Supp Web Exclusives):37–53.

33. Stille CJ, Jerant A, Bell D, Meltzer D, Elmore JG. Coordinating care across diseases, settings, and clinicians: a key role for the generalist in practice. *Ann Intern Med.* 2005;142:700–708.

34. Schillinger D, Bibbins-Domingo K, Vranizan K, Bacchetti P, Luce JM, Bindman AB. Effects of primary care coordination on public hospital patients. *J Gen Intern Med.* 2000;15:329–336.

35. Vale MJ, Jelinek MV, Best JD, Dart AM, Grigg LE, Hare DL, Ho BP, Newman RW, McNeil JJ; COACH Study Group. Coaching patients On Achieving Cardiovascular Health (COACH): a multicenter randomized trial in patients with coronary disease. *Arch Intern Med.* 2003;163: 2775–2783.

36. Lynn J, Adamson DM. Living well at the end of life: adapting health care to serious chronic illness in old age. White Paper, RAND Health WP-137 (2003). Available at: http://www.medicaring.org/whitepaper/. Accessed August 10, 2005.

37. Wagner EH, Austin BT, Davis C, Hindmarsh M, Schaefer J, Bonomi A. Improving chronic illness care: translating evidence into action. *Health Aff (Millwood).* 2001;20:64–78.

38. Wagner EH, Austin BT, Von Korff M. Organizing care for patients with chronic illness. *Milbank Q.* 1996;74:511–544.

39. Bodenheimer T, Wagner EH, Grumbach K. Improving primary care for patients with chronic illness. *JAMA.* 2002;288:1775–1779.

40. Siminerio L, Zgibor J, Solano FX Jr. Implementing the chronic care model for improvement in diabetes practice and outcomes in primary care: the University of Pittsburgh Medical Center experience. *Clin Diabetes.* 2004;22:54–58.

41. Cordisco ME, Benjaminovitz A, Hammond K, Mancini D. Use of telemonitoring to decrease the rate of hospitalization in patients with severe congestive heart failure. *Am J Cardiol.* 1999;84:860–862,A8.

42. Fonarow GC, Stevenson LW, Walden JA, Livingston NA, Steimle AE, Hamilton MA, Moriguchi J, Tillisch JH, Woo MA. Impact of a comprehensive heart failure management program on hospital readmission and functional status of patients with advanced heart failure. *J Am Coll Cardiol.* 1997;30:725–732.

43. Ekman I, Andersson B, Ehnfors M, Matejka G, Persson B, Fagerberg B. Feasibility of a nurse-monitored, outpatient-care programme for elderly patients with moderate-to-severe, chronic heart failure. *Eur Heart J.* 1998;19:1254–1260.

44. Atienza F, Anguita M, Martinez-Alzamora N, Osca J, Ojeda S, Almenar L, Ridocci F, Vallés F, de Velasco JA. Multicenter randomized trial of a comprehensive hospital discharge and outpatient heart failure management program. *Eur J Heart Fail.* 2004;6:643–652.

45. California Medi-Cal Type 2 Diabetes Study Group. Closing the gap: effect of diabetes case management on glycemic control among low-income ethnic minority populations. The California Medi-Cal Type 2 Diabetes Study. *Diabetes Care.* 2004;27:95–103.

46. D'Eramo-Melkus GA, Wylie-Rosett J, Hagan JA. Metabolic impact of education in NIDDM. *Diabetes Care.* 1992;15:864–869.

47. Rothman RL, DeWalt DA, Malone R, Bryant B, Shintani A, Crigler B, Weinberger M, Pignone M. Influence of patient literacy on the effectiveness of a primary care-based diabetes disease management program. *JAMA.* 2004;292:1711–1716.

48. Sadur CN, Moline N, Costa M, Michalik D, Mendlowitz D, Roller S, Watson R, Swain BE, Selby JJ, Javorski WC. Diabetes management in a health maintenance organization: efficacy of care management using cluster visits. *Diabetes Care.* 1999;22:2011–2017.

49. Costantini O, Huck K, Carlson MD, Boyd K, Buchter CM, Raiz P, Cooper GS. Impact of a guideline-based disease management team on outcomes of hospitalized patients with congestive heart failure. *Arch Intern Med.* 2001;161:177–182.

50. Mueller TM, Vuckovic KM, Knox DA, Williams RE. Telemanagement of heart failure: a diuretic treatment algorithm for advanced practice nurses. *Heart Lung.* 2002;31:340–347.

51. Philbin EF, Rocco TA, Lindenmuth NW, Ulrich K, McCall M, Jenkins PL. The results of a randomized trial of a quality improvement intervention in the care of patients with heart failure. The MISCHF Study Investigators. *Am J Med.* 2000;109:443–449.

52. Weingarten S, Henning JM, Badamgarav E, Knight K, Hasselblad V, Gano A Jr, Ofman JJ. Interventions used in disease management programmes for patients with chronic illness—which ones work? Meta-analysis of published reports. *BMJ.* 2002;325:925–932.

53. Integrated care for diabetes: clinical, psychosocial, and economic evaluation. Diabetes Integrated Care Evaluation Team. *BMJ.* 1994;308: 1208–1212.

54. Domenech MI, Assad D, Mazzei ME, Kronsbein P, Gagliardino JJ. Evaluation of the effectiveness of an ambulatory teaching/treatment programme for non-insulin dependent (type 2) diabetic patients. *Acta Diabetol.* 1995;32:143–147.

55. Kinmonth AL, Woodcock A, Griffin S, Spiegal N, Campbell MJ. Randomised controlled trial of patient centred care of diabetes in general practice: impact on current wellbeing and future disease risk. The Diabetes Care From Diagnosis Research Team. *BMJ.* 1998;317: 1201–1208.

56. Kulkarni K, Castle G, Gregory R, Holmes A, Leontos C, Powers M, Snetselaar L, Splett P, Wylie-Rosett J, for the Diabetes Care and Education Dietetic Practice Group. Nutrition Practice Guidelines for Type 1 Diabetes Mellitus positively affect dietitian practices and patient outcomes. The Diabetes Care and Education Dietetic Practice Group. *J Am Diet Assoc.* 1998;98:62–70.

57. O'Connor PJ, Rush WA, Peterson J, Morben P, Cherney L, Keogh C, Lasch S. Continuous quality improvement can improve glycemic control for HMO patients with diabetes. *Arch Fam Med.* 1996;5:502–506.

58. Vinicor F, Cohen SJ, Mazzuca SA, Moorman N, Wheeler M, Kuebler T, Swanson S, Ours P, Fineberg SE, Gordon EE, Duckworth W, Norton JA, Fineberg NS, Clark CM Jr. DIABEDS: a randomized trial of the effects of physician and/or patient education on diabetes patient outcomes. *J Chron Dis.* 1987;40:345–356.

59. Riegel B, Carlson B. Is individual peer support a promising intervention for persons with heart failure? *J Cardiovasc Nurs.* 2004;19:174–183.

60. Aubert RE, Herman WH, Waters J, Moore W, Sutton D, Peterson BL, Bailey CM, Koplan JP. Nurse case management to improve glycemic control in diabetic patients in a health maintenance organization. *Ann Intern Med.* 1998;129:605–612.

61. De Weerdt I, Visser AP, Kok GJ, de Weerdt O, van der Veen EA. Randomized controlled multicentre evaluation of an education programme for insulin-treated diabetic patients: effects on metabolic control, quality of life, and costs of therapy. *Diabet Med.* 1991;8:338–345.

62. Raz I, Soskolne V, Stein P. Influence of small-group education sessions on glucose homeostasis in NIDDM. *Diabetes Care.* 1988;11:67–71.

63. Taylor CB, Miller NH, Reilly KR, Greenwald G, Cunning D, Deeter A, Abascal L. Evaluation of a nurse-care management system to improve outcomes in patients with complicated diabetes. *Diabetes Care.* 2003;26: 1058–1063.

64. Windham BG, Bennett RG, Gottlieb S. Care management interventions for older patients with congestive heart failure. *Am J Manag Care*. 2003;9:447–459.

65. Blue L, Lang E, McMurray JJ, Davie AP, McDonagh TA, Murdoch DR, Petrie MC, Connolly E, Norrie J, Round CE, Ford I, Morrison CE. Randomised controlled trial of specialist nurse intervention in heart failure. *BMJ*. 2001;323:715–718.

66. Stewart S, Pearson S, Horowitz JD. Effects of a home-based intervention among patients with congestive heart failure discharged from acute hospital care. *Arch Intern Med*. 1998;158:1067–1072.

67. Stewart S, Marley JE, Horowitz JD. Effects of a multidisciplinary, home-based intervention on unplanned readmissions and survival among patients with chronic congestive heart failure: a randomised controlled study. *Lancet*. 1999;354:1077–1083.

68. Bouvy ML, Heerdink ER, Urquhart J, Grobbee DE, Hoes AW, Leufkens HG. Effect of a pharmacist-led intervention on diuretic compliance in heart failure patients: a randomized controlled study [published correction in *J Card Fail*. 2003;9:481]. *J Card Fail*. 2003;9:404–411.

69. Gattis WA, Hasselblad V, Whellan DJ, O'Connor C. Reduction in heart failure events by the addition of a clinical pharmacist to the heart failure management team: results of the Pharmacist in Heart Failure Assessment Recommendation and Monitoring (PHARM) study. *Arch Intern Med*. 1999;159:1939–1945.

70. Davidson MB. Effect of nurse-directed diabetes care in a minority population. *Diabetes Care*. 2003;26:2281–2287.

71. Jaber LA, Halapy H, Fernet M, Tummalapalli S, Diwakaran H. Evaluation of a pharmaceutical care model on diabetes management. *Ann Pharmacother*. 1996;30:238–243.

72. Riegel B, Thomason T, Carlson B, Bernasconi B, Hoagland P, Maringer D, Watkins J. Implementation of a multidisciplinary disease management program for heart failure patients. *Congest Heart Fail*. 1999;5:164–170.

73. Hunkeler E, Meresman JF, Hargreaves WA, Fireman B, Berman WH, Kirsch AJ, Groebe J, Hurt SW, Braden P, Getzell M, Feigenbaum PA, Peng T, Salzer M. Efficacy of nurse telehealth care and peer support in augmenting treatment of depression in primary care. *Arch Fam Med*. 2000;9:700–708.

74. Katon W, Von Korff M, Lin E, Walker E, Simon GE, Bush T, Robinson P, Russo J. Collaborative management to achieve treatment guidelines: impact on depression in primary care. *JAMA*. 1995;273:1026–1031.

75. Katon W, Robinson P, Von Korff M, Lin E, Bush T. A multifaceted intervention to improve treatment of depression in primary care. *Arch Gen Psychiatry*. 1996;53:924–932.

76. Benatar D, Bondmass M, Ghitelman J, Avitall B. Outcomes of chronic heart failure. *Arch Intern Med*. 2003;163:347–352.

77. De Lusignan S, Wells S, Johnson P, Meredith K, Leatham E. Compliance and effectiveness of 1 year's home telemonitoring: the report of a pilot study of patients with chronic heart failure. *Eur J Heart Fail*. 2001;3: 723–730.

78. DeBusk RF, Miller NH, Parker KM, Bandura A, Kraemer HC, Cher DJ, West JA, Fowler MB, Greenwald G. Care management for low-risk patients with heart failure: a randomized controlled trial. *Ann Intern Med*. 2004;141:606–613.

79. Goldberg LR, Piette JD, Walsh MN, Frank TA, Jaski BE, Smith AL, Rodriguez R, Mancini DM, Hopton LA, Orav EJ, Loh E; WHARF Investigators. Randomized trial of a daily electronic home monitoring system in patients with advanced heart failure: the Weight Monitoring in Heart Failure (WHARF) trial. *Am Heart J*. 2003;146:705–712.

80. Heidenreich P, Ruggerio CM, Massie BM. Effect of a home monitoring system on hospitalization and resource use for patients with heart failure. *Am Heart J*. 1999;138(4 part 1):663–640.

81. Piette JD, Weinberger M, Kraemer FB, McPhee SJ. Impact of automated calls with nurse follow-up on diabetes treatment outcomes in a Department of Veterans Affairs health care system. *Diabetes Care*. 2001; 24:202–208.

82. Villagra VG, Ahmed T. Effectiveness of a disease management program for patients with diabetes. *Health Aff (Millwood)*. 2004;23:255–266.

83. Gilbody S, Whitty P, Grimshaw J, Thomas R. Education and organizational interventions to improve the management of depression in primary care: a systematic review. *JAMA*. 2003;289:3145–3151.

84. Ledwidge M, Ryan E, O'Loughlin C, Ryder M, Travers B, Kieran E, Walsh A, McDonald K. Heart failure care in a hospital unit: a comparison of standard 3-month and extended 6-month programs. *Eur J Heart Fail*. 2005;7:385–391.

85. Stewart S, Horowitz JD. Home-based intervention in congestive heart failure: long-term implications on readmission and survival. *Circulation*. 2002;105:2861–2866.

86. Krumholz HM, Amatruda J, Smith GL, Mattera JA, Roumanis SA, Radford MJ, Crombie P, Vaccarino V. Randomized trial of an education and support intervention to prevent readmission of patients with heart failure. *J Am Coll Cardiol*. 2002;39:83–89.

87. *Naylor* MD, Brooten D, Campbell R, Jacobsen BS, Mezey MD, Pauly MV, Schwartz JS. Comprehensive discharge planning and home follow-up of hospitalized elders: a randomized clinical trial. *JAMA*. 1999; 281:613–620.

POPULATION HEALTH MANAGEMENT
Volume 11, Number 4, 2008
© Mary Ann Liebert, Inc. DOI: 10.1089/pop.2008.114804

COMMENTARY

Disease Management Outcomes: Are We Asking the Right Questions Yet?

Gordon K. Norman, M.D., M.B.A.

DESPITE COMPOUND ANNUAL GROWTH RATES of 30% to 40% for the disease management (DM) industry over the past decade, the question "Does disease management work?" has persisted. (The older term, "disease management," and its abbreviation, "DM," are used here to denote the wide array of health and DM programs currently referred to as the "population health improvement model" by DMAA: The Care Continuum Alliance.1) Raised to greater public awareness by a skeptical Congressional Budget Office report2 in 2004, the debate was further fueled by a 2007 RAND report3 that surveyed the literature and concluded that the evidence of savings from published DM studies is inconclusive—due partly to the paucity of published evidence, criticisms with study design and rigor, and a mixture of outcomes across different programs, conditions, and populations. Few question the ability of disease and care management programs to improve processes of care, adherence to evidence-based guidelines, and clinical outcomes; even the authors of the RAND review concede the evidence for these DM outcomes is consistently positive.

What remains in dispute is whether DM programs consistently produce return on investment (ROI), meaning short-term net savings for the health plans, self-insured employers, and public sector sponsors who typically pay for these services. The Centers for Medicare and Medic-aid Services (CMS) recently made national headlines[4] and prompted

congressional concern[5] over the decision to curtail the Medicare Health Support (MHS) program for fee-for-service Medicare beneficiaries[6] based on a preliminary analysis that showed no cost savings for the first 6 months of the project.[7] This action—taken midstream during a 3-year, randomized, controlled trial (RCT) designed to evaluate financial and other outcomes[8]—appears to reflect a rush to judgment by CMS. Most DM practitioners appreciate that outcomes take time to achieve, particularly for a population of older and sicker patients, and so would have expected exactly what the early MHS evaluation described. This puzzling action prompted one seasoned observer to pose, "Is CMS the enemy of disease management?"[9]

While financial results for DM programs are important, they are not the only outcomes with which we should be concerned. It is time we start asking the right questions about DM outcomes and seeking answers in ways that reflect a much deeper understanding than just whether DM "works" to save money. Ultimately, there are fundamental things we want to know about any DM program:

- Is it beneficial? What are the specific benefits? For whom, when, and why?
- Are the benefits predictable and durable? Are some early, some later?
- Are the benefits replicable across different contexts, populations, and time?

- Can these benefits be achieved cost-effectively? Where, when, and how?
- Are cost savings possible? How much? When are savings likely? When not?
- What about the intervention seems most directly related to benefits? Is it more about who, what, how, or when it is delivered?
- What contextual factors influence the likelihood of benefits?
- What can we do better to improve these benefits?

These questions do not seem profound or even complicated, so why should they be so challenging to answer? The answer lies partly in the complexity and diversity of these programs, and partly in the different paradigms used by academia and business for evaluating programs and their respective standards for "proof." Academic researchers and policy makers usually seek proof "beyond a reasonable doubt," analogous to the criminal standard of proof with strong internal validity; nothing less than rigorous experimental designs are satisfactory for causal proof with strong internal validity, hence the strong preference for RCTs for evaluating DM programs. In contrast, private employers, some public sector entities, and most health plans apply a "preponderance of evidence" threshold, analogous to the civil standard of proof; quasi-experimental or careful nonexperimental actuarial methods may suffice to compute outcomes with sufficient credibility for their purposes.

Another important difference is the conclusion scope and time frame that different entities apply when evaluating DM outcomes. Policy makers strive to make generalizable assessments based on all the available evidence about DM programs, as they use these judgments to guide policy decisions on the assumption that future performance is best predicted by retrospective evidence of past performance. In essence, they are addressing the complex question, "Do (and will) DM programs always work?" By contrast, private health plans or employers are interested in favorable results for their own experience rather than assurance that all users of similar programs achieve comparable results. (From a competitive perspective, they may actually wish the opposite.) When local analysts, actuaries, and/or chief financial officers have evaluated their own DM programs and found that cost, utilization, quality, and satisfaction measures all correlate in a favorable direction, they are generally satisfied they have answered the question "Do my DM programs work?" in the affirmative.

This is not a subtle distinction if one believes that differing DM programs for different conditions applied to different populations with different interventions will necessarily generate different outcomes.

If substantial heterogeneity exists in the makeup of DM programs and the outcomes from these programs, how are we to know what is best under what circumstances? Are RCTs a panacea for resolving the debate, "Does DM work?" Long-time health care executive Scott MacStravic, PhD, recently pointed out the limitations of scientific studies in assessing DM outcomes.[10] Excerpted from his World Health Care Blog entry from April 14, 2008 is the following:

The same error in logic keeps turning up in evaluations of proactive health management (PHM) efforts, with recent examples relative to both disease management and prevention. It is the attempt to reach an overall conclusion about PHM in general, as well as its various components, as if each is a uniform "solution" to a single "problem." Since this is simply not the case, all such efforts are doomed to failure from the start, but manage to capture headlines when they are reached, nevertheless.

It is an unfortunate reality of the model for evaluation used in such cases that its very rigor in stipulating what is "scientific" works to limit the probability of success in what is evaluated. The best way to succeed in either DM specifically, or prevention in general, is to treat both as a "marketing" challenge—identify which people are the best prospective "customers" for using the proposed "product," specifically in terms of their potential for success. Then, customize the intervention to match both what such prospects are most likely to "buy" and what is most likely to deliver a positive return on the investment involved.

Such a matching process, i.e., making the intervention fit the individual prospect—in terms of both likelihood of their "buying" or engaging in it, and probability of doing so realizing as much as possible of their individual potential for delivering savings—would optimize the return on investment. Unfortunately, it would also violate the "rules" of scientific evaluation from beginning to end. It would not provide a single form of the intervention, but one that varies by individual, and not to a randomly assigned group, but one composed of people who were "self-selected" to different interventions by design.

Even the frequent reports of disappointing or equivocal results from DM and prevention include examples of particular interventions that do work, along with those that do not. It is only the overall picture that is reported, whereas it would make more sense to be delighted by even a few examples that work, in order to determine how to improve interventions, rather than condemn all with the same brush. If the same logic were extended to identifying which are the best prospects, and customizing interventions, the overall picture would probably be considerably more positive.

Moreover, we would learn more about what does work, instead of denying ourselves potential gains because a majority of science-restricted interventions do not. Presumably the idea is to gain success, in reducing sickness care use and expense, improving the quality of life of consumers, saving money and improving performance for employers. The aim for success should be the dominant concern when planning, implementing, and evaluating DM and preventive interventions, not scientific restrictions that reduce the chances of such success.

MacStravic's observations, while perhaps unorthodox to some, are neither radical nor Luddite in nature. They simply point out that methods commonly used for scientific proof in medicine have limitations when applied to complex, multifactorial interventions that are more rooted in epidemiology, quality improvement, and social science than biology or medicine. His insights echo similar themes raised by eminent health quality guru Don Berwick, M.D., in a recent *Journal of the American Medical Association* commentary on "the science of improvement."[11] DM is often characterized as the application of quality improvement principles to population health. Berwick is critical that slavish adherence to principles of evidence-based medicine may not be in our best interest when it comes to improving patient safety and quality of care. In his editorial, Berwick points out why RCTs may be limiting in the quality improvement realm and makes a plea to reevaluate the design and evaluation of DM programs for better learning.

Berwick also cites the work of Pawson and Tilley in *Realistic Evaluation*,[12] which presents the view that for evaluating complex programs (social programs in particular), RCTs seeking to disprove the null hypothesis with high internal validity based on average measures are less useful than what they label the "realistic evaluation" approach that seeks to understand what works for whom under what circumstances, and places equal emphasis on external validity, generalizability, and cumulative learning from evaluating programs. DM is very much a social intervention, the benefits of which will vary by program, by population, by circumstance, and by individual—how to design evaluations that discover what works best for whom and under what conditions is our primary challenge for learning, even as purchasers and policy makers continue to stress short-term ROI "proofs" to justify their investments. Again, classic experimental designs seem ill suited to both tasks, and perhaps less valuable for either one than once expected.

As a physician, quality improvement practitioner, and DM proponent, I have long regarded the question, "Does DM work?" to be as nonsensical as questions such as, "Does medication work?" or "Does surgery work?" The answer to each is, "It all depends." The right medicine taken for the right condition in the right dosage for the right time period surely can improve health (though saving money is highly unlikely). Surgery performed by the right surgeon for the right indication at the right time for the right patient can yield better health (but rarely cost savings).

More relevant and interesting questions are: "For whom does DM produce what outcomes?" "For what conditions?" "Under what circumstances?" DM strategies are not like a pill or a procedure; they are not uniform, standardized health interventions, but rather a complex series of tools and interactions aimed at influencing health behaviors, often personalized down to the individual level, to achieve maximal impact for each participant. Obviously, people with chronic conditions or serious health risks are as heterogeneous a group of experimental subjects as one can find, so differing responses to any intervention would be expected, if not guaranteed.

A strong case can be made that measurement for learning and measurement for judgment, at least for DM, require different perspectives. How we reconcile this with academicians' skepticism, as well as industry efforts to build consensus on pragmatic approaches to evaluating DM, poses a significant challenge. With due respect to the classical hierarchy of evidence used in proving new medical science, it is not clear that the application of the most rigorous of these methods will resolve the ongoing debate; it seems incumbent upon the industry to point out the logical fallacy that only RCTs can prove DM value, while providing a road map for better methods that promote industry learning and quality improvement.

In most cases, DM does not introduce new science. Rather, it strives to narrow the gaps between actual practice and evidence-based medicine by applying best practices to chronic condition management and health improvement. Various pundits have offered the observation that *doing what we know better* often trumps *knowing better what to do* in terms of value to society.[13] Despite this, the National Institutes of Health budget for science discovery is greater than 88-fold of that for the Agency for Healthcare Research and Quality to evaluate the delivery of health services. And what CMS spends on research, demonstration, and evaluation is less than 1.5% of the amount it spends for operations (largely claims payments). It seems our national research priorities are skewed away from learning how best to use existing knowledge of care delivery. We also are relatively unsophisticated in our knowledge of how best to measure health delivery programs.

Most of what we spend in the name of health care is intended to produce a health benefit outcome—longer life, better quality of life, or both. Despite conventional wisdom and recent political rhetoric to the contrary, most prevention and routine health interventions are not cost saving,[14] yet they are widely perceived as beneficial and worthwhile because they improve health in a cost-effective fashion. Cost saving was not the original intent of the DM pioneers in the early 1990s, either; rather, their goal was to apply quality improvement principles to see if patients at risk for avoidable morbidity could lessen those risks by close adherence to evidence-based medicine, better compliance with physician treatment plans and prescribed medications, and more healthful lifestyle behaviors. It just so happened that when targeting certain high-risk, high-cost populations, these interventions not only increased quality of life, but the avoided morbidity costs led to a net reduction in health care cost for payers. Thus was born the expectation for DM ROI, which continues to the present.

Better value for health spending is what we seek, and what our fragmented health care non-system is lacking. Assuming the common representation of value = quality/cost, value is improved whenever we raise quality for the same cost, raise quality and reduce cost simultaneously, or reduce cost for the same quality. Even when DM does not produce net savings for a given circumstance, is it likely that it still achieves notable health quality benefits with attractive cost-effectiveness relative to other health interventions? This is not a question I hear posed by academics or policy makers often, which is surprising, given the preponderance of evidence that demonstrates DM programs increase health care value by raising quality. I suggest that DM should not be held

to a different standard than other common health care interventions. CMS covers new interventions shown to be effective without consideration of cost savings or even cost-effectiveness. The FDA approves new medicines on the basis of safety and effectiveness, not cost or cost-effectiveness. Yet resources are limited, and for a society facing health care costs that now consume more than 16% of the gross domestic product, we cannot ignore cost. It is appropriate to evaluate DM cost-effectiveness; in most cases I believe it will be shown to be highly cost-effective, and under many circumstances it will produce cost savings. That is more than can be said for the vast majority of health interventions for which we now pay without hesitation.

Thanks to Wennberg's prolific research, we have known for more than 35 years that profound and unwarranted variation in the care of patients is ubiquitous in this country.[15] We have been shown repeatedly by McGlynn[16] and others that when it comes to the consistent delivery of health care services known to be beneficial, we are just plain lousy. On average, Americans receive about half of recommended care processes, and the gap between what we know works and what actually is done is substantial and troubling. In their latest Dartmouth Atlas,[17] which focuses on the care chronically ill seniors receive in the last 2 years of life, Wennberg and team have demonstrated yet again that rampant unwarranted variation in care also pervades that segment of the population. Among their recommendations for addressing this problem, the authors suggest care management systems, such as disease registries and DM protocols. Given this dismal status quo and good, albeit imperfect, evidence that DM can raise care quality by closing these gaps in evidence-based care, we must be thoughtful and deliberate about separating the DM "baby" from the chronic care "bathwater." We can ill afford to be cavalier about evaluating such programs or drawing casual inferences, given the promise these approaches hold for efficiently improving population health.

So back to the original question, "Does DM work?" Averaging the successes and failures of different programs for diverse conditions over heterogeneous populations to answer that question seems unhelpful, if not misleading. More important knowledge comes from answering the question, "Does DM ever work?" If DM savings result from any programs, then the circumstances of those programs can be scrutinized to develop a deeper understanding of why, for population X, the specific interventions led to changes that resulted in net savings. Then, by examining more instances of such specific linkages between interventions and their causative mechanisms, applied to specific contexts and their resulting outcomes, we can develop better insight about how to approach novel situations to replicate these outcomes. For social program evaluators, this paradigm is quite familiar and routine, but it is a nuanced and fundamentally different way of viewing the evaluation conundrum for those who engage in the DM ROI debate.

Questions that challenge the DM industry and preoccupy those working across the industry for answers through DMAA: The Care Continuum Alliance include:

- How do we reconcile the demands for more rigorous DM evaluations with the methods we have developed in our consensus Outcomes Guidelines editions that attempt a pragmatic balance between suitability and acceptability?
- If a number of key industry stakeholders continue to maintain that only RCTs constitute compelling evidence for causation, to what extent should the industry be willing to conduct more RCTs, despite the shortcomings described by Berwick, Pawson & Tilley, and others, and despite the disinterest of most current DM purchasers to fund such studies?
- Will more RCTs increase the probability of publication and dissemination of credible outcomes to help resolve the debate, or are they likely to perpetuate "nothing works consistently" conclusions by virtue of an inherent misalignment with the nature of DM as a social experiment with high contextual influence?
- When we cannot conduct RCTs, should we seek "realistic evaluation" approaches using pluralistic quasi-experimental methods as rigorously as we can, then strive for greater dissemination and discussion of those results with iterative learning going forward?
- Is it necessary to divide our thinking about measurement for judgment and measurement for learning? If cumulative learning requires different evaluation approaches from what external stakeholders are expecting for "proof," how do we best resolve this dilemma?

Turning the dialog to these more illuminating questions just may begin to generate more light than heat, unlike the present debate. It is time to start asking better questions in lieu of perpetuating the stalemate over "Does DM work?"

References

1. DMAA: The Care Continuum Alliance. Advancing the population health improvement model. Available at: <www.dmaa.org/phi_definition.asp>. Last accessed June 26, 2008.
2. Holtz-Eakin D. An analysis of the literature on disease management programs, Congressional Budget Office report to Congress, October 13, 2004. Available at: <www.cbo.gov/doc.cfm?index=5909&type=0>. Last accessed June 26, 2008.
3. Mattke S. Evidence for the effect of disease management: is $1 billion a year a good investment? *Am J Manag Care*. 2007;13:670–676.
4. Abelson R. Medicare finds how hard it is to save money. *New York Times*. April 7, 2008. Available at: <www.ny-times.com/2008/04/07/business/07medicare.html?page- wanted=1&_r=1&hp>. Last accessed June 26, 2008.
5. The Henry J. Kaiser Family Foundation, kaisernetwork.org. Senators ask CMS to reconsider decision to delay second phase of disease management pilot program. Available at: <www.kaisernetwork.org/daily_reports/rep_index.cfm?DR_ID=51013>. Last accessed June 26, 2008.
6. Centers for Medicare and Medicaid Services. Completion of phase I of Medicare health support program FAQs. Available at: =www.cms.hhs.gov/CCIP/downloads/MH-SEOPexfaqsfin012808_FINAL.pdf=. Last accessed June 26, 2008.
7. McCall N, Cromwell J, Bernard S. Report to Congress: evaluation of phase I of Medicare health support (formerly voluntary chronic care improvement) pilot program under traditional fee-for-service Medicare. Available at: <www.cms.hhs.gov/Reports/Downloads/McCall.pdf>. Last accessed June 26, 2008.
8. Centers for Medicare & Medicaid Services. Medicare Health Support. Available at: <www.cms.hhs.gov/CCIP/>. Last accessed June 26, 2008.
9. MacStravic S. Is CMS the enemy of disease management? World Health Care Blog. Available at: <www.worldhealth-careblog.org/2008/02/24/is-cms-the-enemy-of-disease-management/>. Last accessed June 26, 2008.

10. MacStravic S. Science vs. success in evaluating health management. World Health Care Blog. Available at: <*www.worldhealthcareblog.org/2008/04/14/science-vs-success-in-evaluating-health-management/*>. Last accessed June 26, 2008.

11. Berwick D. The science of improvement. *JAMA*. 2008;299: 1182-1184.

12. Pawson R, Tilley N. *Realistic Evaluation*. London, England: SAGE Publications, Ltd: 1997.

13. Woolf SH. The break-even point: when medical advances are less important than improving the fidelity with which they are delivered. *Ann Fam Med*. 2005;3:545–552.

14. Cohen JT, Neumann PJ, Weinstein MC. Does preventive care save money? *N Engl J Med*. 2008;358: 661–663.

15. Wennberg J, Gittelsohn A. Small area variation in health care delivery. *Science*. 1973;182:1102–1108.

16. McGlynn EA, Asche SM, Adams J, et al. The quality of health care delivered to adults in the United States. *N Engl J Med*. 2003;348:2635–2645.

17. Wennberg JE, Fisher ES, Goodman DC, Skinner JS. Tracking the care of patients with severe chronic illness. The Dart-mouth Atlas of Health Care 2008. Available at: =*www.dart-mouthatlas.org/atlases/2008_Chronic_Care_Atlas.pdf*=. Last accessed on June 26, 2008.

Address reprint requests to:
Gordon K. Norman, M.D., M.B.A. Chairman-Elect, DMAA:
The Care Continuum Alliance 700 Pennsylvania Ave. N.W.
Suite 700 Washington, D.C. 20004-2694
E-mail: cgraziano@dmaa.org

GLOSSARY

Access—the ability to receive health care when needed.

Accreditation—a standardized program for evaluating health care organizations to ensure a specified level of quality based on standards.

Actuarial data—assumptions with statistical relevance are used to help the third-party payer arrive at the premium rate.

Acute care case management—a case management model that focuses on providing case management services to acute care patients who are at high risk for complications, longer hospital stays, and high-cost care.

Advance directives—living wills and other similar legal documents.

Adverse selection—an insurance characteristic that indicates the enrollee pool includes a higher percentage of high-risk individuals than the percentage of high-risk individuals in the average population, resulting in the potential for greater utilization of health care services.

Advocacy—providing information that is useful to the patient and supporting the patient's decision; representing the patient.

Aid to Families with Dependent Children (AFDC)—a federal government financial program that provides funds to needy children under the age of 21, Old-Age Assistance, Aid to the Blind, persons who are permanently and totally disabled, and the elderly over 65 years and on welfare.

Algorithms—a formatted process in the form of a decision-making tree.

Ambulatory care case management—a case management model that is community-based case management with case management services provided to patients receiving ambulatory care.

Ancillary services—diagnostic and therapeutic services such as radiology, laboratory testing, electrocardiography, invasive imaging, and cardiac testing.

Annual limits—a type of limit on the amount that the employee is required to pay annually for medical services based on the health care insurance plan.

Assessment—collecting data to identify actual and potential problems to establish a plan of care with expected outcomes, interventions, and resources required to meet the outcomes.

Authorization—an insurance method used to control the utilization of ancillary services by requiring approval of health care services.

Balanced Budget Act of 1997 (BBA)—the law that expanded the ability of Medicare to offer managed care options to its beneficiaries.

Benchmarking—a form of measuring outcomes; assessing the quality and cost of health care by comparing performance with similar organizations (healthcare, insurers).

Benefit package—the description of total health services that will be covered under a specific insurance plan for enrollees.

Benefits—medical services included in a health insurance policy to which the insured person or enrollee is entitled.

Beyond the walls—case management that is provided in the community or in payer-based settings such as a managed care organization.

Bonuses—financial performance-based rewards paid to health care providers by insurers.

Capitation—a payment method in which a prepaid dollar amount is established to cover the cost of health care delivered to a person, per year, regardless of the number or nature of services provided.

Care management—a collaborative process of assessment, planning, facilitation, and advocacy for options and services to meet an individual's health needs through communication and available resources to promote quality cost-effective outcomes (CMSA); generally focuses on specifically identified patients' (high risk, high volume, high cost) care needs across the episode or continuum of an illness.

Carve-outs—a third-party payer strategy used to control reimbursement costs by separating out specific medical services from other services for special reimbursement review or special interventions.

Case management plan—the plan of care developed by the case manager, describing services the patient requires, when they should be provided, and by whom.

Case management process—four phases used to assist in coordinating effective care for patients: assessment and problem identification, patient and environmental interventions, discharge planning and transitional planning, and evaluation.

Case manager—a health care professional, typically a nurse or social worker, who provides case management services.

Case rate—a prospective, pre-established rate based on the type of case (e.g., a flat fee is paid for a vaginal delivery).

Cherry picking—insurer recruiting that focuses on getting healthy beneficiaries to control costs.

Claims processing—the process of determining whether an insurance claim meets all the covered services requirements.

Clinical guidelines—systematically developed statements to assist practitioner and patient decisions about appropriate health care for specific clinical circumstances; ideally based on evidence (EBP).

Clinical pathways—a written guide that provides specific direction for the care required to meet the needs of specific medical problems, including sequencing and timing of interventions.

Closed-panel HMOs—a type of managed health plan that contracts with physicians on an exclusive basis, limiting physicians in contracting to work with other health plans.

Collaborative care—recognition of the expertise of others within and outside the profession and referral to those other providers when appropriate; health care providers work together to reach goal in a more successful and usually more efficient way.

Communication—transmission of information and understanding takes place on many different levels: individual to individual, in small teams or groups, in large organizations, and between large organizations.

Community rating—a method of determining the cost of health insurance by determining the average cost for all covered individuals in a geographic area.

Comorbidities—more than one coexisting medical condition.

Conflict—two or more people or organizations disagree or have opposing views about a problem or solution.

Consent—agreement to receive a health care intervention or treatment after receiving sufficient information about the intervention of treatment.

Consolidated Omnibus Budget Reconciliation Act of 1985 (COBRA)—provides certain former employees, retirees, spouses, former spouses, and dependent children the right to temporary continuation of health coverage for up to 18 months at group rates. This coverage, however, is only available when coverage is lost due to certain specific events.

Consumer—the patient who receives the care, or it can also be the person or organization that purchases or pays for health care, such as an employer who contributes to health care payment.

Consumer rights—now a major issue in health care policy, particularly owing to dissatisfaction with managed care.

Continuity of care—to ensure that all services required are provided at the appropriate time, over time, across multiple health care providers and settings, and across the illness spectrum.

Continuous reassessment—multiple assessments throughout the care process to adjust patient's treatment plan and needs as required.

Coordination—organizing, securing, integrating, modifying, and documenting the resources necessary to accomplish the goals set forth in the case management plan.

Copayment/Coinsurance—a specified flat amount per unit of service or unit of time paid my enrollees in a health plan at the time of the service, with the insurer paying the rest of the cost.

Cost shifting—offsetting losses from treating one group of patients by charging other patients more.

Covered services—the written benefit plan describing the benefits that are provided to the enrollee as well as the financial coverage for those benefits.

Credentialing—an in-depth professional review process that includes evaluation of licenses, certification if required in a specialty area, evidence of malpractice insurance as required, history of involvement in malpractice suits, and education.

Critical thinking—purposeful, informed, outcome-focused (results-oriented) thinking that requires careful identification of key problems, issues, and risks involved.

Deductible—the initial amount that a consumer must first pay before the health insurer begins to pay for covered health services.

Delegation—transferring to a competent individual authority to perform a selected task in a selected situation.

Demand management—focusing on services or support that assist the consumer (member or enrollee) such as self-help tools, nurse advice lines, and preventive services with the goal of decreasing demand for services.

Diagnosis-related groups (DRGs)—a statistical system that classifies acute care into groups used to determine health care reimbursement developed by the Centers for Medicare and Medicaid Services.

Discharge planning—plans that are made to assist a patient with discharge from one type of care to another; typically acute care to ambulatory or community care.

Discounted fee-for-service—an insurance payment method that pays the provider a specific percentage of the provider's usual charge or a reduced rate.

Disease management programs—a system of coordinated health care interventions and communications for populations with conditions in which patient self-care efforts are significant (DMMA).

Durable power of attorney—a legal method that allows an individual to represent another to determine type of care the individual will receive when the individual is unable to represent himself or herself.

Enrollee—a member, subscriber, or beneficiary eligible for health plan services.

Entrepreneur—a person who sees things differently and takes the opportunity to make a difference.

Environmental intervention—the part of a case management plan that include activities such as linkage with community resources, consultation with families and caregivers, education, maintenance and expansion of social networks, collaboration with health care providers, and advocacy.

Episode of care—the period of time when a patient is under the direct care of health care providers.

Evaluation—clarifies performance expectations, reinforces constructive behavior, corrects unsatisfactory behavior, provides recognition, increases self-awareness, and promotes growth and change.

Evidence-based practice (EBP)—A method to improve the quality of care based on evidence: clinically relevant research that can be applied to clinical practice, clinical expertise, patient values and preferences, and patient history and assessment data.

Exclusions—services that are not covered by a health plan.

Exclusive provider organizations (EPOs)—a type of preferred provider organization (PPO) that requires the insured to use only designated providers.

Experience rating—a rating system used to determine health care costs that considers the actual medical claims history or utilization history of the employees as well as anticipated care based on such factors as age and gender.

Fee-for-service (FFS)—an insurance payment method that offers to pay the provider a specific percentage of the provider's usual charge or a reduced rate.

Formulary—an insurer's or health care facility's listing of approved drugs for reimbursement or prescription.

Gatekeeper—a physician or other designated health care professional who coordinates and directs the patient's care and is responsible for referrals to specialists.

Government benefit plans—the federal government benefit plans are Medicare, Medicaid, the Federal Employees Health Benefit Program (FEHBP), TriCare, and the Civilian Health and Medical Program of the Uniform Services (CHAMPUS). In addition, states provide health care coverage for state employees.

Group model HMO—a type of health maintenance organization (HMO) that owns or partly owns or contracts with medical centers where many different health services are provided to members in a central location. A large physician practice may also contract to provide care exclusively to members of an HMO.

Health maintenaince organization (HMO)—a managed care model that pays the bills for its members' health services but also manages and provides care to its members; the original model or prototype of managed care.

Health Maintenance Organization Act of 1973—stipulates that HMOs are organized entities that ensure health care service delivery in a specific geographic area; provide basic and optional benefits; and members join voluntarily.

Health Plan Employer Data and Information Set (HEDIS)—a core set of performance measures to assist employers and other health purchasers in understanding the value of health care purchases and evaluating health plan performance; administered by the National Committee for Quality Assurance (NCQA).

Healthcare Financing Administration (HCFA)—the federal agency responsible for administering Medicare and overseeing states' administration of Medicaid; part of the U.S. Department of Health and Human Services.

Home care case management—a case management model that focuses on case management services for patients receiving home care.

Hospitalist—a health care provider, typically a physician but could be a clinical nurse specialist, who provides the overall medical coverage for patients rather than having the patient's primary care provider meet these responsibilities.

Indemnity insurance—a traditional health plan in which the patient submits the provider's bill to the insurer with the insurer paying a predetermined amount to the provider.

Indicator—a descriptor to define a measurable dimension of quality.

Informed consent—consent given by a patient, next of kin, legal guardian, or designated person for a kind of intervention, treatment, or service after the provision of sufficient information by the provider.

Insurance—the written benefit plan that provides the enrollee financial coverage for health care benefits.

Insurance commission—the state organization responsible for regulating both the solvency of insurers and the marketing of insurance.

Intensivist—a health care provider, typically a physician, who provides the overall medical coverage for patients in intensive care.

Intervention phase—coordination and monitoring to ensure that all needs are met in a timely manner by the appropriate provider.

Level of care—the description of the amount of care a patient may require based on the patient's needs, e.g., acute (hospital); subacute (requires high level of nursing, medical, and therapy services and can be provided in a hospital unit or a separate organization) (may also be referred to as transitional care); skilled nursing facility (SNF) providing 24-hour nursing care and rehabilitation, social services either short term or long term; home health; and hospice.

Liability—legal responsibility for failure to act appropriately or for actions that do not meet the standard of care.

Macroconsumer—the consumer who is a large purchaser of health care (e.g., employers, government); also called the customer.

Malpractice—professional misconduct, and negligent care or failure to meet the standard of care, that results in patient harm.

Medical/social case management—model that focuses on a long-term care patient population who are at risk for hospitalization and who require coordination, assessment of resource utilization, planning, outcomes, and so on.

Medicare Catastrophic Coverage Act of 1988—the law that initiated the Medicare program.

Medicare Part A—Medicare Part A covers inpatient hospital costs and limited skilled posthospital costs, based on DRGs.

Medicare Part B—Medicare Part B, supplementary medical insurance program covering the cost of physician services and some outpatient services and medical supplies not covered by Part A.

Medicare Part C—provides health coverage choice administered by private companies approved by Medicare with the beneficiary paying extra costs.

Medicare Part D—Medicare prescription drug coverage.

Medigap plans—special nongovernmental supplemental insurance plans for Medicare beneficiaries.

Member—enrollees to benefit/insurance plans.

Member services—customer services or consumer affairs, focusing on helping the enrollee or member with problems and grievances, tracking consumer issues and resolutions, and improving member satisfaction.

Microconsumer—the employee and the employee's family and people who buy insurance as individuals.

National Committee for Quality Assurance (NCQA)—a private, not-for-profit organization that evaluates and awards accreditation and certification for health insurance plans including managed care organizations, disease management programs, and wellness and health promotion programs.

Negligence—conduct lacking due care; legal criteria for negligence are: a duty owed to the patient; a breach of duty or standard by the health care professional; harm caused by the breach of duty or standard; and the person (plaintiff) experienced damages or injuries.

Negotiation—to resolve conflict; those in involved in the conflict must discuss how to resolve it in a way that is acceptable to all of the persons involved.

Open-access HMOs—a type of HMO in which members are allowed to see a specialist in the provider network without first seeing a primary care provider, but they require that the member pay an additional copayment.

Outcomes-oriented care delivery—focuses on monitoring and measurement of patient safety, continuity, and quality of care.

Outliers—patients whose cost of care or length-of-stay are outside the expected.

Out-of-pocket expenses—the portion of payments for health services required to be paid by the enrollee, including copayments, coinsurance, and deductibles.

Patient navigation—a type of care management that encompasses a wide range of advocacy and coordination activities.

Payer mix—the proportion of total revenues that the provider expects from different payers.

Per diem—a reimbursement that is fixed based on each day in a health care facility (e.g., $600 per day).

Performance-based reimbursement evaluation—reimbursement to providers based on performance evaluation results.

Point-of-service (POS)—a health plan that allows the covered person to choose to receive a service from a participating or nonparticipating provider at the time of service, paying additional costs if using a nonparticipating provider.

Population-based care management (PCM)—a case management model based on the idea that persons must be cared for in the context of their health status, in consideration of the interplay between existing conditions, or risk for conditions.

Practice guidelines—focus on general treatment for a specific illness or condition, whereas pathways are more specific and are unique to the health care agency or insurer.

Preexisting conditions—any medical condition that has been diagnosed within a specified period immediately preceding the covered person's effective date of coverage under the group health insurance plan.

Preferred provider organization (PPO)—a type of managed care organization in which contracts are established with providers of medical care.

Premium rate setting—third-party payer determination of the premiums (prices or rate) for its products or services that paid by the insurance member or enrollee.

Premium—rate that a plan subscriber pays for coverage of health services.

Primary care—general entry-level health care delivered by a physician or nurse practitioner.

Primary prevention—health promotion by maintaining or improving general health in individuals and communities through, for example, immunization and education.

Provider panel (also called provider directory)—an insurer's list of approved providers, individuals and health care organizations.

Providers—physician, advanced practice nurse or nurse practitioner, nurse midwife, registered nurse, physician assistant, nurse anesthetist, pharmacist, dentist, optometrist, chiropractor, podiatrist, hospital, home health agency, hospice, long-term care facility, psychiatric hospital, skilled nursing home, infusion therapy agency, and so on, who provides care to patients.

Quality—in this context, quality in the health care delivery system, health care reimbursement, and case management.

Quality improvement (QI)—identify errors and hazards in care; understand and implement basic safety design principles, such as standardization and simplification; continually understand and measure quality of care in terms of structure, process, and outcomes in relation to patient an community needs; and design and test interventions to change processes an systems of care, with the objective of improving quality, as defined by the Institute of Medicine (IOM).

Red flags—identification of patients at high risk for complications and higher costs and who could benefit from case management.

Reimbursement—payment for health care services.

Reimbursement strategies—insurer methods used to control cost and ensure effective care (e.g., capitation, withholds, bonuses, authorization, formularies).

Report cards—reports of specific performance data about an organization at specific intervals with a focus on quality and safety.

Retrospective payment system—paying for care after it is received.

Risk management—strategies used by health care providers to reduce liability costs through reducing actions that may lead to liability or by responding quickly to actions that may increase liability risk.

Secondary prevention—focuses on early diagnosis of symptoms and treatment after the onset of disease or illness and recognizes that early treatment may decrease complications. Examples are mammograms and diabetes screening.

Service benefit plan—a plan that pays the provider directly.

Service strategies—methods used by insurers to manage delivery of care in all types of health care settings with the goal of decreasing cost and provide quality care.

Social case management—a case management model that emphasizes comprehensive long-term community care services to delay hospitalization; usually provided by a social worker.

Social Security Act of 1935—the federal law that established Medicare and Medicaid.

Staff model HMOs—an HMO model (managed care) that relies on employee or salaried staff physicians to provide most of the medical care to its members.

Standards of care—statements that describe the minimum requirements for effective care.

Structure—the environment in which services are provided.

Subscriber—an enrollee or member of an insurance plan.

Targeted patient population—populations that will receive case management services.

Tax Equity and Fiscal Responsibility Act of 1982 (TEFRA)—the federal law that created the current risk and cost contract provisions under which health plans contract with the HCFA and which defined the primary and secondary coverage responsibilities of the Medicare program.

Telephonic case management—a case management model that uses telephone, e-mail, and other forms of electronic communication to assist in delivering case management.

Tertiary prevention—focuses on rehabilitative strategies to decrease disability from a disease or illness. Examples of interventions are chemotherapy education for a cancer patient and bladder training for a stroke patient.

Third-party payer—public or private insurance providers paying for health care (not the patient).

Transformation leadership—leadership style that developes a vision of what could be and working toward it, viewing the total picture, accepting change and seeing it as an opportunity, guiding and rewarding staff you work with, and encouraging the team to be self-aware and to take risks; to learn from mistakes.

Transitional planning—focuses on moving a patient from the most complex to less complex care settings, or in some cases the reverse, should the patient require more intense services.

Underwriting—the assessment method in which insurance companies project what the expected covered health costs will be for a particular person or group.

Utilization management (UM)—the process of evaluating necessity, appropriateness, and efficiency of health care services for specific patients or patient populations.

Utilization Review Accreditation Commission (URAC)—a private, nonprofit, independent accrediting and certification organization for utilization management programs.

Variances—deviations from expected outcomes.

Withholds—the dollar amount that a managed care organization deducts from a provider's fees; setting aside the amount in a risk-sharing fund, which may be returned to the provider if certain preset goals are met.

Within the walls—case management models that provide services within a hospital or acute care setting.

Workers' compensation—a type of insurance for employees that provides medical benefits and replacement of lost wages that result from injuries or illnesses that arise from the workplace; in turn, the employee cannot normally sue the employer unless true negligence exists.

INDEX